SEXUAL ECOLOGY

SEXUAL
ECOLOGY

AIDS
AND THE DESTINY
OF GAY MEN

GABRIEL ROTELLO

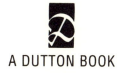

A DUTTON BOOK

DUTTON
Published by the Penguin Group
Penguin Books USA Inc., 375 Hudson Street,
New York, New York 10014, U.S.A.
Penguin Books Ltd, 27 Wrights Lane, London W8 5TZ, England
Penguin Books Australia Ltd, Ringwood, Victoria, Australia
Penguin Books Canada Ltd, 10 Alcorn Avenue, Toronto, Ontario, Canada M4V 3B2
Penguin Books (N.Z.) Ltd, 182–190 Wairau Road, Auckland 10, New Zealand

Penguin Books Ltd, Registered Offices:
Harmondsworth, Middlesex, England

First published by Dutton, an imprint of Dutton Signet,
a division of Penguin Books USA Inc.
Distributed in Canada by McClelland & Stewart Inc.

First Printing, April, 1997
10 9 8 7 6 5 4 3 2 1

 REGISTERED TRADEMARK—MARCA REGISTRADA

LIBRARY OF CONGRESS CATALOGING-IN-PUBLICATION DATA:
Rotello, Gabriel
    Sexual ecology: AIDS and the destiny of gay men/Gabriel Rotello.
        p.   cm.
    Includes bibliographical references and index.
    ISBN 0-525-94164-9
    1. AIDS (Disease)   2. Gay men—Health and hygiene.   I. Title.
RA644.A25R68   1997
362.1'969792'0086642—dc21   96-49706
                                                                CIP

Printed in the United States of America
Set in Garamond Light

This book is printed on acid-free paper.

In Memory of Hap Hatton

The truth that is suppressed by friends is the readiest weapon of the enemy.
—ROBERT LOUIS STEVENSON

Contents

Acknowledgments xi

Introduction: AIDS and the Destiny of Gay Men 1

Chapter 1. The Birth of AIDS 19

Chapter 2. Gay Sexual Ecology 38

Chapter 3. The Synergy of Plagues 65

Chapter 4. The Birth of the Condom Code 91

Chapter 5. The "Second Wave" 118

Chapter 6. Surfing the Second Wave 135

Chapter 7. The Ecology of "Heterosexual AIDS" 163

Chapter 8. Holistic Prevention 184

Chapter 9. Imagining a Sustainable Culture 211

Chapter 10. Building Incentives into Gay Culture 233

Chapter 11. The Stakes 262

Notes 292

Selected Bibliography 306

Index 311

Acknowledgments

This book would not have been possible without the generous support of many epidemiologists and researchers who made themselves available to discuss and critique these ideas. I wish to particularly thank the directors and researchers of the Center for AIDS Prevention Studies in San Francisco for offering to conduct a peer review of the unedited manuscript. That review was invaluable in helping to shape this volume. In particular, CAPS epidemiologist Ron Stall provided great insight into the issues raised here, and I am also indebted to Tom Coates, Susan Kegeles, Pam DeCarlo, Katherine Haynes Sanstad, Maria Elkstrand, Raphael Diaz, Katherine Wood, Dan Wohlfeiler, Chris Collins, Jeff Stryker, Bob Hayes, Don Barrett, Jay Paul, Kevin Filocamo and all of those at CAPS who attended the review and commented on the manuscript.

Other epidemiologists, researchers and health officials who assisted by granting interviews, making studies available, pointing out additional areas of inquiry or candidly discussing and critiquing ideas in this book include Mark Barnes, Ronald Bayer, Bernard Bihari, Wayne Blakenship, Sally Blower, Ralph Bolton, Mary Ann Chiasson, John Cladwell, Marcus Conant, Sally Cooper, Jim Curran, William Darrow, Laura Dean, Linda Doll, Max Essex, Paul Ewald, Alvin Freidman-Kein, Chuck Frutchey, John Gagnon, Robert Gallo, Jerome Groopman, Margaret Hamburg, Scott Hammer, Gerard Illaria, Harold Jaffe, John James, Ronald Johnson, Mitchell

Katz, Jeffrey Kelly, James Koopman, Mathilde Krim, Jeffrey Lawrence, Alan Lifson, Jonathan Mann, Lawrence Mass, Francine McCutchan, Leon McKusick, the late John Martin, Kenneth Mayer, Vickie Mays, Luc Montagnier, Martina Morris, Stephen Morse, Gerald Myers, Paul O'Malley, David Ostrow, Nancy Padian, Tom Peterman, Jeffrey Pudney, Alison Quayle, Mark Rapoport, Robert Root-Bernstein, Michael Samuel, Peter Schlager, Sharon Schneider, Mervyn Silverman, Cladd E. Stevens, Kent Taylor, James Thompson, Rodrick Wallace, Warren Winkelstein, and Rebecca Young.

Although we have never met in person, I wish to thank medical historian Mirko Grmek for his seminal book *History of AIDS* and for his enligthening telephone interviews, which first raised many of the questions examined in this volume. I am also grateful to my *New York Newsday* colleague Laurie Garrett, whose book *The Coming Plague*, and whose articles and conversations, also originally raised many of the questions discussed here.

The New York Academy of Medicine Library and librarian Peter Wansor were extremely helpful in locating studies, papers, and sources.

Some material in this book originally appeared as an article in *Out* magazine, edited by Ann D'Adesky. Certain other portions grew from my *New York Newsday* columns, edited by Ken Emerson, Kate McCormick and Mary Suh.

Many friends contributed thoughts and were invaluable in simply listening. I wish to particularly thank Michelangelo Signorile for his insightful contributions and criticisms, as well as Roger Jacobs, David Kirby, Dr. Frank Lipton, Kendall Morrison, Richard Ottens, and Evan Wolfson.

I also wish to thank the many others who, sometimes by sharing ideas and sometimes by forcefully disagreeing with ideas presented here, contributed to this book. Among them are Virginia Appuzzo, David Barr, Mike Barr, Andrew Beaver, Brian Beloviotch, Brenda Bergman, Richard Berkowitz, Allan Bérubé, Tom Blewitt, Jay Blotcher, Darren Britten, Michael Bronski, Frank Browning, Elinore Burkett, the late Michael Callen, Jonathan Capehart, Mel Cheren, Carlos Cordero, Spencer Cox, Denis deLeon, Martin Delaney, Bill Dobbs, Martin Duberman, Jim Eigo, Richard Elovich, Jim Fouratt, Liz Galst, Stephen Gendin, Michael Goff, David Gold, Jewelle Gomez, the late Robin Hardy, Mark Harrington, the late Essex Hemphill, Derek Hodel, Amber Hollibaugh, Tim Horn, Andy

Humm, Richard Isay, Michael Isbell, Alan Klein, Larry Kramer, Troy Masters, Roger McFarlane, Len McNally, Mark Milano, Scott Morgan, Michael Nesline, Joe Nicholson, Dave Nimmons, Ann Northrop, Alvin Novick, Walt Odets, Torrie Osborn, Duncan Osborne, Tim Rasta, Eric Rofes, Douglas Sadownick, Benjamin Schatz, Michael Shernoff, Mark Schoofs, Sarah Schulman, Greg Scott, Charles Silverstein, Sean Strub, Stephen Soba, Tom Stoddard, Urvashi Vaid, Dana Van Gorder, Carmen Vasquez, Joyce Wallace, Michael Warner, and Daniel Wolfe.

I owe an enormous debt of gratitude to editorial assistant Alex Swenson, to my agent, Jed Mattes, who provided supportive guidance and thoughtful suggestions throughout, and to my editor, Carole DeSanti, who believed in and supported this project from the beginning.

Finally I wish to thank my parents, Christine and Louis Rotello, whose consistent and unstinting support have made all the difference.

INTRODUCTION

AIDS and the Destiny of Gay Men

Why did AIDS happen to gay men?

The answer may seem so obvious that this question barely merits asking, yet different people have different "obvious" answers. To some, particularly in the gay community, the gay AIDS epidemic is often considered a result of social and governmental homophobia and neglect, even an act of genocide. To others, particularly conservatives, it's considered the fault of gay male promiscuity, even proof of the inherent unhealthiness of gay sex. To still others, particularly those who take public health warnings to heart, AIDS was simply an accident that just happened to sideswipe gay men first on its way to careening through the entire population. Each person's obvious answer tends to reveal that person's views on a host of subjects, many of them unrelated to AIDS itself.

It therefore might surprise many people to know that researchers who study the epidemic are almost unanimous in their understanding of why AIDS spread so disastrously among gay men, and their explanations have little to do with those mentioned above. AIDS, they say, is like all epidemics: an ecological disturbance that resulted when human behaviors created a niche for a particular microbe. To understand how the HIV epidemic occurred in a given population, we have to study how that population's behavior patterns changed in ways that provided HIV with its ecological opportunity.

The first portion of this book explores that topic. As a result, it is not about how homophobia contributed to the epidemic, or about what the government or the media did or did not do to exacerbate it. It is not about the failings of the medical establishment, or the ego of scientists, or the greed of drug companies. There have already been a number of excellent books on those subjects, and there will undoubtedly be many more in the years to come. Instead, what I seek to explore here is how gay behavior itself interacted with HIV to contribute to the epidemic. I will try to look at AIDS as an ecological rather than as a political or social event, and attempt to shed light on the process of the epidemic from what might be called the virus's point of view. To do so, I will try to place the epidemic firmly in the context of the previous sexually transmitted epidemics that struck gay men in the seventies, thereby questioning the "AIDS exceptionalism" that would have this epidemic stand as a unique and unfathomable event. I will examine theories of why, despite widespread knowledge about safer sex, the epidemic has continued to rage among gay men. And I will attempt to explore why many experts believe that if AIDS is ever partially or completely cured and gay men return to the behavior patterns of the past, the same kind of disaster will almost certainly happen again.

I am a gay man. I live in New York City, ground zero of the epidemic, one of the urban environments most devastated by AIDS. I arrived here almost a full decade before the epidemic began, and was an enthusiastic participant in the gay sexual culture I will shortly describe. I believed then, as I believe now, that homosexuals have been terribly oppressed by both the wider society and by our own legacy of self-hatred, and that gay liberation offers genuine hope of changing our lives for the better. Throughout the seventies I came to believe that gay people were making genuine progress toward building a world where future generations would not have to suffer as we had.

Then I watched with horror as a plague descended and much of my world sickened and died. It is almost impossible to overstate the impact of the AIDS epidemic on gay men, to exaggerate what happened when a group of people deeply stigmatized for the way they make love finally emerged from the shadows, proclaimed that Gay Is Good, and then were struck down by a disease spread through the very behavior that was the focus of their stigma. The overwhelming shock of this was something many gay men could scarcely deal with, but then we scarcely had time. We had work to do. We had to discover and fix whatever was causing the epidemic, a task we thought was quickly accomplished with the invention of safer sex. We had to aid the stricken, which we did with the creation of a vast network of personal and institutional caregiving and volunteerism. And we had to fight for a cure, which we did with everything from inside-the-Beltway lobbying to tenacious street activism.

I participated in all of these efforts. I practiced and promoted safer sex. I volunteered and cared for friends and bore witness to their suffering and their deaths. I wielded the tools of activism and advocacy journalism to help fight a desperate, and in many ways successful, guerrilla war against the pernicious agenda of blame. I worked for a cure, a struggle now bearing fruit in new drugs that are prolonging the lives of people with HIV. I believed, as most of my activist colleagues believed, that AIDS was an accident, that we were its heroes as well as its innocent victims (as, in many ways, we were and are), and that if there was any grain of truth to the idea that gay male behavior had played some role in AIDS, there was no point dwelling on it, since that would play dangerously into the hands of our enemies and since the problem had been solved by safer sex. In all these respects, I not only followed the party line, I helped write it.

But as the years have passed I have also followed the epidemic with a growing sense of foreboding. AIDS is not living up to our activist expectations. Despite the fact that by now virtually everyone knows how AIDS is spread and how to avoid it, it is continuing to saturate the gay male population at the same levels it always has. It is also continuing to devastate IV drug users who share needles, and their sexual partners, and, often, their children. But—and this is a very major but—it is not producing a self-sustaining heterosexual epidemic in the middle-class, mainstream American population. True, there are growing cases of what is sometimes called "heterosexual AIDS," but virtually all of these cases occur when HIV is passed from IV drug users to their sexual partners and children. While this is a tragedy for those concerned, and an additional blight on the poorest in America, it is a very different thing from a self-sustaining heterosexual epidemic, which would, by definition, be fueled by heterosexual transmission alone. Twenty years into the AIDS epidemic among gays, the absence of such a self-sustaining heterosexual epidemic can no longer be explained by the fact that it hasn't had time to occur. It is not happening because, as we will see, the sexual ecology of middle-class Western heterosexuals does not promote the efficient spread of HIV, and it will not occur unless there are major changes either in the biology of HIV or the behavior of heterosexuals or both. So something is happening on one side of the AIDS equation, among gay men and IV drug users, that is not happening on the other side, among the surrounding middle-class majority. Something potentially disastrous to both the prospects of the inner-city poor and the gay male community. And for me, by extension, something with enormously troubling implications for the future of gay liberation.

In my case, then, René Dubos's famous ecological injunction to "think globally, act locally" has convinced me to search more deeply for the roots of AIDS where I find them: here in my own environment. The word *ecology* comes from the Greek words for "home," *oikos*, and "knowledge," *logia*, and is sometimes translated as "home wisdom." This book is my attempt, as an AIDS activist and a gay journalist, to seek a home wisdom in the age of AIDS by taking an unblinking, and admittedly painful, look at the means by which an invader was able to roll like a Trojan Horse into the center of our home.

An ancient adage is "Know your enemy." Most of us in the age of AIDS have thought of the enemy as HIV itself. We have generally failed to recognize that an equal if not greater enemy is the complex set of conditions that favor HIV's transmission. Without those conditions, HIV would stand outside of our bodies and our lives like a million other potentially deadly viruses that swirl about the earth and would kill us if they could, but cannot because they cannot infect us. So while it is unquestionably important to know everything we can about the biology of HIV, it is equally crucial that we learn everything we can about the ecology, the process, the condition, that allows this particular virus entree into our lives. Only by knowing that enemy can we fight it.

When it comes to epidemiology, our ignorance stands in stark contrast to our often intensive study of other aspects of AIDS. Gay men have become reluctant experts at virology and immunology. We study the fluctuations of pharmaceutical stocks, are conversant with the ins and outs of the federal health bureaucracy, and often know more than our own doctors about the resourceful mutations of a tiny retrovirus whose very existence was unknown to the most advanced biologists less than a generation ago. But we have generally failed to recognize that the epidemic is itself an organism, a macroparasite that operates by laws as elegant as Einstein's and as discernible as Mendel's. Although it is now possible to understand the larger ways of the epidemic as surely as we understand the predations of HIV on the cellular level, we gay men, as citizens and victims, have generally chosen not to. And that is no accident.

HIV truly strikes us where we live. Its means of transmission—sex—is the very thing that to many of us defines us as gay men, drives our politics and our erotics, gives us our modern identity, provides the mortar of much of our philosophy and community, animates much of our lives. For these reasons we have good cause to shy away from a close examination of how certain key elements of our identity contributed to the disaster that now engulfs us. We have another good cause as well: Gay men have been blamed for AIDS since the disease appeared in mid 1981, and our reflexive response has been to resist being made scapegoats for a scourge that counted us among its primary victims. It has seemed politically wise instead to shift the focus to the substantial failings of government and media and the scientific establishment. Those failings were so egregious, and contributed so seriously to the epidemic in the early years, that it was hardly a stretch of the imagination to believe that AIDS was the result of factors wholly outside the gay world.

Someone has remarked that if you want to tell a really convincing lie, you have to believe it yourself. If so, AIDS activists must sound very convincing when we argue that "sex does not cause AIDS, a virus does." Or when we say, "There are no risk groups, only risky behaviors." Or when we insist, "It's not who you have sex with or where you have it that counts, it's what you do." Fighting the soundbites of blame with our own soundbites of self-defense has seemed essential to the goal of convincing ourselves of the absolute justice of our cause. And once gay men came to believe in the mid eighties that we had largely solved the problem of HIV transmission through the invention of safer sex—an invention, by the way, that society at large did little to encourage and much to

hinder—further discussion of our own role seemed not only politically unwise, but pointless, self-loathing, downright mean. And so
we have thrown up a fog of half-truths, and in the process we have
blinded ourselves.

Such was already the situation in 1987 when Randy Shilts published *And the Band Played On*. In that seminal work he described
the epidemic as a result of a series of failures by the government,
the health and research establishments, the media, and, importantly, the gay community. Yet he was vilified by many gay and
AIDS activists who felt that any discussion of gay men's role was too
much discussion. Many felt then, and many still feel, with some justification, that it is better to circle the wagons, fight off the hate
mongers, and leave any theoretical discussions of our own possible
role in AIDS to the ponderings of future generations.

Those who disliked Shilts's book for those reasons may absolutely
hate this one. For here I have deliberately omitted almost all mention of the role of government, the research establishment, and the
media in the genesis of the gay AIDS epidemic, and have focused
almost exclusively on the ways that gay men ourselves—inadvertently and innocently but nonetheless decisively—facilitated the epidemic. I have done so not because the failures of government and
media and science were not important. They were very important.
But there are several pressing reasons why our own behavioral role
must be explored and understood, especially now, as new drug
therapies open up the possibility of a paradigm shift in the epidemic.

For one thing, it has become increasingly clear that our failure to
delve into sexual ecology is itself contributing to the epidemic's
longevity. Strategies for dealing with the so-called Second Wave are
hobbled by a distorted, incomplete, and thoroughly unecological
view of the processes of epidemics generally, and this one in particular. In the most literal sense, our self-enforced ignorance about
sexual ecology is killing us.

Some might argue that while this may have been true in the past,
new advances in drug therapy are rendering traditional approaches
to prevention moot and even promising to end the epidemic. Why
stir things up now? But, if anything, sexual ecology is more important now than ever before, precisely because now, for the first time
since the epidemic began, there is both genuine hope of ending it
and a genuine danger of derailing that opportunity forever. The
next several years will be particularly decisive for the future of

AIDS. Newly developed antiviral drugs are becoming available, and newer and better formulations are promised. But these drugs do not immediately or completely eliminate the virus from the body. Instead, they suppress viral replication, placing HIV under intensive evolutionary pressure. We fondly hope that this pressure will be too much for HIV and that it will succumb. But HIV is without question the most mutable virus yet encountered, and there remains a very real danger that it will somehow manage to elude even the most potent drug combinations and emerge in drug-resistant forms. If it does, that would obviously be tragic for the unlucky individuals in whom it occurs. But if gay men mistakenly believe that the epidemic is waning and return to the habits of the past, rapidly transmitting new, drug-resistant strains of HIV across newly reconstituted viral highways, the potential for tragedy is almost unthinkable. It is altogether possible that over the next several years gay men's failure to comprehend and modify our sexual ecology could lead to a decisive Third Wave of the epidemic, this time with drug-resistant strains of HIV that can never be treated by the drugs otherwise most likely to work. So failure to understand sexual ecology could result in the squandering of our last best hope of ending the epidemic.

HIV aside, there are powerful additional reasons why we need to face the facts of why AIDS happened to gay men. Almost every researcher studying the epidemic is convinced of one overarching fact: that if gay men ever re-create the sexual conditions of the seventies, the same kind of thing will happen again with other microbes. There are already drug-resistant or incurable diseases circulating in the gay population—things like hepatitis C, antibiotic-resistant gonorrhea, various strains of herpes—and they all stand poised to sweep through the gay population the moment we provide them an opportunity to spread. There are still others that, as of this writing, are only dimly understood, such as the viral cause of Kaposi's sarcoma. And, say the experts, there are probably many more microbes whose existence we know nothing about, just as we once knew nothing about HIV. If gay men re-create the right conditions, such pathogens would almost certainly thrive and spread. So a key challenge facing us in a post-AIDS world, if there is one, is to prevent old diseases from mutating and spreading, and entirely new ones from sprouting from the same fertile soil that germinated AIDS.

Finally, an understanding of how AIDS happened to gay men

transcends AIDS itself. We live in a world of rapidly emerging diseases where our faith in the power of drugs to tame infectious illness has been humbled by the wiliness of microbes, their ability to evolve into drug-resistant strains, and the brilliantly adaptive way they exploit the niches we provide them. The story of gay men and AIDS is a telling parable of modern life, an example of how a mistaken belief in the powers of medicine contributed to a lifestyle of intrinsic risk. To understand that story is important for all people, because it challenges the pervasive myth that humans have somehow transcended the limits of the biological world. The extinction gay men have faced is a prologue to what may ultimately face everyone on the planet if we do not learn from the lessons all around us.

Myths

Our reluctance to examine the epidemiology of AIDS has helped perpetuate a number of myths about the epidemic, at least within the gay world, and so the first chapters of this book will attempt to walk the reader through AIDS as it is now understood by researchers, challenging the misconceptions that have become ingrained in the public imagination of the disease.

Myth: The epidemic occurred primarily because HIV is a new disease in humans, one that crossed from simians to people very recently and found a hospitable niche. In fact, while HIV clearly evolved from a simian virus or viruses, it appears to have existed in humans for at least several decades before the epidemic began in the seventies. It may even have occurred, although rarely, for centuries. It now seems likely that the primary reason the epidemic began when it did was not that a microbe jumped from animals to people, but that large-scale changes in human behavior provided HIV with radically new opportunities to spread.

Myth: It was essentially an accident that the epidemic struck gay men. In fact HIV is extremely selective and only produces epidemics when a population's behavior provides it with a niche. Without favorable conditions, HIV cannot spread in a given population. Among gay men in the seventies, our sexual behavior was extraordinarily conducive to the transmission of HIV.

Myth: These kinds of behavioral explanations cannot really explain why AIDS hit gay men when it did, because gay men have always behaved essentially the same. In fact, gay history provides compelling evidence that there were very significant changes in gay male behavior in the years preceding the epidemic, the very kinds of changes needed to facilitate the rapid spread of HIV. These included a sharp increase in anal sex with multiple partners, the appearance of so-called core groups of men who engaged in extraordinary levels of risky sexual behavior, and a rapid increase in the amount of sexual mixing between people in those core groups and the rest of the gay population. Indeed, few groups in history appear to have changed their overall sexual behavior as rapidly and profoundly as homosexual American men in the decades before AIDS.

Myth: It is homophobic to implicate aspects of gay behavior in the epidemic because straight people behave essentially the same. In fact, HIV will soon sweep the heterosexual population in the United States the same way it swept through gay men. In fact, twenty years after HIV began its relentless decimation of the gay population, it remains largely confined to the same heterosexual groups in the developed world that it infected from the start: hemophiliacs, intravenous drug users, and their female sexual partners and children. The only self-sustaining heterosexual HIV epidemic in the United States appears to be among crack cocaine addicts, who share many factors of sexual ecology with gay men.

Myth: While the above might be true here in the developed world, HIV is a heterosexual disease in the rest of the world, proving that gay behavior is irrelevant. In fact, HIV is spreading in an extremely selective way in the wider world, causing disastrous epidemics in places where heterosexual ecology favors its spread, and causing no epidemic at all in places where heterosexual behavior is less conducive. If anything, the highly selective spread of HIV around the world shows that AIDS is neither a gay nor a straight epidemic, but an ecological epidemic that exploits certain behaviors, chief among them the practice of having large numbers of partners, straight or gay.

Myth: Multiple partners don't matter, because gay men's promotion of condoms created a workable version of safe sex that allows people to continue to have multiple partners safely. In fact, the condom code does not seem ever to have been very successful in containing the epidemic. The drop in new infections in the mid-eighties, for example, probably occurred because most of the susceptible gay men were already infected. Now that a new generation of susceptible young men have entered the gay world, they are getting infected at rates that indicate that about half will eventually get AIDS, which is about the same ratio as in the older generation. The fact is that many people do not seem able to use condoms consistently enough to stem the epidemic.

Condoms are very important in the battle against AIDS, but total reliance on the condom code blinds us to the fact that condoms are just one narrow possibility in the possible arsenal of responses to AIDS. The condom code in the gay world is, in many ways, as much a political as a medical construction. Its dual purpose has been to prevent HIV transmission while preserving the "sex positivity" of gay male culture, thereby proving that the gay sexual revolution of the seventies can continue during a fatal epidemic of a sexually transmitted disease. But it provides virtually no room for error, and is in many respects anti-ecological, a classic "technological fix," because it has never addressed the larger factors in the gay environment that helped spread HIV. Since it is not working to contain the epidemic, we need to explore more holistic possibilities, which involve challenging and changing larger factors of gay life that encourage unsafe behavior.

Finally, we have the most potentially dangerous myth of all:

Myth: If AIDS is cured or contained by drug treatments, gay men can return to the sexual lifestyle of the seventies. Ultimately, to understand sexual ecology is to understand that the gay sexual revolution of the seventies was profoundly anti-ecological. Gay men can never go back.

In the final portion of this volume I will discuss how ecological thinking might help gay men create a new gay culture that could lower overall risk. The goal is a sustainable gay culture that both affirms gay identity and sexuality and, at the same time, provides a built-in measure of safety that would prevent the resurgence of AIDS or the emergence of new epidemics. I will draw parallels between the challenge facing gay men and that of other ecological movements, particularly the quest for population control, which shares many areas of common concern with AIDS prevention. But before we delve into these issues in more detail, it's important first to draw connections among the basic concepts of ecology, disease transmission, and sexual behavior that will appear again and again throughout this book.

A Primer on Ecology

Most people associate ecology with efforts to preserve nature, to recycle waste products and conserve resources and heal or prevent the wounds people inflict upon the world's ecosystems. But although these are important results of ecological thinking, ecology itself is much more. In its original sense, it is the science of connections. It seeks to describe the vast web of interrelationships that tie living things to their environments, its fundamental premise being that a change in any part of one of the "tangled banks" of life we call ecosystems can have broad and often unexpected implications for any living thing seeking to survive within them.

In some ways ecology is not a science so much as a way of looking at life itself. Its perspective begins with the tiniest systems that constitute life—atoms, molecules, energy—and radiates out in widening circles of complexity until it arrives at its basic units of study, which are populations. How does a given population survive and evolve? How does it interact with other populations? How does it adapt to the challenges before it? To answer these questions ecology widens its scope to consider the ecosystems in which populations live, an ecosystem being the combination of a population and its environment, functioning together as a unit.

Charles Darwin is often called the first great ecologist. His seminal observation that evolution proceeds through natural selection provided the essential underpinning upon which all of modern ecology is based. Natural selection is the chief animator of ecology, and the primary engine of natural selection is adaptation, the process by which a population changes and adjusts to meet its constant challenges. In one of the most significant of all biological insights, Darwin realized that genetic adaptation, or evolution, occurs for two basic reasons: Organisms are always struggling for survival, and random mutations sometimes occur that give an individual organism an edge in survival. Whenever such a mutation occurs, its possessor has an increased ability to reproduce and pass the mutation along. If the mutation continues to provide an edge in survival and reproduction, it may eventually predominate in the species, or help create a new species altogether.

Humans share genetic evolution with other organisms, but we possess an ecological trait unique to us: cultural adaptation. This is the process by which people consciously develop modes of living to meet the challenges of their environments, and then pass them down to succeeding generations through culture and education. From an ecological perspective, human cultures are far more than just "lifestyles" comprised of rituals and rules with symbolic meanings for their members. Cultures are adaptive strategies for survival, ways of life that allow their members to cope with the complex obstacles that nature, and other people, place in their way.

Medical Ecology

Modern ecology has produced subdisciplines called "human ecology" and "medical ecology" that view human health the way ecologists in general view the processes of life—as part of the interconnectedness of everything with everything else. To medical ecologists, human disease is more than just the tiny workings of microscopic or toxic invaders on the body, although it certainly includes that. Human disease, and the more difficult to measure entity called human health, are reflections of the complex relationships between human populations and their habitats, which include neighboring human populations, other populations of animals and plants and microscopic fellow travelers, and the inanimate world of elements and energy and earth.

The health of a given human population is a measure of adaptation: how well that population has adapted to its constantly changing habitat. Populations in good health are considered to be successfully adapted to the world they find themselves in. Those in precarious health have not found, or have somehow lost, the most advantageous accommodation with their habitats. And populations afflicted with chronic illness, or in the grip of plagues, have for the moment failed to find a successful niche and are, in the lingo of environmentalism, committing "ecocide," self-destruction via ecological catastrophe. If such a failure goes unchecked, that population faces oblivion by the same relentless law that has led to the disappearance of over 99 percent of all of the species that have ever lived on earth: extinction via natural selection.

To medical ecologists, no infectious disease simply happens. If one of the great biological and medical triumphs of the nineteenth century was the discovery that infectious diseases are largely caused by specific microbes, an equally important insight of the twentieth century is that diseases are more than the simple sum of their microbial causes. Almost as soon as medicine discovered "germs" it was faced with a corollary question: Why do some people, and some populations, succumb to some germs while others do not? Why is cholera typical of Bengal but not Brittany? Why does sleeping sickness affect Africans but not Austrians? Why does one person exposed to influenza become ill and another person not? If diseases are caused by germs, why do some germs affect some people and pass others by? From these questions the science of epidemiology was born, and the explanations it produces often complicate, if not undermine, the simple idea that germs cause disease. It seems that germs need help, and we humans are often the ones who provide it.

Take, for example, the story of schistosomiasis in modern Egypt. When epidemiologists look at this medical debacle that now afflicts up to 58 percent of the rural Egyptian population, they do not simply see a nasty, debilitating parasitic disease spread by water-borne snails. They see that, of course, because that's what schistosomiasis is. But beyond that they see a wider web of ecological—and therefore in a sense preventable—causes and effects.

The immediate cause of schistosomiasis is a parasite called a schistosome, whose intermediate hosts are snails that thrive in slow-moving streams and stagnant ponds. Each infected snail can produce thousands of male and female sporocysts that are released from the snail and swim out into the water, free to infect any humans they come into contact with. Once those sporocysts infect their unfortunate human hosts, they migrate to the heart, lungs, and liver, where they mate and reproduce, causing debilitation, weakness, weight loss, lassitude, and decreased resistance to other diseases.

For thousands of years the snails that serve this terrible intermediate function were kept in check by two notable factors of Egyptian ecology: One, the snails do not thrive in fast-moving streams or rivers, and the Nile flows swiftly; and two, Egypt was irrigated each year by the flooding Nile, which deposited silt and water (and snails) on the land and then soaked in, giving nourishment to the soil but leaving any stranded snails to die in the disappearing puddles and ponds. So there was schistosomiasis throughout the ages in Egypt—we see its biological record in the tissue of mummies and its cultural record in the carvings of the hieroglyphs—but apparently not very much. Indeed, it's doubtful that Egypt could have sustained its millennial glory if a majority of its people had been stricken with such a debilitating disease.

Then, in the mid twentieth century, came the momentous decision to build the Aswan High Dam, the greatest engineering project in North Africa since the pyramids. The Aswan Dam ended the annual rhythm of the Nile's floods and replaced it with thousands of miles of stagnant irrigation ditches, canals, and holding ponds covering the length and breadth of the country, waterworks that remain submerged for much of the year. These were ideal habitats for the snails, and their population exploded. As went the snails, so went the prevalence of schistosomes. And since rural Egyptians routinely wade in these irrigation projects as part of their daily work, so went the prevalence of schistosomiasis in Egyptians. Suddenly, almost overnight, this disease came to infect a majority of the population, a modern catastrophe from which there is, at present anyway, no way out.

From a narrow medical perspective, schistosomiasis is, and remains, a simple disease caused by a parasite long native to, and "natural" to, the Nile. In the lingo of AIDS activism, we might say, "Irrigation doesn't cause schistosomiasis; a sporocyst does." But from a broader ecological perspective, the calamity of schistosomiasis in modern Egypt is part of a complex web in which sporocysts, agriculture, engineering, a desire to tame the annual floods of the Nile, economic development, overpopulation, the politics of the Cold War, techniques of irrigation farming, and numerous other factors combined to create a human disaster.

All Diseases Are Ecological

When looked at in this way, every infectious ailment is both narrowly biological and broadly ecological. The difference between the health of the people of Katmandu, who typically suffer from chronic intestinal parasites caused by drinking water contaminated with fecal matter, and the health of their counterparts in Paris, where such diseases are virtually unknown, is an example. Katmandu has no modern sewage system and no uncontaminated source of potable water, while Paris constructed such systems over centuries.

The two biggest killers of Americans—heart disease and

cancer—are both deeply embedded in behavior and environment. Heart disease is primarily caused by the lifestyle of too little exercise, too much obesity, too much salt and fat in the diet, and smoking. Many of the contributing factors that affect the development of cancer are related to our ingestion of carcinogenic pollutants unknown to our ancestors.

Across the planet and throughout our lives, the diseases that buffet us, from the most trivial to the most fatal, all have environmental components. Think of the toddler afflicted with a continuous stream of minor colds that circulate in the sneezy environment of the day-care center. The sub-Saharan nomad, weakened by a famine caused by overgrazing and desertification, succumbing to a simple infection she might otherwise have survived. The non-smoking bartender dying of lung cancer from a lifetime of breathing other people's smoke. The person felled by *E. coli* poisoning after eating a tainted hamburger. The former resident of Love Canal dying of cancer caused by toxic wastes leaching from the backyard. In the broad purview of medical ecology nothing in our varied biosphere just happens, especially not disease. The microbial world, the chemical world, the realm of toxins and pollutants, parasites and microbes, are intimately connected to our behavior, our physical condition, our diet, all of which are intimately connected to the economic world, the cultural world, the social and religious and technological world around us. All ebb and flow in a seamless web of cause and effect. It remains for us to seek, so far as we are able, to understand these processes. Or, if we cannot or will not, to suffer the consequences.

Sexually Transmitted Diseases

Most human diseases are infectious or contagious; that is, they are caused by microscopic entities passed to their human hosts from previously infected persons, insects, animals, or plants. Whether through air, water or food, a rabid dog or a hungry tick, a sneeze or a kiss or a curse, living beings transmit diseases among ourselves in endless chains of cause and effect.

One specific group of infectious diseases are those transmitted by the physical act of love. Sexually transmitted diseases (STDs) differ from other infectious diseases in that their transmission generally requires the exchange of bodily fluids—semen, preejacu-latory fluid, cervical/vaginal fluids, saliva, mucus, blood, feces—during sex. No one knows precisely when sexually transmitted diseases first appeared in human populations. There are early records contained in Hippocratic treatises from the fifth century B.C. that refer directly to genital herpes and indirectly to lym-phogranuloma venereum, and other ancient texts, including the Bible, mention STDs. Certainly since human societies grew ad-vanced enough to sustain urban populations in the thousands and tens of thousands, people have been afflicted to varying degrees with serious diseases spread through sex. The more common are syphilis; gonnorhea; genital herpes; genital warts; and chlamydia; but the list also includes hepatitis A, B and C; cytomegalovirus; Epstein-Barr virus mononucleosis; nongonococal urethritis for men; pelvis inflammatory disease for women; and several others, undoubtedly including some not yet recognized. (Researchers now believe, for example, that a previously unknown sexually trans-mitted herpes virus is responsible for Kaposi's sarcoma. This undoubtedly would not have been noticed were it not for its close association with the AIDS epidemic.)

At certain times, among certain populations, STDs were rare or unknown. At other times they were more common but still largely limited to certain core groups within the population: prostitutes and those who patronized them, soldiers, prisoners, the young, the very poor, and so on. At still other times they were pervasive dan-gers that were considered background threats to the health of almost anyone. And at still other times they burst into epidemics, plunging whole societies into medical, cultural, economic, and reli-gious crisis and altering the course of history. Some historians now argue, for example, that the vast syphilis epidemic that swept Europe from the 1490s onward may have contributed to the Refor-mation and the rise of Puritanism, a development that still has echoes in our own time. There are, it bears repeating, no accidents in nature. If differing rates of diseases among populations are largely the result of different human ecologies, differing rates of sexually transmitted diseases are largely the result of different sexual ecologies.

Sexual ecology, then, consists of the entire spectrum of causes and effects that influence the spread of sexually transmitted dis-eases. It includes the direct microbial cause of an STD, the way it enters the body, and the ways it reproduces and interferes with the normal working of cells, thereby causing disease. It includes the role specific sexual behaviors play in transmitting microbes from one person to another. It includes any biological cofactors that determine whether, once exposed, infection takes place, and once infected, illness results. And it includes the way in which the course of illness itself impairs or enhances a person's ability to pass the infection on to others.

Sexual ecology also includes the ways in which human behaviors affect disease transmission, including the mysteries of why individuals and entire societies behave in ways that place them at sharply different risks for certain STDs. Beyond beliefs and ideologies and group behaviors, it includes the ways that human technologies impact STD transmission. How do diseases travel from one part of the world to another: slowly on horseback, more swiftly on steamship, instantly on jumbo jets? How does the availability of treatments, cures, or vaccines, or the lack of them, affect transmission, or the mutation of old diseases into new strains? How do the cultural values that stem from access to certain technologies or medicines affect our beliefs about disease, thereby affecting our behavior?

It is high time to apply the fundamental questions of ecology to the terrible event of AIDS in the gay world, to ask the tough questions and to follow wherever they lead. How, for example, were the behaviors that favored HIV in the gay world created? How were our ecosystems altered in ways that facilitated HIV? What were those changes? And if the epidemic can be explained in terms of altered ecology, does that suggest ways it can be curbed or ended? Can the gay male community use the basic knowledge of medical ecology and human adaptation to readapt our sexual behavior, to undo the changes that have almost destroyed us? And can we do so in ways that preserve the vital human gains of gay liberation? Just as environmentalists ponder the creation of "sustainable" economic growth that doesn't destroy the planet, or "sustainable" cities that don't pollute, can we create a *sustainable gay culture*, one in which people are free to be homosexual, but one that does not destroy the very souls it liberates?

Some may object to this discussion, fearing that it will damage the reputation of gay men. But here is the quandary: Containing the epidemic requires a full, open understanding of its mechanisms.

Precisely such an understanding, especially an open public discussion of it, seems to play into the hands of anti-gay forces. In a cruel irony, the only public discussion likely to save gay men from further saturation with AIDS is the very public discussion we least want to have, one almost guaranteed to embarrass many of us.

But I believe that there is little that a Jesse Helms or a Pat Robertson can do to gay men that approaches the damage wrought by the endless continuation of AIDS. The application of ecology to AIDS has importance not only for the lives that stand to be saved, but for the social and political movement that stands to be rescued. AIDS and the series of epidemics that preceded it in the seventies have cast a pall over the entire edifice of gay liberation. The appearance of a multitude of epidemic diseases almost immediately after gay men had carved out zones of sexual freedom has opened up the grim, almost unthinkable possibility that for gay men, sexual freedom leads inexorably to disease. As time goes on and the epidemic continues to rage among gay men while largely sparing the rest of the population, that nightmare grows only more plausible. It was one thing to believe we were accidental victims who would soon be joined in our sorrow by everyone else. It is quite another to discover that we will not be joined, that we stand almost alone, consumed with disease. Ultimately the only way to refute this nightmarish connection is to prove it wrong, and the only way to do that is by creating a sustainable gay culture in which gay men are both sexual and healthy, free to love, and free from plague.

The first step in imagining that sustainable future is to go back in time and seek answers to how we got to this terrible impasse in the first place. Where did HIV come from? How did it enter our world? And are there clues in the story of the birth of AIDS that can help us bring about its end?

CHAPTER 1

The Birth of AIDS

Except for one detail, the twenty-eight-year-old Tennessee man was a typical AIDS patient. He had been healthy and robust until a shortness of breath turned suddenly to pneumonia and he had to be rushed, gasping for air, to Baptist Memorial Hospital in Memphis. Then over the next few months he suffered one debilitating infection after another, well-known milestones along the *via dolorosa* of AIDS: enlarged lymph nodes and depressed lymphocyte counts, fevers, repeated bouts of pneumonia, chronic inflammatory reaction, growing malaise, and finally an uncontrollable cytomegalovirus infection that spread throughout his system and snuffed out his life.

But although the acquired immunodeficiency syndrome that afflicted R.G. (as medical history knows him) was depressingly typical from a symptomatic point of view, there was something very unusual about his case, something that would earn it, and him, a lasting place in medical history: the date.

It was February 1952.

We have long been accustomed to considering AIDS a new disease, a scourge sent from God or the deepest jungles of Africa sometime in the 1970s to fatally disrupt the established patterns of our lives. But scientists increasingly suspect that the order of that equation was reversed: that first we ourselves disrupted the patterns of our lives, and only then did a scourge descend. It now seems likely that although the epidemic of AIDS is certainly new, HIV itself is probably old in humans. It burst into epidemic proportions when and where it did not simply because of changes in the natural world but because of changes in human behaviors. More ominously, wherever those newly altered behaviors flourish, the AIDS epidemic has relentlessly spread.

Combining the hypotheses of the various disciplines working on this question yields an emerging general theory of AIDS history that goes something like this: HIV-1, the virus that causes AIDS in most of the world, has existed in humans in Europe and America as well as in Africa since at least the mid-fifties and possibly for decades longer or even centuries. For however long it has harbored in humans, HIV easily eluded notice. It was rare, it had no uniform set of symptoms to mark it as a single disease, and it never sparked a noticeable epidemic, primarily because it is dozens or even hundreds of times more difficult to transmit than any other known venereal pathogen. To stir up an epidemic with such a germ would require a level of sexual partner change far higher than that practiced by most societies for most of history.

Unlike other STDs that often pass directly through mucous membranes of sexual organs to infect new hosts, HIV generally does not (although it can). It prefers a direct line to the host's bloodstream: a hole, a lesion, a puncture, a tear. In addition, it prefers a host whose immunity is suppressed by additional active infections. And even then it usually requires repeated exposures before it finally steps aboard. So back in a world before blood transfusions, the theory goes, before injection drugs, before mass immunization programs, before sexual revolutions, what chance did HIV have? Among our ancestors it was the Sisyphus of germs, barely able to maintain the essential ratio that marks a microbe's survival: one new host infected for every old host killed. Until the creation of vast new sexual and blood-sharing ecosystems, very few people could have been infected with HIV. Some virologists have ventured a guess that the prevalence level might have ranged from 1 in 100,000 to 1 in a 1,000,000.

Then in the sixties and early seventies came a series of revolutions affecting what is sometimes called the "socioecology" of the world. A huge increase in urbanization. A revolution in the use of blood transfusions and blood products. An explosion in the use of injection drugs. A sexual revolution. A gay revolution. These changes brought about new global ecosystems in which the blood and sexual fluids of millions of people flowed into one another, and flowed the way HIV likes to travel: nonstop, straight to the vein.

What happened in the seventies, the theory goes, was this: Eventually some HIV-infected person came along. Perhaps a man tempted by the emerging culture of sexual liberation in Uganda or gay New York or San Francisco. Perhaps a youth tempted by injection drugs. That HIV-infected person saw something enticing about one of these sexual or needle-sharing ecosystems and dived in, mixing his rare infection in a vast communal pool.

In that instant, probably sometime in the early seventies, the die was cast. HIV had found what it was looking for, the answer to its viral dreams. The rest was epidemic history.

The Recent Crossover Theory

AFRICAN AIDS "DEADLY THREAT TO BRITAIN" shrieked a London *Daily Telegraph* headline in 1986, accurately summing up mid-1980s thinking in Europe and the United States about where the new disease of AIDS had come from. Even though the earliest known cases of the new syndrome occurred in Americans and Europeans—AIDS was discovered because of its appearance in American gay men—from almost the very beginning it was assumed that AIDS could not have arisen in the West. Renee Sabatier writes in *Blaming Others* that it was "thought unlikely that such an unusual disease could have gone unnoticed for long in the United States." Despite recent epidemics of Legionnaires' disease and toxic shock syndrome, many experts still felt that new diseases simply don't arise in the shiny, healthy cities of the West. So when a few early AIDS cases also appeared in Africans residing in Europe, scientists immediately suspected Africa.

That suspicion seemed confirmed in the mid-1980s when an HIV antibody test was developed and the first batches of stored African blood were found to have a 50 percent HIV seropositivity rate. Scientists and journalists quickly announced that their suspicions had been confirmed. Later, however, it turned out their announcement was premature. Cindy Patton writes in *Inventing AIDS* that researchers found that "the HIV antibody test developed in the U.S. could not distinguish between antibodies to HIV and antibodies to malaria, which is endemic to rural, equatorial Africa."

Further confirmation of Africa as the fount of plague seemed to come when a team of scientists in California led by Murray Gardner examined the blood of captive macaques who were suffering from an AIDS-like ailment and discovered the first simian immunodeficiency virus (SIV), a member of the same clade, or family, of viruses as HIV. Eventually several strains of SIV were found in wild African monkeys, and the molecular structure of a particular strain found in sooty mangabeys proved almost identical to the molecular structure of HIV-2, which causes a relatively mild form of AIDS in the same region of west Africa that the mangabeys inhabit. This seemed to confirm that the HIVs began as SIVs in monkeys and then, as Robert Gallo wrote in *Scientific American* in 1987, "somehow entered human beings, initiating a series of mutations that yielded the intermediary viruses before termination in the fierce pathology" of HIV.

The date of the crossover was fiercely debated. Gerald Myers, head of an HIV research team at the Los Alamos National Laboratory, believes the event occurred in the late sixties or even the seventies. Others, like Gallo and HIV co-discoverer Luc Montagnier, have publicly speculated that the crossover may have occurred longer ago in remote African villages, and that human infection then smoldered in tribal isolation until postcolonial trade and travel patterns spread it to the outside world. But whatever the date, almost everyone seemed to agree: HIV had begun in African monkeys and crossed over to humans. And most agreed that the crossover was probably recent.

The only remaining question, and a subject of hot international debate, was why the two different forms of the virus, HIV-1 and HIV-2, burst into epidemic forms when they did. Did the huge international vaccination programs of the sixties spread monkey blood, and possibly HIV, to millions of unsuspecting patients? Did the World Health Organization's smallpox vaccination drive in the late 1960s somehow transform an already widely disseminated but nonlethal form of HIV into a newly virulent and deadly form? Some felt that no particular explanation was needed, that the timing of the epidemic was linked to the timing of the cross-species transmission. As Los Alamos researcher Myers put it, "If this was a fairly recent cross species transmission, it's not surprising that a virus that was well adapted to the animal population would not be virulent by the fact that it was now in a foreign host." Microbes that have recently passed from animals to humans, he noted, can be inherently unstable.

The idea soon became entrenched that AIDS was not just a new epidemic but a new human disease, one that passed from simians to humans in Africa, then swiftly crossed the Atlantic to America. Randy Shilts helped popularize this concept in his 1987 book *And the Band Played On* by speculating on the exact moment of arrival: the Bicentennial celebration of 1976, when the stately Tall Ships regatta brought thousands of foreign sailors, including many from Africa, into contact with gay New Yorkers. Shilts opens the book by picturing the Bicentennial bacchanal as a modern-day Masque of the Red Death:

> Deep into the morning, bars all over the city were crammed with sailors. . . . That was the part the epidemiologists would later note, when they stayed up late at night and the conversation drifted toward where it had started and when. They would remember that glorious night in New York Harbor, all those sailors, and recall: From all over the world they came to New York.

African Anomalies

From the very beginning, however, problems arose with the recent simian crossover hypothesis. The major one was that although HIV-2 is closely related to the SIVs, HIV-1, the killer virus we call AIDS, is not. The only strain of SIV that even remotely resembles HIV-1 was found in a single wild chimpanzee in Gabon and has never been found in any other chimps. Most experts believe that it's far more likely that this particular chimp was infected by humans than the other way around.

Genetic analysis indicates that HIV-1 is distantly descended from some simian retrovirus. But, as Rockefeller University virologist Stephen Morse told me, "There is no known virus that looks even closely ancestral to HIV-1 in the wild. It's a genuine missing link." If so, it's a whopper. After all, if HIV-1 is a monkey virus that recently jumped to humans, where are the infected monkeys?

A second problem might be called the HIV-2 paradox. Medical historian Mirko Grmek puts it this way: "You can suppose some kind of cross species transmission as a single event, but how can you make a theory to account for two contemporary transmissions of two completely different viruses that both cause the same disease?" The idea that HIV-1 and HIV-2, only 40 percent genetically related and therefore distant cousins from a viral point of view, both just happened to cross over accidentally to the same species (us) at the same time is, according to Grmek, "extremely improbable, even impossible, if held to be the result of chance biological mutation." And Robert Gallo's initial theory, that HIV-2 crossed over from simians to humans and then evolved into HIV-1, was decisively debunked by genetic analyses of their structures. It is now universally agreed that HIV-2 cannot have given birth to HIV-1.

Unfortunately, the quick acceptance of the recent crossover thesis by the Western scientific establishment precluded the exploration of other possibilities. Everybody agreed that HIV was new in humans and pronounced the mystery solved. Without adequate examination of alternatives, modern scientists made the same kind of mistake their predecessors did in presuming the earth was flat, or that maggots spontaneously generated from rotting meat, because things looked that way; the mistake of favoring the simple over the complex. In the case of HIV, as we have repeatedly learned to our woe, the subtle and complex almost always turn out to be closest to the truth.

Politicizing the Source

By the late 1980s there were ample reasons why researchers were generally not eager to investigate complex theories about the origin of AIDS. The question had become intensely political. Defensiveness about "causing" AIDS had originally led several African governments to deny that an AIDS problem even existed within their borders, which in turn delayed prevention measures and contributed to the growing disaster. So partly out of fear of giving further offense to African officials on whose cooperation they increasingly relied, and partly because it was difficult to justify spending scarce AIDS dollars on what some scornfully termed "butterfly collecting," scientists shied away from launching full-scale investigations to find HIV-1's direct ancestors.

Here in the West research into the origins of the epidemic was discouraged by chauvinists unwilling to conceptualize that any new disease could possibly be spawned in industrialized countries. Gay men and AIDS activists, too, were less than eager to pull closely at the threads of AIDS history. Blamed by the Right for that worst of biblical crimes—the bringing down of plague—many felt that the stigma of causing an epidemic was so politically damaging that it rendered open discussion of the epidemic's origin extremely unwise. At ACT UP meetings in New York, activists hissed when anyone even raised the subject of the epidemic's origin.

Into this potent politicization of what remained, at heart, a medical mystery, scientists ventured at their peril. But a few ventured anyway. A breakthrough event occurred in 1989 with the French publication of Mirko Grmek's landmark *History of AIDS*, in which one of the world's leading authorities on medical history presented the startling hypothesis that HIV has long existed in human populations, not just in Africa but in the West as well. Grmek's book was hailed by critics for its thorough scholarship, its cautious, unsensational approach to the subject, and for the fact that someone of Grmek's stature was willing to tackle the subject at all, much less challenge traditional thinking about it.

Grmek described three basic ways to test the hypothesis that HIV is old in humans: Search old medical records for retrospective diagnoses of AIDS; test old blood and tissue samples to see if they contain traces of HIV or antibodies to HIV; and genetically sequence different samples of the virus to attempt to reconstruct its past.

Retrospective Diagnosis

Using the first technique, researchers found dozens of possible AIDS cases from medical records dating back to the 1930s. Formerly healthy people had, with no discernible underlying cause, suddenly developed fulminant Kaposi's sarcoma or unexplained pneumonia combined with cytomegalovirus infection, or fatal bouts of other opportunistic infections typical of AIDS. In the United States alone, writes Grmek, specialists consider at least sixteen of these once baffling deaths to what he termed "accepted cases" of pre-epidemic AIDS, the earliest dating to 1940. Many more cases seem suspiciously like AIDS but are not as fully accepted by experts like Grmek because the records are less precise. Medical records in Europe also contain a large number of AIDS-like cases dating back to the forties. Cases are twice as common among men as among women, and records on both continents reveal apparent examples of male-to-female transmission.

But retrospective diagnosis has obvious drawbacks. Doctors began describing atypical cases only at the end of the last century, and accurate modern records date to only about the 1930s. Even then you can't be too sure. "Anytime you start to work with old medical charts there's so many factors you could be misreading," points out Laurie Garrett, author of *The Coming Plague.* "Starting with: what did the doctors write down and not write down; what tests did they do and not do? A perfectly good doctor could have overlooked a perfectly obvious diagnosis."

Also undermining the usefulness of retrospective diagnosis is "non-HIV AIDS." A small number of people in the world today have the low T-cell counts and opportunistic infections indicative of AIDS, but are not infected with HIV-1. At the 1992 International AIDS Conference in Amsterdam the announcement of this syndrome created a media sensation that completely overshadowed the conference's work. When the dust settled it was shown that the syndrome, dubbed ICL (idiopathic CD4 T-lymphocytopenia), afflicts far fewer people than some originally claimed, and the cases occur sporadically rather than being linked together, indicating that the syndrome is not passed from person to person. Researchers now feel that individual cases of ICL have little or nothing in common with each other and are probably caused by a diverse spectrum of bacteria, toxins, parasites, and fungi.

Nevertheless, there's strong justification for diagnosing AIDS by its symptoms alone. After all, that's how the CDC itself diagnosed AIDS before HIV was discovered. Back in the early eighties if a patient had any of the official opportunistic infections associated with AIDS, that patient was considered to have AIDS. When such symptom-diagnosed patients were subsequently tested for HIV antibodies, virtually all were found to be HIV infected, thus confirming the value of symptom diagnosis. So to apply symptom diagnosis to long-dead patients is not so far-fetched.

Beyond these individual cases lies another intriguing phenomenon. Medical historians speculate that if virulent strains of HIV had occasionally emerged and sparked quasi-epidemics in America and

Europe, the main documentary artifact would be unexplained increases in the number of people who died of opportunistic infections, particularly tuberculosis, one of the most common opportunistic infections associated with AIDS and one of the most closely monitored diseases throughout the nineteenth and early twentieth centuries. Medical historians have found what Grmek calls "curious changing" in past rates of TB. And TB is not the only AIDS-related illness whose historic incidence unaccountably rose and fell. Some of the oddest fluctuations in disease rates have occurred in that most telltale of AIDS-related diseases among gay men, Kaposi's sarcoma.

In 1868 a brilliant young Viennese dermatologist received a visit from a middle-aged male patient who sought his help for a strange skin cancer, one neither the doctor, Moritz Kaposi, nor any of his colleagues had ever seen. As this strange malignancy spread to the patient's internal organs, Kaposi kept a careful record of the unusual malady, confident he'd never see another case. A few months after the patient died, though, a second patient appeared with the same condition. Then a third patient, and a fourth and a fifth, all middle-aged men, all soon dead. Via an autopsy, one of them was found to have strange lesions in his lungs which, from today's perspective, sound suspiciously like Pneumocystis carinii pneumonia, another of the most common AIDS afflictions. This cluster of KS cases—ending as abruptly as it began—provided Kaposi with the opportunity to describe the cancer that now bears his name.

In the late 1870s and early 1880s another physician, Tommaso De Amicis, stumbled across another cluster of twelve cases of Kaposi's sarcoma. Except for one small child, all were Neapolitan men between the ages of thirty-nine and forty-four. A third recorded outbreak occurred among European men in the early twentieth century, and a fourth in postwar Africa was serious enough to warrant convening an international symposium in Kampala in 1961 to discuss the problem. Writing in the *Journal of the National Medical Association*, researchers Harold P. Katner and George A. Pankey argued that by using KS as a "probable marker" of pre-epidemic AIDS, they were able to identify tentative AIDS cases back to 1902.

It is now believed that KS is transmitted by a herpes virus, and patterns of KS in gay men strongly suggest that this virus is, like HIV, sexually transmitted. One study suggests it may be spread in saliva. But the cancer itself virtually never appears in gay men in the absence of HIV. Whatever causes the cancer appears to require HIV's additional immune suppressive infection to produce disease. So it is theoretically possible that what Kaposi and others observed in decades past was quasi-epidemic clusters of HIV and the KS virus, clusters that died out for lack of the kind of multipartner sexual networks needed to kindle a full-fledged epidemic.

Stored Tissue Samples

Most of these retrospective cases are missing the preserved tissue or blood that would confirm an AIDS diagnosis, but not all. In rare cases doctors, mystified by a dying patient's unusual or bizarre symptoms, harvested and froze that patient's blood or tissue, hoping that future medical advances might solve the mystery. As a result, doctors have occasionally been able to test their suspicions by giving HIV tests to long-deceased patients.

Perhaps the most widely known example is the case of "Robert R." He was a fifteen-year-old African-American youth who checked into St. Louis City Hospital in 1968 with edema of the lower body and various other afflictions and died the next year, beset with Kaposi's sarcoma, Chlamydia trachomatis, STDs, and intestinal disorders. After he died physicians collected and froze samples of his blood and lymph nodes for future study. In 1987 the samples were examined by microbiologist Robert Garry at Tulane University, who published his results in the *Journal of the American Medical Association*. To the surprise of the AIDS medical community, Robert R. had tested HIV-antibody positive, two decades after his death.

An even earlier case provides the first confirmed example of transmission from a husband to his wife, and from the wife to their infant child. In 1966 a twenty-year-old Norwegian man checked into Oslo's Rikshospitalet complaining of recurrent colds, lymphadenopathy, and Kaposi's-like dark spots on his skin. He did not improve, and the next year his wife came down with candidiasis, cystitis, and other afflictions. A child born to the couple that same year seemed healthy at first, but by age two was suffering from severe bronchial candidiasis. They all died within months of each other, and serum samples were collected and frozen. In 1988 the long-dead family all tested HIV seropositive.

Of course, such testing can never fully solve the issue of HIV's longevity in humans. For one thing, no one knows whether even today's highly accurate tests such as PCR would be able to detect HIV that has been inactivated for decades. More importantly, few if any stored samples go back farther than the mid fifties. Researchers have discussed hunting for HIV among preserved human tissue in pathological museums and even among mummies from ancient Egypt, but the prognosis is not great. "People who run pathological museums are very protective of their samples," says Rockefeller University's Stephen Morse. Even if they weren't, and even if long-dead HIV were detectable, the search might still prove futile. If pre-epidemic HIV infected only 1 in 100,000 to 1 in 1,000,000 people, researchers would have to test hundreds of thousands or millions of samples, or else get incredibly lucky, before they could expect to stumble across a rare, random case.

Genetic Sequencing

Was there an explosive evolutionary event thirty years ago when today's major subtypes of HIV-1 burst from a common ancestor? Or have those types existed in humans for centuries? Those are the questions facing geneticists who employ the third technique for understanding the history of AIDS: genetic sequencing. By analyzing the genetic structure of HIV, geneticists believe they can estimate how far and for how long its various strains have evolved away from a common ancestor. The process is similar to the way the age of the universe is dated. Astronomers measure how far apart galaxies are and how fast they are traveling, then extrapolate backward in time to the point at which they must have emanated from a single event: the Big Bang. Likewise, geneticists can measure the differences between the major subtypes of HIV, estimate how fast the viruses are evolving, and then extrapolate backward in time to a point at which they all may have emanated from a single common parent. In the case of HIV it is presumed that this point was the moment when the virus leapt from its original animal host into the human population.

For several years the main problem with this technique was that genetic estimates varied widely depending on how fast scientists presumed the virus's genetic clock was ticking. Much of the disagreement stemmed from the fact that different researchers were basing their estimates on different proteins of the virus's surface. Analyzing one such protein, for example, Japanese researcher S. Yokoyama estimated that HIV broke from its common ancestors no less than 280 years ago. Using another, a different team estimated that the break occurred about 900 years ago. Research in this area gained momentum in the mid nineties as scientists prepared to mount large-scale vaccine trials and sought to pinpoint which strains of HIV-1 exist in which geographic populations so that they could prepare appropriate vaccines. As a result of this effort, however, the entire question of how quickly different subtypes of HIV are evolving away from each other received an unexpected jolt. Researchers at the 1996 International AIDS Conference in Vancouver presented data indicating that instead of evolving away from each other, some global strains of HIV are evolving toward each other, joining together in a process researchers call recombination. *Recombination* refers to the unique and frightening ability of retroviruses to fuse together. When a person is infected with two or more strains of a retrovirus like HIV, those strains can literally merge, fusing characteristics of both into a wholly new strain. In collecting samples of HIV from around the world in the nineties and comparing them to earlier samples, the researchers discovered that some of the most troublesome strains on the planet, including virulent subtype E, are recombinants that have only recently emerged. "Recombinant HIV [strains] have already established a global reservoir and are responsible for the rapidly expanding epidemic in Southeast Asia," one group of researchers wrote, and they concluded that exchanges of genetic material between HIV subtypes from around the world may represent "a common adaptive strategy with significant functional and epidemiological implications."

While the researchers did not say so in their paper, their discovery provided evidence that AIDS is an old disease in humans. The reason is simple. If, under the jet-age conditions of the modern world, the different global strains of HIV are combining with each other, then how and under what conditions could those strains have evolved separately in the first place? A logical answer, some say the only logical answer, is that their evolution must have occurred before the jet-age conditions of the modern world, when Africans, Asians, Americans, and Europeans lived in relative isolation from each other. Under those conditions, the theory goes, HIV was able to evolve into the major subtypes that existed when the epidemic was first noticed. Now, however, under current conditions, they have begun to recombine. Some researchers suspect that eventually the global viral pool of HIV may merge into entirely new recombinant strains, mixing characteristics of all the older strains that had evolved before the modern age. By analogy, we can see much the same process in our own human species, both biologically and culturally. The different races of humankind arose, it is believed, when populations on various continents were virtually cut off from each other, allowing Homo sapiens time and space to evolve into physically and culturally distinct races and groups. Now, as humans from all over the planet travel, emigrate, mix, and intermarry, the global races and global cultures are very slowly combining. If this process continues for millennia, human populations may eventually become culturally and even genetically homogenized.

The discovery that global strains of HIV are recombining not only added to the evidence that HIV may be old in humans, it also raised the possibility that modern HIV itself is a product of the recombination of several primate viruses and lentiviruses. According to this idea, scientists will never discover a direct ancestor of HIV in the wild because one does not exist. Rather, modern HIV may have come into existence when an individual or individuals became infected by several different viruses which then recombined into the ancestor of modern HIV.

The Camouflaged Killer

If HIV has been among us for decades or longer, how did AIDS manage to evade discovery for so long? One obvious answer is that its symptoms were too diverse to be recognized as a single disease. Another is that its incubation period is so long that people were unable to connect one case with another. Still another answer is that until the epidemic broke, the disease existed at a level too low and sporadic to be noticed.

Even if AIDS had raged as an epidemic in the past, would it have been recognized as such in the days before the immune system and retroviruses were understood? Cindy Patton writes in *Inventing AIDS* that the epidemic happened to arise "at the moment when advanced technology could relate a primary causative agent to a set of extremely diverse symptoms. Had AIDS occurred fifty years ago, it would probably have been considered inexplicably untreatable forms of a dozen different diseases rather than the symptoms of an under-lying immune disorder." Underscoring this notion is the fact that other diseases continue to go unnoticed under the very nose of modern medicine. In 1994, for example, a mysterious and often fatal respiratory ailment caused by a hantavirus appeared in the American Southwest, seemingly from nowhere. Eventually researchers from the CDC's Special Pathogens Branch announced their belief that this particular hantavirus has been killing Americans for ages, and that only a conflation of unusual events—heavy rains causing an over-abundant piñon crop causing an overabundance of piñon-eating, virus-carrying mice causing an explosion of mice-to-human transmis-sion—caused it to be noticed.

"No biologist worth his salt is going to tell you that we've identi-fied all the lethal microbes out there," says Laurie Garrett. "There are thousands of unsolved deaths every year, even in the U.S." If there are today, there certainly were in the past.

Why Now?

One final, explosive question remains: Why did a virus that was once so rare suddenly burst into a global pandemic? Although the question is medical, many fear that the answer has frighteningly political implications. If the behaviors of certain groups played a role in bringing about the epidemic, such information would be a potent weapon against them. That concern has contributed to a general silence on the subject, one that effectively prevents society, including gay society, from considering the probability that the seeds of future epidemics lie in the history of the current one.

In *The Coming Plague*, Garrett describes a crucial phase needed to transform a low level of virus into outright epidemic. She calls that phase "amplification." Some thing or things have to happen for a microbe to escape its previously harmless ecological niche and reach critical mass. The history of epidemics shows that such factors are almost always related to human behaviors. Looking at the subject from a slightly different angle, virologist Stephen Morse says that most epidemics result from changes in "viral traffic patterns," either between animals and humans or among humans ourselves. Again, these changes almost always occur when humans inadvertently pave new pathways for the microbial world. Both hypotheses fit neatly with what we know of the emergence of HIV.

As you'd expect, given the ways of the world, we know much more about the precise mechanisms that amplified AIDS in America than in Africa, but we know that in both places enormous social and sexual revolutions occurred just before the epidemics broke out. In Africa decolonization was followed by social shocks so profound that many cultures experienced greater change in a single generation than in the previous thousand years. Industrialization was crammed into five-year plans. Displaced farmers flocked by the millions to cities that mushroomed where villages had recently stood. Highways plunged through jungles and across deserts, connecting ancient neighbors who had barely guessed each other's existence. Catastrophic wars dislocated millions. Mass communications exposed millions more to the powerful, prosperous—and sexually liberated—models of the Western world.

New viral trails were blazed as a result of all these phenomena. Male villagers in Third World countries, now laboring for much of the year in cities far from wives and family, replaced traditional village monogamy or polygamy with multipartner urban sexuality. In many cases in Africa, the wives left behind were compelled to turn to casual, part-time prostitution to supplement their incomes. There was a post-colonial explosion of unsterile needle use by ill-trained, or even untrained, "needle doctors," as well as poorly executed mass immunization programs. Military conflicts were marked by incidences of mass rape that facilitated the dissemination of many venereal pathogens.

These and other forces led to explosions of sexually transmitted diseases, which often went untreated, causing festering venereal sores and ulcerations that appear to have contributed in several ways to the vastly higher incidences of female-to-male HIV transmission in Africa and other Third World lands. One reason is that HIV prefers a direct pathway to the bloodstream, and an untreated venereal ulcer on the penis presents just such a pathway. Another is that untreated STDs such as syphilis produce large quantities of white blood cells—the very cells that HIV initially infects—which collect in the genital area, the very spot most likely to come into contact with HIV during sex with an infected partner. Conversely, HIV-positive people with untreated STDs are more likely to transmit their HIV infection because they produce increased amounts of white blood cells in their semen or vaginal secretions, again the very cells that harbor the highest concentrations of HIV. At the Ninth International Conference on AIDS in Berlin, Belgian researcher Marie Laga demonstrated that an untreated STD in either partner can increase the risk of HIV transmission by up to a hundredfold.

Given the lack of medical resources devoted to many Third World nations, we may never know all the reasons why AIDS there behaves differently from AIDS in developed lands, and especially why transmission from women to men is so much easier. But though mysteries abound, one fact seems clear: If small amounts of HIV had been present for generations in Africa, says Grmek, "the dynamics of the postcolonial medical and social revolutions were, by themselves, most probably sufficient to amplify it to epidemic proportions."

First-World Behavior Shifts

In the developed world, and particularly in America, HIV's golden opportunities are obvious to anyone monitoring the epidemic, if for no other reason than that the American epidemic began among people who received blood transfusions and clotting factors, injected drugs, or engaged in male-to-male anal sex. Tellingly, huge increases in those behaviors were all launched at around the same time, the era of Woodstock and Stonewall.

Blood transfusions became a regular part of the medical regimen as far back as World War I, but for several decades afterward they consisted of one donor to one recipient; not a terribly efficient way to disseminate disease. In the sixties medical advances led to the culling of blood products from multiple donors, and clotting factors developed from the blood of thousands of donors were introduced only in 1970. During the seventies foreign blood products began flowing into the United States from Third World countries to feed this new technology, and the international exchange of blood and blood products in general exploded. So did transfusion-related diseases. As Grmek writes, what had been a "narrow path . . . for the transmission of some sporadic infections . . . has become the royal road."

Nevertheless, as a source of disease amplification, blood exchange has sharp restrictions. Whereas blood recipients can easily receive infectious agents, passing them on is difficult. Many blood recipients die shortly after their transfusions. Many who survive are elderly or chronically ill and often do not donate blood or engage in drug use or sexual activity that might spread their infections. From HIV's point of view, they represent a viral dead end: Microbes can get in but can't get out. The main exceptions are young and otherwise healthy hemophiliacs, but there is a built-in limitation to how much viral amplification can occur within the hemophiliac population: its size. According to the CDC, there are only fifteen thousand hemophiliacs in the United States. As of this writing, the CDC reports that only 3 percent of all U.S. AIDS cases result from transfused blood or blood products.

As for injected drugs, although needles and syringes were developed in the nineteenth century, they were expensive and complicated metal-and-glass contraptions until World War II, when their widespread medicinal use began. Even after the war, few recreational drug users bothered with the still-clumsy needles, instead preferring to sniff or swallow their drugs. Self-injection of heroin began its meteoric rise only in the mid sixties, spurred in part by the easy availability of heroin among GIs in Vietnam, and really exploded when cheap, dispensable plastic syringes were introduced in 1970.

Still, sharing needles creates a somewhat limited viral highway. For one thing, transmission has been geographically limited because patterns of drug use and heroin marketing strongly affect the spread of HIV. Most injection drug users (IDUs) on the West Coast buy their drugs from dealers and then go home to inject, whereas in many East Coast cities dealers sell their drugs through shooting galleries that also provide needles and a common setting to inject. As a result, while infection rates have soared above 50 percent among some East Coast IDUs, among West Coast users rates have rarely exceeded 20 percent.

Socioeconomic factors also come into play. Large shooting galleries, where a needle may be passed among dozens, are most common among the poorest users, who are also the least likely to travel and spread their infections beyond their immediate circle. In *The Social Impact of AIDS in the United States*, demographers from the National Research Council described IDUs and their partners as "a relatively immobile population that depends on a strong network of neighborhood residential and social ties to maintain contacts with 'running buddies' and drug suppliers." In addition, IDUs often share needles with the same small cluster of people, keeping infection within a limited circle. Indeed, in one celebrated instance, a small group of IDUs was found amid a larger population of IDUs whose level of HIV infection was far above 50 percent, yet no one in this circle was HIV infected. The reason? They had all shared needles for years, but only among themselves.

Finally, the spread of AIDS beyond core groups of drug users is limited by the tight social networks such people form. Most IDUs have sex with women who reside in their neighborhoods, but as we will see, these women rarely spread infection beyond their immediate circles. As a result, injection drug use has created a catastrophe of HIV transmission within certain communities already burdened with a synergy of poverty, discrimination, and disease, but has not created conditions that would spread infection far beyond the initial cores. New York City health authorities, for example, recognize that that city's current TB epidemic, which is driven by HIV infection, began surfacing among IV drug users in the mid 1970s, indicating that HIV existed among that population for years without amplifying into a broader epidemic.

In the end, one thing seems clear. No matter how long HIV has harbored in humans, be it decades or centuries, the virus did not have the means to become an epidemic in most of the world until the vast liberalization of human behavior combined with the vast increase in technology in the mid to late twentieth century. Without these fundamental changes, the best HIV could hope for was a sporadic blossoming, not the impressive global pandemic it now so perversely enjoys.

But what about the piece of the puzzle we have so far omitted? AIDS was discovered first in North American gay men. If environmental factors were primarily responsible for its emergence among other populations, can the same be said for male homosexuals? In a sense, the ecological pathogenesis of AIDS might be said to stand or fall on the evidence of this, its first population, its most saturated population, and the population in the Western world that has, for perhaps most people, come to be identified most closely with the epidemic. So it is to that subject that we now turn—the birth of AIDS in the gay population.

CHAPTER 2

Gay Sexual Ecology

I f the history of sexuality indicates anything, it is that human sexual behavior is not a constant. Humans possess powerful biological impulses that propel our sexual desires, but those impulses are shaped by social forces in very significant and often completely unconscious ways. A man who has, say, an intense attraction to women's lingerie may consider this wholly natural and certainly involuntary, and it is. But if that man had been raised in a Neolithic culture where lingerie did not exist, such an attraction would be impossible. Not only are sexual desires and behaviors shaped by culture, they change over time within cultures. Anyone living in our anorexic era who strolls through an art museum is aware that a revolution in male taste has occurred since plump young beauties posed for Reubens. And anyone who came of age prior to the sixties can attest to major changes that have swept Americans' sex lives and habits since that tumultuous decade.

In the case of gay men and AIDS, were there significant changes in gay behavior in the years before the epidemic that might explain its rise? And if so, what were they and how did they interact with the virus to produce an epidemic?

These are controversial questions, and many people might not want to see them answered. Some are convinced that the gay AIDS epidemic happened simply because gay men were "promiscuous," or because homosexuality is "unnatural," or because anal intercourse is inherently "dirty." They might be discomfited to know that earlier generations of gay men, even those who had lots of partners, do not appear to have been mired in disease, and that historically speaking homosexuality and disease do not seem any more closely related than heterosexuality and disease, perhaps even less so. Others, mostly in the gay world, cling to the idea that the epidemic was an accident that first struck our community by chance. To this way of thinking there is no fire wall in nature to demarcate the collective sexual destinies of gay and straight, or for that matter, rich and poor, Third World and Western. We all face the same risk, say proponents of this theory, just on different timetables. And so they sometimes feel pressured to contend that there were no significant changes in gay behavior that might have given rise to AIDS, to argue that although gay life was rocked by social and political revolutions just before the epidemic, gay sex has remained roughly the same since time immemorial.

If this were true, then the hypothesis that AIDS emerged like other epidemics largely because of changes in human behaviors could not apply to gay men, and we would have to look elsewhere for answers. But it does not appear to be true. Evidence convincingly argues that before the middle of the century gay sexual behavior was vastly different from what it later became, that from mid century onward there were fundamental changes not only in gay male self-perceptions and beliefs, but also in sexual habits, kinds and numbers of partners, even ways of making love. These revolutions reached a fever pitch just at the moment when HIV exploded like a series of time bombs across the archipelago of gay America. When gay experience is viewed collectively, it appears that the simultaneous introduction of new behaviors and a dramatic rise in the scale of old ones produced one of the greatest shifts in sexual ecology ever recorded. There is convincing evidence that this shift had a decisive impact on the transmission of virtually every sexually transmitted disease, of which HIV was merely one, albeit the most deadly.

The Ecology of the Closet

Nowhere, it seems, have sexual attitudes and behaviors changed more dramatically than among gay men. The very idea that defines

gay men—the idea that people are naturally divided into homosexuals and heterosexuals—is now thought to be a recent cultural
creation. In *Gay New York*, his brilliant examination of New York
City homosexuals from the 1890s to the 1930s, George Chauncey
describes a preliberation culture in which this distinction did not
yet exist. For most working-class Americans, Chauncey writes,
"homosexual behavior per se became the primary basis for labeling
and self-identification of men as 'queer' only around the middle of
the twentieth century; before then, most men were so labeled only
if they displayed a much broader inversion of their ascribed gender
status by assuming the sexual and other cultural roles ascribed to
women." In other words, only men who acted and dressed effeminately were presumed to be, as they often called themselves,
"fairies" and "queers." It apparently did not seem logical, or even
possible, that a man could be masculine and homosexual at the
same time, and so a desire for same-sex relations was considered
just one facet of a much larger complex of effeminate characteristics that caused men to be labeled deviant and, at least in urban
centers like New York, sometimes propelled them into a demimonde of their own.

This particular "social construction" of same-sex desire influenced not just the way straight people viewed gays, but also the
way gay men viewed themselves. Not only did it help foster a very
different kind of self-identification than the one gay men have
today, but even different ways of having sex. For one thing, homosexuals back then did not necessarily seek or desire sex with each
other. Instead, they often sought sex with those whom they themselves termed "normal" men.

"Many fairies and queers socialized into the dominant prewar
homosexual culture," writes Chauncey, "considered the ideal
sexual partner to be 'trade,' a 'real man,' that is, ideally, a sailor, a
soldier, or some other embodiment of the aggressive masculine
ideal, who was neither homosexually interested nor effeminately
gendered himself but who would accept the sexual advances of a
queer. The centrality of effeminacy to the definition of the fairy in
the dominant culture enabled trade to have sex with both the
queers and fairies without risking being labeled queer themselves,
so long as they maintained a masculine demeanor and sexual role."

Chauncey quotes Dick Addison, a gay man who came out in the
1930s: "Most of my crowd [in the 1930s and 1940s] wanted to have

sex with a straight man. There was something very hot about a married man! And a lot of straight boys let us have sex with them. People don't believe it now. People say now that they must have been gay. But they weren't. They wouldn't look for [it] or suck a guy's thing, but they'd let you suck theirs."

For many "fairies" and "queers" of this era, having sex with (ideally) straight partners was so much what being queer was about that they were turned off at the very thought of having sex with each other. They "looked down on having sex with other gay men," writes Allan Bérubé, another prominent gay historian. "They had learned to prefer 'servicing' straight men in semipublic places," and they often considered the masculinity and butchness of their partners one of the most appealing aspects of sex.

Many gay men today cringe at the thought that this was a major component of the sexuality of our precursors. It seems so debasing, emotionally empty, self-loathing. Yet the ubiquitous classified ads in gay publications today seeking "straight-acting" partners indicates that for whatever reason, masculinity has remained a sexual ideal for a large proportion of gay men. Now, of course, masculine men can be found within gay culture itself, but in an era when most people thought it was impossible for a homosexual to be masculine, gay men's attraction to straight men seems logical, even inevitable.

Many people today can't imagine why so many heterosexual men in the past were willing to be serviced—usually fellated or masturbated—by homosexuals. But Chauncey points out that among young, working-class straights there appears to have been little or no stigma attached to such activity, as long as you remained sexually disinterested in your "fairy" partner and were never penetrated. Whereas today anyone engaging in male-to-male sexual activity is suspected of being homosexual, in those days the stigma was entirely attached to the partner who supposedly relinquished his masculinity by adopting the sexually receptive role. In addition, very little was expected of the trade partner except merely to consent to lie back and enjoy the experience. Indeed, even open consent was not always required, since one of the more typical conventions of such liaisons was that the gay seducer plied the trade with alcohol, enabling the trade to pretend he was only semiconscious or even unconscious during the encounter.

Oral Sex. Not only did the ideal object of gay desire differ from today's, there is also considerable evidence that there was a different emphasis on sexual acts themselves. Most accounts of male-on-male sex from the early decades of this century cite oral sex, and less often masturbation, as the predominant forms of activity, with the acknowledged homosexual fellating or masturbating his partner. Comparatively fewer accounts refer to anal sex. My own informal survey of older gay men who were sexually active prior to World War II gives credence to the idea that anal sex, especially anal sex with multiple partners, was considerably less common than it later became.

This question must be approached with caution, since there are no studies comparing the practices. Nor should this suggest that anal sex was unknown or even rare. Many gay men in long-standing couples had anal sex, and from at least the late nineteenth century onward there was a nascent gay community in New York and possibly other cities within which men had affairs that certainly included fucking. The fact that anal sex was also sometimes practiced in anonymous encounters is evidenced by the fact that one New York cruising area popular in gay circles was named "Vaseline Alley." But long-standing gay male couples were relatively rare in an era when few men lived openly as homosexuals, and from the scarce evidence it seems that gay sex was more likely to occur on a lark in a big city, often with a sailor or workingman and in dangerous circumstances, than with a long-term lover or another gay-identified partner. In such cases, it seems more likely to have been a blow job or masturbation than anal sex.

It's not hard to understand why. In places like parks, rest rooms, and other public or semipublic places where participants could be easily interrupted, oral sex is safer because it's less entangling. Even today, gay sex in public or semipublic places like parks and tea rooms tends to be oral rather than anal, although anal sex is not unknown in such venues. And to many straight-identified men, an offer to be sucked or masturbated must have seemed more enticing than an offer of anal sex, since to be penetrated was unthinkable and to penetrate a male partner would tend to imply some interest in that partner. In that sense a major advantage of oral sex was that it required virtually no reciprocation from the (supposedly) "disinterested" party except to lie back and enjoy it.

For whatever combination of reasons, oral sex seems to have

been predominate enough that when gay men from that era speak of sex itself, that's often what they mean. For his 1980 book *Alienated Affections,* for example, Seymour Kleinberg interviewed a seventy-five-year-old gay man about his youthful sexual life. He found that this man reserved a special vocabulary for anal sex, using the terms "browning" and "up the back." But "[w]hen he said he had sex, he took for granted that we meant oral sex and that being affectionate implied oral reciprocation." In histories of sex scandals such as the famous Newport scandal after World War I, in which older gay men were accused of forming a "sex ring" to seduce young sailors and soldiers, oral sex was virtually their sole activity. (The scandal, by the way, arose not so much because of the sex itself, but because navy investigators sent young servicemen in as undercover agents to be seduced and often fellated by the men in the ring. When this came to light at the subsequent trials, it shocked the nation, ended several navy careers, and briefly threatened the career of young Secretary of the Navy Franklin D. Roosevelt.) The belief that expertise in oral sex was a basic trait of homosexuals seems to have influenced medical perceptions of homosexuality as well. Allan Bérubé reports in *Coming Out Under Fire* that army doctors in World War II developed a test to screen out gays based on the apparent assumption that homosexuals were expert fellators. The doctors would insert tongue depressors into the throats of suspected queers, believing that the heterosexuals would gag and the homosexuals would not.

How Epidemics Work

If this general description of homosexual activity prior to World War II is reasonably accurate, such activity would not have been very efficient in spreading most STDs. It certainly would not have been sufficient to induce an epidemic of a difficult-to-transmit virus like HIV. To better understand why, we need to take a brief look at the theory of how epidemics spread, and particularly at the topic of "core groups" and how they contribute to that process.

By definition, an epidemic is any disease that is increasing in size within a population. This can happen with sexually transmitted diseases only if the average infected person infects more than one other person. The rate at which one person infects others is called the "reproductive rate" of the disease, or r. When r is precisely at one, each infected person infects precisely one other person, and the disease is said to lie on the "epidemic threshold" or "tipping point" at which it neither grows nor shrinks. But when r exceeds one, even just by a fraction, the disease "tips" into epidemic growth. If r exceeds one for an extended time the epidemic can grow until eventually virtually all the "susceptibles" in the population—those whose behavior or biology puts them at risk—have become infected. At that point the number of new infections will rapidly decline because the epidemic will have devoured its fuel faster than it could be replaced. If no new susceptibles become available, the disease can entirely die out within the population. If new susceptibles enter the population, the disease can sometimes sustain itself indefinitely, although usually at much lower rates than the original explosion.

Whether or not an STD will rise above the epidemic tipping point is governed by several factors, the most basic being infectivity, prevalence, and rate of partner change. *Infectivity* describes the likelihood that a particular microbe will be transmitted under particular circumstances. It is influenced by the basic properties of the microbe, by the susceptibility of the uninfected person—what biological factors make that individual more or less likely to become infected once exposed—and by the kinds of acts people perform. Both gonorrhea and chlamydia, for example, have an estimated 20 percent chance of being passed from an infected woman to her male partner in a single act of unprotected vaginal intercourse, but a 90 percent chance of passing from an infected man to his female partner in a single act, since both microbes have a much easier time penetrating the membranes of the vagina than the penis. These kinds of differences abound in STD transmission, and they form the basis of many public health interventions and safer sex strategies. In the context of AIDS, for example, the central purpose of condoms is to reduce infectivity per sex act by blocking the exchange of infectious fluids.

Prevalence is defined as the percentage of a population that is currently infected, and it also affects risk in a basic way. If people choose their partners from a population with a gonorrhea prevalence of 0.001 percent, for example, their risk of getting gonorrhea is vanishingly low regardless of gonorrhea's infectivity, whether condoms are used and whether they have lots of partners. If, however, they choose their partners from a population with a 50 per-cent prevalence of gonorrhea, they may have a much higher risk of infection even if they use condoms and have few partners, since condoms provide less than complete protection and since there's a much higher chance that any partner will be infected.

Rate of partner change, or contact rate, is the third significant factor that influences risk. Simply put, without partner change no STD can spread. Partner A may infect partner B, but things will end there. In a thoroughly monogamous population there would be no STDs at all, no matter how infectious certain microbes might theo-retically be. Conversely, the higher the level of partner change, the more likely that even microbes that are relatively hard to transmit will have an opportunity to spread.

A crucial point about epidemics is that not all members of a given population behave in a uniform way. There are sexual ecosys-tems in every population consisting of groups of people who gen-erally choose their sexual partners from among people very similar to themselves. Princes do not often marry paupers. Physicists do not generally choose their mates from among subsistence farmers. For that matter, blacks rarely marry whites, Moslems rarely mate with Presbyterians, and twentysomethings don't generally mate with octogenarians. Within each society, each city, each town, dis-tinct sexual cultures—sexual ecosystems—live side by side.

In a typical American city, for example, the students at the local university mostly date each other, and in general their sexual activity is characterized by fairly high levels of casual partner change. Most consider this perfectly acceptable, thanks to a wide array of cultural influences, from the music they listen to and the magazines they read to what their older siblings told them about college life. Because they mostly have the same kind of sexual rela-tions within the same pool of partners, their sexual ecosystem is characterized by relatively high levels of fast-moving STDs like syphilis and gonorrhea, which have an opportunity to spread in an environment where people often switch partners before they dis-cover they are infected and get treatment.

For the fortysomething married professionals on the other side of our hypothetical town, partner change occurs mostly in the form of occasional adultery, divorce, and remarriage. Since the social costs of adultery, divorce, and remarriage are far more onerous than the casual partner switching among college students, there is understandably less of it. Fewer than half of all partners engage in even a limited episode of adultery during their marriage, and fewer than 5 percent engage in a continuous pattern of adultery with multiple partners. As a result, in this ecosystem there is less opportunity for short-term, curable STDs like syphilis or gonorrhea to gain a foothold. Most STDs here will consist of lifelong and incurable infections such as herpes and HPV, diseases that most people acquired when they were college age and have never gotten rid of.

Members of the very conservative religious community across town endorse lifelong marriage without divorce, but accept a moderate amount of male infidelity provided it does not destabilize marriage and is extremely discreet. As a result there is significant male adultery with female prostitutes, and here the infections that enter this population generally flow one way, from husbands to their wives, and tend to stop there.

There might be dozens more examples of discreet sexual ecosystems in our hypothetical town—the military base, the gay neighborhood, the retirement home, the adult singles scene. Each "lifestyle" in the population is mirrored by an invisible but very real sexual ecology. These social communities form the critical "populations" of sexual ecology, and the invisible pools they form constitute the critical "sexual ecosystems" that matter most in terms of STD transmission. This is just as true with AIDS as with any other STD. The Global AIDS Policy Coalition notes, for example, that "[e]ven within a single city or population area, several different [AIDS] epidemics are usually underway, each with its own rate of spread, intensity, and special characteristics."

Core Groups

While all sexual ecosystems play a role in overall ecology, some are far more significant than others. By far the most significant in terms of epidemics are the ecosystems researchers call "core groups" or "risk groups." In epidemiological terms a core group or risk group is a collection of people who, because of a variety of circumstances, suffer from and transmit STDs at much higher rates than the rest of the population. Researchers have long noticed, for example, that as much as 80 percent of certain STDs can be concentrated in fewer than 20 percent of the people who contract them, while the remaining 20 percent of infections are widely diffused among the remaining 80 percent of those who get the disease. In the 1970s researchers developed models that seemed to confirm that core groups can, by themselves, generate or sustain diseases that would otherwise never have a chance to maintain themselves in the wider population. James Yorke and Herbert Hethcote's work implied that such cores can be quite small and can remain clearly definable within tight geographic locations. In examining gonorrhea transmission in Denver, for example, field investigators discovered that the vast majority of infections were focused in just four small neighborhoods: around a military base, in an African-American neighborhood, in a largely Hispanic neighborhood, and in a gay neighborhood. Similar patterns have since been observed around the world. Groups that form self-sustaining cores of STD infection include college students, gay men, crack cocaine users, people who live in pockets of urban poverty, and prostitutes and their customers, who often include cores of military men and long-distance truck drivers.

Core Dynamics. The dynamics of transmission vary from core to core, but there are a number of factors that many core groups have in common. First and foremost, people in cores have significantly higher numbers of partners than those outside. Second, and perhaps equally importantly, those partners also have significantly higher numbers of partners *within the core*, creating a kind of biological feedback loop that is primed to magnify disease. Third, core members tend to engage in forms of sex that are conducive to transmission, which generally requires some kind of fluid exchange. (A core in which everyone uses condoms or engages only in masturbation is not going to amplify disease.) And finally, members of cores also tend to suffer from what researchers sometimes call the "synergism of plagues," a complex of health problems related to poverty, substance abuse, lack of adequate medical care, and heightened exposure to diseases like tuberculosis as well as repeated STD infections. This synergy lowers the "group immunity" or "herd immunity" of people in the core, so that not only are they more frequently exposed to infections, they are also more likely to become infected when exposed. The triple whammy of having a large number of partners within a high prevalence group, of engaging in high-risk sexual acts with those partners, and of suffering heightened susceptibility because of a synergy of other factors, can multiply risk tremendously. Because of this, pathogens that are difficult to transmit and might never gain a foothold in a healthy population can enter and become entrenched in a core group relatively easily.

Of course, it's impossible for people in cores to spread STDs beyond their immediate group unless they have sex with people outside. So after a disease becomes endemic in a core, the key factor that influences its outward spread is how much *sexual mixing* or *bridging* goes on between core group members and those outside. The amount of such mixing can vary greatly from population to population. Within disadvantaged inner-city neighborhoods, for example, crack cocaine users and injection drug users sometimes engage in significant sexual mixing with neighbors who don't take drugs, which has contributed to a serious HIV crisis among people in the inner city who are not themselves drug users. By contrast, there appears to be very little mixing between drug users and middle-class suburbanites, a fact that has sharply limited the spread of HIV outside of economically disadvantaged populations.

The idea of core groups is one of the most politically challenging and least understood concepts in sexual ecology. Throughout the AIDS epidemic the very existence of such groups has been hotly disputed by activists who argue that there are no such things as risk groups, just risky behaviors. This is an understandable defense against blame, but it is dangerously misleading. No sophisticated understanding of the dynamics of the AIDS epidemic is possible without noting the crucial role played by core group dynamics.

It is important, however, to tread carefully around the concept of core groups. The categorization is useful and important in understanding epidemics, and as such it would be highly dangerous to ignore, but it is also easy to misunderstand and abuse. To accuse a group of people of contributing to the spread of disease is a powerful way to stigmatize, placing that group in the position of the contaminating Other. This is particularly troubling when the group in question is already marginalized and disadvantaged, as is often the case. Such accusations have often preceded some of the worst chapters in history. In the case of gay men and AIDS, there have been continuous attempts to treat the entire gay male population as a contaminating core, and even within the gay world there has sometimes been a tendency to "blame" the AIDS epidemic on the promiscuous, the denizens of sex clubs, the HIV positive, and so on. So strong was the original belief in the gay world that AIDS would only strike the most promiscuous that for the first several years of the epidemic many gay men who did not consider themselves particularly promiscuous simply did not consider themselves at risk. That turned out to be a dangerous and often fatal myth. Any attempts to exploit the concept of core groups to make oneself feel better, or safer, is likely to lead to similar woeful results. So in many ways misinterpreting the concept of core groups can be just as dangerous as ignoring their reality. Still, if we want to understand the dynamics of STD epidemics and how they might be contained, ways must be found to incorporate the important concept of core groups while resisting attempts to distort that concept to demonize.

Before Stonewall. Returning to the historical evidence, it seems unlikely that homosexual men in the early part of this century formed very efficient core groups. While some men had multiple partners, few seem to have had multiple partners within their own circle of gay-identified men, and fewer still seem to have had multiple partners who themselves also had multiple partners within the same circle. Instead, many of the most sexually active gay men tended to concentrate their attentions on so-called "normal" partners who themselves had few male sexual contacts. The famous Newport scandal seems a typical example. The gay men arrested at Newport often had sex with lots of young sailors, but for most of those sailors it seems to have been a onetime experience.

Second, most of those who did have multiple partners seem to have engaged more often in oral than anal sex, and oral sex is considerably less conducive to transmission of many STDs, including HIV. That is not to say that earlier generations of gays did not get STDs. They surely did. But it seems telling that some people at the time assumed that promiscuous homosexuals were *less* likely to transmit disease than comparable heterosexuals. Chauncey reports, for example, that after World War I the chief of New York's vice squad halted a crackdown on homosexual activity because he "grew concerned that the campaign had diverted too much attention from the squad's efforts against prostitutes, who, he apparently feared, posed a medical, as well as moral, danger to their customers. . . . Telling his men that 'one prostitute was more dangerous than five degenerates,' he ordered them to give more attention to the former." Obviously this chief's primitive attempt at epidemiological risk assessment may simply have been wrong. But his basic belief was so widespread that gay men themselves sometimes used it as a come-on. Chauncey reports that "some gay men interested in sex with 'straight' men also portrayed themselves as less dangerous than women by arguing that there was no chance they would infect the men with the venereal diseases women were thought to carry." The elderly gay man Kleinberg interviewed, for whom the word *sex* automatically meant *oral* sex, may have been fairly typical when he reported that he had "never had any form of V.D., never contracted a sexually related disease."

Of course, it is speculative to argue that gay life before World War II did not produce significant disease amplification. The fact is that data on gay male sexual behavior is extremely scarce, and deduction has to be based on very limited evidence. But there is at least one further bit of evidence that bolsters this conclusion. For most of the century, records from both public and private medical sources indicate that there was a rough balance in STD rates between males and females. If gay men had been forming efficient cores, this would almost certainly not have been the case. As we will soon see, once gay men in the sixties and seventies did create efficient cores, the balance in STD rates between men and women shifted dramatically. The rates for men showed enormous increases while those for women remained stable or rose very slowly. Eventually some diseases afflicted men at rates of from 10 to 100 times higher than they afflicted women, a discrepancy caused almost completely by men having sex with men in highly efficient core groups. The fact that no such discrepancy was observed before the sixties strongly argues that the sexual ecology of gay men was not particularly conducive to epidemic amplification.

The Mid-Century Shift

By the mid century, however, the ecology of homosexuality began to undergo a profound evolution. Prompted largely by developments in psychiatry, a change occurred in the very definition of deviance. The old idea was that the temptation to commit sin was inherent in all individuals, and that certain people simply chose to give in to that temptation. This was slowly replaced with the new idea that there are two basic "sexual orientations" in the world, homosexual and heterosexual, defined by whether one is attracted to the same or the opposite sex. Originating among Germans such as jurist Karl Heinrich Ulrichs in the 1860s and Magnus Hirschfeld at the turn of the century, this concept was reinforced by Freud and his successors, and made major inroads in American popular consciousness in the thirties, forties, and fifties. According to the popular version, any man who desires sex with another man is inherently "homosexual" no matter what role he plays during sex and regardless of his gender identity or outward mannerisms. "Only in the 1930s, 1940s and 1950s," Chauncey writes, "did the now conventional division of men into 'homosexuals' and 'heterosexuals,' based on the sex of their sexual partners, replace the division of men into 'fairies' and 'normal men.'" This represented a sea change in the public perception of homosexuality. In Foucault's famous phrase, "The sodomite has been a temporary aberration; the homosexual was now a species." And a deviant and mentally diseased species as well.

It may seem odd, but this deviant definition of homosexuality contributed greatly to the rise of gay liberation. Historians argue that it was pivotal in prompting gay men and lesbians to begin forging a positive identity, because they could now stop thinking of themselves as isolated individuals inexplicably prone to weakness and sin, and argue instead that they were being oppressed for an illness they could not control. Since society does not generally punish people for their illnesses, it followed that society should not persecute gays.

Just as this new idea was gaining currency, World War II threw vast numbers of gay men and lesbians together in the military service, where they faced intense discrimination. The military establishment had enthusiastically embraced the medical view of homosexuality, and used it to detect, punish, and discharge service members. Yet even as they faced humiliation and discharge, lesbian and gay service members participated in an unparalleled experience of self-discovery, evolving a new pride and self-awareness from which the modern gay world would coalesce. After the war, discharged by the tens of thousands into cosmopolitan cities such as San Francisco, communities of lesbian and gay veterans formed the rudiments of a new culture. It was a culture strongly shaped by the experiences of wartime, from which it retained a powerful sense of camaraderie as well as distinctive social customs and folklore—camp sensibility, drag, diva worship, and so on—that served as unifying forces. This nascent community stretched across the nation in an archipelago of budding gay and lesbian communities that served as magnets and examples for those who remained closeted.

Amid these social and demographic shifts, gay male sex life began changing as well. As the distinction between straight and gay solidified in the popular imagination, working-class straight men who had once felt no stigma being served by "fairies" now started worrying that participating in such liaisons might indicate that they themselves were homosexual. As a result they drew away, helping to precipitate a profound change in gay sexual patterns. Chauncey writes that by the sixties and seventies the category of trade had "virtually disappeared as a sexual identity (if not a sexual role) within the gay world, as men began to regard anyone who participated in a homosexual encounter as 'gay,' and, conversely, to insist that men could be defined as 'straight' only on the basis of a total absence of homosexual interest and behavior." Eventually, he writes, the lines were "drawn between the heterosexual and the homosexual so sharply and publicly that men were no longer able to participate in a homosexual encounter without suspecting it meant (to the outside world, and to themselves) that they were gay."

This growing sexual iron curtain cut many homosexuals off from their traditional objects of desire, and created a dilemma for those who had grown used to such partners. Some later reported that it seriously interrupted their sexual lives, at least for a while. But at the same time, and largely based on the same developments, nascent gay liberationists began calling on gay men and lesbians to throw off the shackles of shame and to feel pride in their sexual orientation. And part of that, they argued cogently, was to end the self-debasement implicit in fairy-trade encounters. An ideological pillar of gay liberation was that gay men should stop playing the effeminate weakling begging sexual favors from straight icons of masculinity. In other words, they should stop idealizing straights and begin idealizing each other.

Unfortunately, the very psychiatric definition of identity that helped fuel this affirming development also helped fuel a rising prejudice against gays. So just as gay men and lesbians began to build genuine communities and distinctive cultures, and as gay men began turning more and more to each other for sexual partnership, they faced a steep rise in stigmatization and official repression. The moral crusaders of the McCarthy era sought to stamp out the gay "lifestyle" that was emerging in large cities by targeting its visible, and particularly its sexual, manifestations. Raids of gay bars, baths, and sexual meeting places increased, and sexual entrapment by plainclothes police became a growing occupational hazard of gay life. You could be arrested for wearing drag, arrested for dancing with members of the same sex, arrested for holding hands in public. As a result, the sexual culture of the emerging gay communities in many respects developed as an outlaw culture. Having gay sex was seen by many as an act of defiance. Gays were considered, and often considered themselves, sexual renegades. To be sure, plenty of homosexuals rejected this characterization, just as many had rejected the earlier characterization of sin. But it permeated both gay and straight society and had a profound impact on the forms that gay male sexual relations took.

A number of excellent studies have described the contradictory lifestyle that emerged in the fifties and sixties prior to Stonewall, as growing pride and self-esteem collided with increased repression. Books like John D'Emilio's *Sexual Politics, Sexual Communities* and Esther Newton's *Cherry Grove* describe a world marked by camaraderie, camp, humor, brotherhood and sisterhood, wit, self-help, and growing indignation at injustice. But this society was also marked by secrets and double lives, by stress and sexual repression and guilt, in which emotionally intimate and long-term sexual relationships between men appear to have been considerably more rare than they were among lesbians or heterosexuals. The central institutions of emerging gay male culture were bars and bathhouses where community-building, self-esteem, and sexual self-discovery were closely associated with alcohol and drug consumption, sexual adventurism, and sensation-seeking. Many gay men rejected these connections and found long-term partners, often away from the hubbub of the emerging gay fast lane. But for many others, sexual freedom became synonymous with adventure and conquest.

Stonewall. Then, in June of 1969, came the acknowledged turning point, the Stonewall Riots. The period of intense organizing and theorizing that followed Stonewall borrowed much from the black civil rights struggle, the women's movement, and the antiwar movement. Those earlier struggles had helped sensitize many gay and lesbian Americans to social injustice and to the idea that such injustice did not have to be borne. To varying degrees they also successfully challenged the same primarily male, white, and heterosexual power structure that energetically sought to oppress gay men and lesbians.

Throughout this era a simultaneous and interconnected movement awakened Americans of both sexes and all races to the possibility of a different kind of liberation. The sexual revolution proclaimed that the long connection in Western culture between sex and sin could and should be challenged, and that the pursuit of sexual happiness was legitimate and important in itself. Throughout the mid and late sixties gay men and lesbians were presented with the fabulous spectacle of various groups demanding not only equality, justice, and fairness, but pleasure. Why should homosexuals be left out? In many ways gay liberation was the culmination of the era's other struggles, combining the demand for human dignity inherent in the civil rights movement, the challenge to the sexual patriarchy articulated by feminism, the assault on colonialism and militarism that was part of the antiwar movement, and the quest for pleasure of the sexual revolution. When New York City police raiders entered the Stonewall Inn to arrest its patrons that June night in 1969, the stage had been well set indeed.

In the aftermath of the Stonewall Riots a vastly different gay society arose on the foundations of the closeted, semisecret past. At the psychic core of this new world was the bold idea that Gay Is Good, and the bolder imperative to Come Out and proudly proclaim your homosexuality. Lesbians and gay men heeded that call by the thousands, determined to smash the edifice of secrecy and shame that had blighted previous generations of gay lives. They quickly succeeded in fostering a proudly open gay culture in cities like San Francisco and New York, utilizing the political savvy garnered in the antiwar, women's, and civil rights movements to establish a small but potent political power base. This base, solidified first through the street actions and protest movements and later through the more traditional methods of reform politics, created a zone of safety around gay social and sexual spaces where at last people could assemble without harassment.

The securing of such freedoms was liberation's first, and for many activists its primary, focus. From the point of view of this study it is telling that these demands met with a significant degree of success almost immediately in cities with large gay populations, particularly San Francisco and New York. Only a short time after Stonewall, the official police harassment of gay social and sexual spaces abated. Suddenly people were free to dance together without fear of arrest, to cruise openly in bars, to patronize bathhouses without fear of raids, even to have sex in certain semipublic locations—parks, piers, alleys, public rest rooms—without fear of invasion by the authorities. The number of openly gay businesses exploded, and the most visible among them were bars, discos, and sexually oriented enterprises like baths, sex clubs, and porn shops whose primary function was to profit from the newly released sexual energies of gay men. Not only were these the most visible enterprises in the gay world, they became the very embodiment of gay male liberation for many of their patrons and for much of society at large.

Different Strokes

The era immediately after Stonewall was a time of intense theoretical and behavioral contradictions. Some gay thinkers, particularly those most closely associated with the left wing and hippie movements, argued for a nonconsumerist approach to gay sexual life. Gay men, they warned, were in danger of slipping into self-oppressive modes of behavior where they were prone to treat each other cruelly based on looks and age, class and race. Many started consciousness-raising groups, advocated experiments with communal living, and generally appealed for a transformative gay lifestyle based on love and self-respect. Others, however, accustomed to secrecy and furtive sex, easily convinced themselves that liberation involved not the abolition of furtiveness, but the freedom to be as furtive as possible. These thinkers argued that restraint and self-control were inherently "sex-negative," that if liberation meant rejecting constraints, then to be more liberated meant to reject even more constraints, and the most liberated (meaning the most gay) were those without any constraints whatsoever. "Promiscuity," trumpeted one prominent gay newspaper, "knits together the social fabric of the gay male community," and as such it was to be celebrated and defended. Those gay idealists and hippies who envisioned a nurturing, nonmasculinist and noncompetitive sexual culture frequently found themselves denounced as assimilationist and self-loathing by a new generation of self-proclaimed sex-positive radicals who encouraged an ideology in which the very forms of sexual behavior imposed on gay men by a despising majority ought to be now taken up as virtues by the victims themselves. Having come of age in the pre-Stonewall era when gay sex was considered illicit and deviant, many gay men could hardly be expected to reject this ingrained conviction overnight. As Ian Young writes in *The Stonewall Experiment*, his searing psycho-history of gay culture, "Centuries of sexual repression and distortion are not quickly or simply overcome, though they can be easily repackaged and labeled Pleasure or Freedom. A society that had made heterosexuality into an absolute had provided no rules, no guidelines, no ways for men to relate affectionately and erotically with one another. . . . Only an insistent sexual need persisted."

The post-Stonewall philosophical division was mirrored in very real divisions in gay male patterns of behavior. Many men, for whom love and companionship seemed more important than sexual freedom, settled down with long-term lovers in monogamous relationships. Such men often chose to avoid large cities where a tempting fast-lane lifestyle was emerging, but rather carved out quiet niches for themselves in smaller towns and cities far from the limelight. Others, however, raced to test the limits of their newfound freedoms in bedrooms and bathhouses, in discos and sex clubs, parks and alleys. Still others, perhaps the majority, vacillated between these two worlds, sometimes committing themselves to relationships, sometimes indulging in the intoxicating freedoms that beckoned in the large gay communities. But whatever their opinions or behaviors, most gay men tended to presume that this grand experiment in human liberation was unaffected by the wider web of nature around them. Just as economists often analyze industrial activity without a thought to its impact on the environment, gay theorists analyzed the new economy of sex without a mention of ecological or microbial perils. Most, if they gave such perils a thought, probably believed they had been conquered long before.

Scale Is Everything

And so, without most gay men noticing it, a revolution in disease transmission began almost as soon as the steady disco beat filled the air. The rise of gay core groups in which men combined anal sex with very large numbers of partners profoundly altered the microbial landscape and created entirely new opportunities for a host of diseases that until then had been held in check.

Scale is crucial to ecology. Behaviors that are safe on a small scale can become catastrophic on larger ones. Perhaps the classic example is that in the sparsely settled American frontier of a century ago it was basically harmless to toss household refuse in a river, or burn the family trash in a bonfire. In a crowded modern city, however, pouring millions of gallons of untreated sewage into a river, or burning tons of municipal refuse in open incinerators, is the very essence of ecological irresponsibility. In his influential essay "The Tragedy of the Commons," Garrett Hardin remarked that "the morality of an act is a function of the state of the system at the time it is performed." Different states and different scales create vastly different effects across the ecological spectrum. For gay men, behaviors that were once engaged in on a limited scale by a few participants appear to have been either harmless or produced problems that were so minor they passed unnoticed. But the mass adoption of those behaviors by large numbers of gay men, particularly in concentrated core groups, created an entirely different situation, the consequences of which are even yet not fully understood.

As the gay version of the sexual revolution took hold among certain groups of gay men in America's largest cities, it precipitated a change in sexual behaviors. Perhaps the most significant change was the fact that some core groups of gay men began practicing anal intercourse with dozens or even hundreds of partners a year. Also significant was a growing emphasis on "versatile" anal sex, in which partners alternately played both receptive and insertive roles, and on new behaviors such as analingus, or rimming, that facilitated the spread of otherwise difficult-to-transmit microbes. Important, too, was a shift in patterns of partnership, from diffuse systems in which a lot of gay sex was with non-gay-identified partners who themselves had few contacts, to fairly closed systems in which most sexual activity was within a circle of other gay men. Also important was a general decline in "group immunity" caused by repeated infections of various STDs, repeated inoculations of antibiotics and other drugs to combat them, as well as recreational substance abuse, stress, and other behaviors that compromised immunity.

But of perhaps greatest significance to epidemiologists later on were two salient facts about the way gay male sexual culture was emerging. One was the fact that these behaviors were not spread evenly throughout the gay world, but were concentrated in relatively small but biologically significant subsets of gay men who formed intensely active core groups that could readily amplify any disease that entered them. The other was that there was a very high level of sexual *mixing* or *bridging* between gay men in those cores and the rest of the gay population. The net result, as we will see, is that, unlike almost any other group in the developed world, gay men created almost laboratory conditions both to amplify STDs within highly active cores of individuals and then to spread those diseases throughout the gay population, including those who were not particularly active at all.

Both core group activity and mixing were facilitated by a new institution that became central to gay life in the sixties and seventies, and it is to that institution that we now turn. In many ways, both the most liberating and the most tragic aspects of the gay sexual revolution were, quite literally, born at the baths.

The Ecology of the Tubs

Gay baths and sex clubs were not exactly new in the sixties and seventies. As early as 1903 New York City boasted a gay bathhouse, which we know about because when the authorities got wind of it, they promptly raided it and shut it down. But throughout the first half of the century baths remained rare, and since scale is so crucial to ecology, it seems doubtful that these scattered institutions had much biological impact. As they increased in popularity in the mid century, however, they proved immensely significant in the development of a new gay consciousness and sexual ecology. Partly because of the all-gay nature of these bathhouses, many men first became aware there of the option of having sex with other self-avowed homosexuals rather than with so-called normal men.

"Many men who came out before there were any gay baths looked down on having sex with other gay men," writes historian Allan Bérubé. "It was a later generation of gay men who, partly by using the bathhouses, learned to enjoy having sex with and loving other gay men. At a time when no one was saying 'gay is good,' the creation of an institution in which gay men were encouraged to appreciate each other was a major step toward gay pride. Since then, several generations of gay men . . . have learned to prefer sexual partners who are also gay. The bathhouses, thus, are partly responsible for this major change in the sexual behavior and self-acceptance of gay men."

That change became much more noticeable in the fifties and sixties when the first truly modern gay bathhouses emerged. Unlike earlier Turkish bath–style institutions where gay men mingled with straights, these newer places were designed to cater to an exclusively homosexual clientele. Patrons would pay a fee to rent a locker or a small cubicle with a bed, check their clothes in the locker or cubicle, then don a towel and roam the dimly lit halls, enjoy the steam rooms and saunas, or relax in the recreational areas, which often provided couches and TVs and sold snacks. There was a tremendous amount of socializing in the baths, and for many men they provided their only haven from the homophobic world outside. Many patrons were far more attracted by the sense of safety and community they experienced than by the purely sexual opportunities, and these institutions were crucial in fostering pride in men's gay identities. Yet the baths were primarily designed with sex in mind, and they maximized sexual partnering and sexual mixing in a way no other institutions could possibly match. People had sex in virtually all areas of the baths, from private cubicles to the showers, saunas, hallways, and rec rooms. In the communal spirit of the Summer of Love in 1967, "orgy rooms" were installed in some bathhouses to facilitate group sex. Soon orgy rooms, mazes, and other spaces devoted to communal sex spread to most institutions, providing venues for the easiest kinds of anonymous encounters. Many orgy rooms were almost pitch dark, so that men could couple without knowing or speaking with each other, indeed often without seeing each other.

Although baths slowly proliferated in the decade before Stonewall, patrons in most cities still knew that they entered at some risk of arrest and exposure, a fact that tended to keep attendance fairly low and the number of such institutions fairly small. But after Stonewall came a relaxation of persecution and a subsequent surge in demand as gay men realized that the baths now constituted truly safe sexual spaces. Entrepreneurs made millions creating chains of opulent pleasure palaces that became among the largest and most prominent commercial institutions in the gay world. In the process the owners themselves became prominent community leaders and among the biggest advertisers in the emerging gay press. By the early eighties there were more than 200 major baths across the nation, and they had spawned a $100-million-per-year industry. Many gay men had no interest in such places, and quite a few openly disapproved. But whether you loved bathhouses or hated them, few gay men were more than a few hours' drive from one no matter where they lived. The baths were instrumental in creating a new sexual culture characterized by enhanced self-esteem and a genuine sense of community. But they were also instrumental in bonding that new culture with a very high level of partner change. And in part because of their safety, privacy, and relative cleanliness, in part because their clientele was now exclusively gay, much of that partner change now involved anal sex.

Other Venues

The baths were not the only institutions that commercialized sex and encouraged a connection between pride and promiscuity. At the same time there was a proliferation of sex clubs, peep shows, movie theaters, and bars with dark back rooms that provided patrons with a safe haven and simultaneously encouraged them to enjoy anonymous sex on the premises. By the early eighties even huge discos like New York's Saint set aside sections for public love-making. With the diminution of legal harassment, outdoor sex in parks, piers, and in other isolated places also increased, although the danger from homophobic cops and thugs, and in northern climates the problem of inclement weather, tended to limit the appeal of outdoor sex.

The bar scene greatly expanded in the seventies as well. By the middle of the decade even many medium-sized cities had at least a few gay bars, and they too were crucial venues for gay men to socialize and build a sense of community. For many men their very first experience of gay life was in a bar, and despite popular stereotypes that depict bars as merely sexual haunts, most were far more: They were psychic centers of community where people could be with friends and escape the crushing pressure of homophobia and danger they experienced throughout much of their lives. But bar culture also helped reinforce the bridge that connected gay life to both alcohol consumption and sexual multipartnerism, just as singles bars did for young urban straights of that era.

The Eco-Significance of the Baths

Still, the level of sexual partner change made possible by the existence of gay bars was dwarfed by the number of partners most men could have at commercial sex establishments, particularly the baths. You might spend all night at a bar and end up with nobody; at best you'd likely end up with a single partner. But nobody ended up with nobody at the tubs, unless of course they wanted to. On the contrary, it was quite possible to have sex with a dozen or more partners in a single visit. In one study of gay male New Yorkers in the pre-AIDS era, for example, the average man had five partners per year at home, which was not that different from the average young heterosexual on the singles scene. But the average gay man also had thirty-six additional partners per year in baths, back rooms, and cinemas. And since this average includes occasional attendees and even people who never went to baths, the numbers for the most sexually active core group members would be vastly higher.

Some have attempted to downplay the role of these establishments in the epidemic by arguing that if baths had not existed, the same amount of partner change would have occurred elsewhere. Logic, however, argues against this. Aside from the obvious fact that one cannot generally have sex at home with a dozen passersby in a single evening, many men reported that they visited a bath or sex club precisely because they had failed to find a partner any other way. Almost every night of the week baths and sex clubs experienced a surge of business immediately after the bars closed, fueled by disappointed men who flocked from the scene of their frustration to one that virtually guaranteed fulfillment. "Now where did you go after you had spent the night on the dance floor of desperate optimism, waiting for the partner that failed to appear?" asked a former self-described "circuit queen" years later in an essay in the *People with AIDS Newsline*. "Well, you could go home to a lonely apartment to take a Quaalude and some vitamins (ridiculous!) and sleep through the day, or you went to seek love at the baths."

During the heyday of the seventies it is estimated that 15,000 men visited the baths every weekend in San Francisco, and probably far more in New York. Since many gay men in each city never attended these institutions at all, and since most of those who did seem to have visited them only occasionally, these huge numbers imply that many of the men who frequented baths were repeat customers, creating an intense core group whose ecological characteristics will be discussed below. Each of these men could easily have sex with several partners per visit, so that someone who patronized the baths several times a week could easily rack up as many as a thousand partners per year. It was among this core that AIDS first appeared. According to CDC interviews, the first several hundred gay men with the disease had an *average* of 1,100 lifetime partners, which means that some reported far more. For most, this level of activity was possible only because of commercial sex institutions.

So precipitous was the rise in the numbers of partners among the most sexually active core of gay men that researchers had to keep revising the definition of multipartnerism to keep up. Laurie Garrett reports that Dr. June Osborn, an NIH researcher who was one of the first to sound the alarm about STD transmission in gay core groups, had a hard time maintaining a handle on the level of multipartnerism. "Every time we do an NIH site visit, the definition of 'multiple sex partners' has changed," Osborn said in 1980. "First it was ten to twenty partners a year. That was nineteen seventy-five. Then in nineteen seventy-six it was fifty partners a year. By nineteen seventy-eight we were talking about a hundred sexual partners a year and now we're using the term to describe five hundred partners in a single year.

"I am," pronounced Osborn, "duly in awe."

Escalation

Many gay men observed a curious social process in the second half of the decade. "The '70s seemed like a rocket ride up in the first half of the decade and a slow emotional descent in the second," writes Doug Sadownick in *Sex Between Men*. "There was an attempt to cushion the coming down with the engineering of drugs—a little marijuana, some mescaline, mixed with a Quaalude or a Valium. But even the presumably 'high' places began to rub the wrong way." Some attempted to fill the void with increasingly exotic sexual behaviors. This "escalation" process is familiar to anyone hooked on addictive substances where, over time, increasing doses are required to achieve the same high. But escalation is not usually associated with adult sexuality. If anything, people tend to settle down as they grow older and integrate their sexual drives into the larger fabric of life.

For many gay men such integration certainly took place. But many others in fast-lane urban populations seemed to grow more jaded and extreme as they grew older. This process did not just involve individuals but seemed to involve the entire fast-lane culture as a whole. As the seventies progressed, the center of gravity of much of urban life seemed to shift. The late gay writer John Preston described the "Black Party" at New York's Mineshaft in 1981, at the historical high-water mark of the gay sexual revolution. Bus loads of "hungry men," he wrote, descended on New York to enjoy the "wallowing" experience:

> The fist fuckers, the piss drinkers, the cock suckers . . . the sadists, the pigs, all of them line up at the door and use the obligatory black masks to get ready to shed even one more layer of American respectability and approach one more step toward sexual fulfillment of their obsessive desires. [This Black Party seems] sleazier than ever. More cock, more piss, more flesh, more leather, more groans, more sex, more Crisco, more men. As its reputation grows and its attendance continues

to climb higher and higher, its life gets longer and longer, we all wonder: Where can this end?

Preston's question was on many minds in the early eighties. Among a dedicated and significant core of urban gay men, the spiraling escalation of the seventies had produced a culture of unprecedented sexual extremism. But rather than sating desires, it seemed to fuel them toward even more escalation. Where would it end, indeed?

CHAPTER 3

The Synergy of Plagues

Some readers, especially gay male readers, may find the following account insensitive, even offensive. Any clinical description of the waves of STD infections that swept over the gay male population seems, to many at least, to reduce gay sexual behavior to mere disease transmission. For that reason, some may fault this account for failing to temper clinical description with the unquestioned good that gay liberation was accomplishing during this period, or for not discussing the many psychological and cultural and spiritual reasons why certain segments of the gay population behaved in ways that were so prone to disease amplification.

I and many others have written at length about the brave and stirring strides that lesbians and gay men made in the decade between Stonewall and AIDS. The creation of a new community, the challenge to oppression, the building of a brilliant, caring culture, have been discussed by writers and activists and historians such as Allan Bérubé, Martin Duberman, Esther Newton, Cindy Patton, and many more, with far more detail and historical, psychological, and spiritual insight than I could possibly present in this essentially medical account. The point here is to do what few have done before: to examine the events that led to the gay AIDS epidemic from a biological perspective, to look at the rise of AIDS in the gay population from the virus's point of view. It is precisely because such a biological approach seems insensitive that we have shied away from it, and it is largely because we have shied away from it that we often retain such a distorted and sometimes even romanticized view of what occurred.

So let me simply say at the outset that what I describe below are biological, not moral, events. Some readers may give them a moralistic spin, arguing that they prove something essential about gay men or homosexuality or promiscuity. Some may see them entirely differently, arguing that they prove something about homophobia or how gay men react to anti-gay oppression. Still others may argue that they prove nothing at all and are, in fact, insignificant, the occupational hazards of living in a century of rapid change and emerging diseases. But the following story exists apart from such interpretations. It happened. We live with its consequences today. And it is vitally important for the future of gay men and all people on our shrinking planet that we look at this history unblinkingly. Not to condemn but to learn, and to use the insights gained to discover ways to save future generations from repeating the same mistakes, and from suffering the same fate.

Distant Thunder

As the ecosystems of gay sexual life burst into bloom in the late sixties and early seventies, they created highly efficient new routes for the epidemic spread of virtually all sexually transmitted diseases. Yet it took a while for many STDs to begin the process of epidemic amplification, and this is to be expected. In mathematical models of such amplification, the most common and easy-to-transmit pathogens will tend to be the first to spread when conditions become favorable, followed by rarer and more difficult to transmit varieties, and, if conditions remain favorable, followed at last by diseases that are extremely rare and extremely hard to transmit.

The combination of multiple sex partners and anal sex in relatively intense core groups had already created an unstable sexual ecology for some gay men even before Stonewall. An article in the *American Journal of Tropical Medical Hygiene* published in 1968 noted that certain pockets of Manhattan's growing gay community had begun to display the medical profiles of a Third World slum or a "tropical isle," with far higher than average rates of traditional

STDs and gastrointestinal parasites. After Stonewall this process sharply accelerated, creating a radical new medical situation in the gay world.

Syphilis and Gonorrhea. It would stand to reason that syphilis and gonorrhea, the most common and among the most easily transmitted STDs, would be the first to take advantage of the new gay sexual ecology, and that appears to have occurred. By the early seventies both were considered unremarkable occupational hazards of life in the gay fast lane. By the end of the seventies, gay men accounted for 80 percent of the 70,000 cases of syphilis treated by San Francisco's public health clinics per year. While gonorrhea also exploded in a similar way among gay men, its preponderance was significant not only numerically but genetically. Strains of gonorrhea began to mutate into ever nastier variants that traveled quickly around the world in a process that illustrates the confluence of the global STD pool.

In 1976 the CDC announced that a frightening new strain of gonorrhea, PPNG, had suddenly appeared that not only resisted penicillin but actually consumed and destroyed the drug. PPNG first appeared in the Philippines among a sexually active core group of prostitutes and servicemen in and around U.S. military bases where many women habitually took black market penicillin as a prophylactic treatment, a practice that almost surely prompted the mutation. At first health experts hoped PPNG could be contained in the Philippines, but once it reached the American gay population it spread like wildfire. In 1977 another new strain of gonorrhea appeared that was resistant to spectinomycin and ampicillin, and a few years later still another that resisted tetracycline. In the past all of these strains might have lingered in their original habitats for decades, but now jet travel transported them into the global sexual ecosystem almost immediately, where they became rampant among gay and, in many cases, minority men in American cities. Overall cases of gonorrhea in the United States grew from 259,000 in 1960 to 600,000 in 1970 and, including the newly resistant varieties, to 1 million in 1980, and most of that growth occurred within the core groups formed by gay men and the urban poor. By the early eighties, just as AIDS was first being noticed, the prevalence of both syphilis and gonorrhea among gay men was several hundred times that among comparable straights.

Herpes. Herpes simplex Type II also quickly penetrated the gay male population. A viral infection that can hide in the body for years, then break through the skin and mucous membranes in a blizzard of shedding in which billions of viral particles are released at once, HSV-II had generally been thought of as an occupational hazard of prostitution. But its prevalence began to increase in the seventies and it reached epidemic proportions among hetero-sexual young people in the early eighties, when studies showed that up to 15 percent of young, middle-class adults were infected. This caused a sensation in Western countries where the threat of serious infectious disease had come to be considered remote. At-tendance at singles bars dropped precipitously, and amid a great wringing of hands over the excesses of the sexual revolution many young people reined in their activities. What went largely unre-ported, however, was the fact that most of the people getting infected were gay men.

A study of the incidence of herpes simplex viruses between 1960 and 1980 by Dr. Andre Nahmias of Emory University revealed that while the prevalence of HSV-II doubled among women during the period, it rose seven times in men. Since HSV-II is equally transmissible between women and men, such a lopsided prepon-derance reflects men having sex with men. According to one study, by 1978, "the incidence of HSV-II infections was ten times higher in homosexual men in the United States than in compa-rable women, and the incidence among gay men nearly doubled during the next seven years. By 1985 homosexual men in their early twenties had an incidence of genital herpes infections eight to twenty times that of heterosexual males of the same age and socioeconomic status."

Intestinal Parasites. Even those differences pale beside gay men's rates of parasitic infections, primarily giardiasis, shigellosis, and amebiasis. These debilitating and hard-to-treat intestinal ail-ments are common in many Third World countries, where they spread through food and water contaminated by fecal matter. But in modern Western countries with indoor plumbing and chlorina-tion, such diseases were virtually unknown until the rising popu-larity of anal sex and analingus with multiple partners provided the parasites with efficient new modes of transmission.

"Rimming," or analingus, was almost unknown before Stonewall, but in the relaxed and presumably hygienic environment of the seventies it spread rapidly among cores of gay men who had lots of partners. Older gay men often report that they had never heard of the practice before the sixties, but by 1980 it was ubiquitous. "That gay men are exuberant in their practice is now verified," Seymour Kleinberg wrote in *Alienated Affections* in 1980, "in the epidemic proportion of amebiasis in recent years," which not only demonstrated the widespread practice of rimming, "but also the fact that its popularity is recent." Oral-anal sex provides an easy route for the transmission of a host of diseases, including hepatitis and intestinal parasites. As with anal sex, it was significant in gay sexual ecology not merely because of its adoption by some gay men, but because of its adoption by men who practiced it with multiple partners.

The parasites that were spread in this way had never before been considered sexually transmitted. Randy Shilts reports that public health departments were caught so completely unawares by the situation that at one point New York health inspectors diligently searched the Greenwich Village water supply for the source of a surge in amoeba cases in the neighborhood, convinced that such parasitic outbreaks had to result from contaminated water. Just how fast these intestinal parasites penetrated certain segments of the gay population is illustrated by the spread of *Entameoba histolytica*. In the mid seventies the only reported cases in the United States were in travelers returning from abroad—there was not a single locally acquired case anywhere in the nation. By 1980, however, a mere five years later, more than 20 percent of all gay men in America were estimated to be infected.

The combination of these and other intestinal infections led doctors to identify a new disease syndrome in 1976. It consisted of any or all of the three above mentioned parasites as well as some combination of condyloma acuminata; anal syphilis or gonorrhea; bleeding hemorrhoids; anal fissures, abscesses, and ulcers; hepatitis; and pruritis ani. Since virtually all of the patients of this syndrome were young urban gay men, doctors named it "Gay Bowel Syndrome." The tag drew protests from some gay community leaders, who considered it an insulting "remedicalization" of homosexuality. But others were not upset at all. The naming of Gay Bowel Syndrome was, in some quarters, "almost a matter of pride," wrote Michael Callen. "Now we even had our own *diseases*, just like we had our own plumbers and tax advisors."

Hepatitis B. Far more dangerous was the growing epidemic of hepatitis B in the gay population. Hepatitis B can cause either chronic or acute disease, can lead to markedly higher risk of liver cancer, and it can kill. Approximately one out of ten persons infected with hepatitis B becomes a chronic carrier, able to infect others for decades. Prior to the seventies it was spread primarily through blood transfusions, and as such was relatively rare. But it spread so rapidly in the gay population of the late seventies that by 1981 health officials in San Francisco estimated that 73 percent of all gay men in the city were infected. In another study, 60 percent of gay men from 5 cities had evidence of hepatitis B infection, as opposed to about 5 percent of heterosexual men.

Other Infections. It was the same story for virtually every sexually transmittable agent then known, and probably for a few that were not then known, like the virus now suspected of causing Kaposi's sarcoma. The rate of cytomegalovirus infection jumped from under 10 percent to over 94 percent of all gay men in less than 10 years. In some cohorts of gay men the Epstein-Barr virus was found in up to 98 percent, and in one case 100 percent, of the study subjects. From rare viruses such as HTLV, to more common infections such as hepatitis A, every sexually transmitted infection that entered the gay male ecosystem rose to unprecedented levels, so that by the end of the decade homosexual men had by far the highest sexually transmitted disease load of any social group in America. In many instances it was dozens or even, as with intestinal parasites, hundreds of times higher than average.

In biological terms this had occurred virtually overnight. If a collective microbial snapshot had been taken of American gay men on the eve of Stonewall in 1969, and another taken on Gay Pride Day a decade later, the difference would have been startling. Those in small cities and towns and in rural areas would have looked relatively unchanged, as would those who had sharply limited their partners or engaged only in nonpenetrative forms of sex. But for the portion of the gay population that engaged in core group activity on a regular or fairly frequent basis, those who had been healthy and vigorous ten years before would now often display the kind of stressed disease profile more typical of the poorer residents of Uganda or Bangladesh.

Multiple Reinfection. A significant aspect of this cascade of infection was that many of these diseases, and in some cases most of them, struck the same core group individuals repeatedly. Michael Callen's self-reported medical history was typical of a gay man in the most active core group frequenting New York's sex clubs and bathhouses.

"It wasn't until I was officially diagnosed with AIDS that I faced squarely just how much sex, and how much disease, I'd had," he wrote in *Surviving AIDS:*

> I calculated that since becoming sexually active in 1973, I had racked up more than three thousand different sex partners in bathhouses, back rooms, meat racks, and tearooms. As a consequence, I had also had the following sexually transmitted diseases, many more than once: hepatitis A, hepatitis B, hepatitis non-A/non-B [now called hepatitis C]; herpes simplex types I and II; venereal warts; amebiasis, including giardia lamblia and entamoeba histolytica; shigella flexneri and salmonella; syphilis; gonorrhea; nonspecific urethritis; chlamydia; cytomegalovirus and Epstein-Barr virus mononucleosis; and eventually cryptosporidiosis.

Callen's history of three thousand partners puts him smack-dab in the center of the highly active core group of gay men who first contracted AIDS.

The Global Connection. It is important to note that this wave of STD infections did not occur in a vacuum. The newfound sexual freedom formed only one part of a vast pattern of rapid change that reconfigured much of the sexual ecology of the planet in the seventies. Laurie Garrett summed up the changes in *The Coming Plague*:

> Worldwide, the seventies were a time of sexual liberation and experimentation for young adults—straight as well as gay—who poured into trendy metropolises from Nairobi to Amsterdam in search of the excitement and anonymity of urban nightlife. The birth control pill gave young women freedom from concern about unwanted pregnancy, and, for the first time in history, heterosexual exploration seemed safe. . . . [T]he scale of multiple-partnering during the late twentieth century was unprecedented. With over five billion people on the planet, an ever increasing percentage of whom were urban residents; with air travel and

mass transit available to allow people from all over the world to go to cities of their choice; with mass youth movements at their zenith, advocating, among other things, sexual freedom; with a feminist spirit alive in much of the industrialized world, promoting female sexual freedom; and with the entire planet bottom-heavy with people under twenty-five—there could be no doubt that the size and drama of this worldwide urban sexual energy was unparalleled.

The Dam Breaks

The rapid spread of HIV infection in the gay male community, then, was hardly accidental or surprising. In a culture so prone to amplifying sexually transmitted infections, including many that were previously rare or even unknown, it was only natural that anything entering this disease pool would undergo rapid and efficient transmission. What makes HIV different from these other infections is not anything about how or why it spread, but simply its generally fatal outcome. In all other ways it was just another bug along for the ride.

Ironically, the reason epidemiologists have such a precise map of the inroads HIV made in the gay world was due to another sexually transmitted disease that was decimating gay men at this time. Prior to the hepatitis B outbreak, most public health officials had ignored the danger signs in gay male epidemiology. A few researchers, like San Francisco's Selma Dritz, the NIH's June Osborn, and the CDC's Don Francis, vainly tried to warn their colleagues that something catastrophic was bound to occur if things continued as they were, but most researchers seemed uncomfortable with the subject and shied away from it. Some were hostile to gay men, others embarrassed by what they considered the exotic intensity of gay sexual culture. Ironically, those who were more kindly disposed, or at least more objective, feared that by focusing on the diseases spawned by the gay sexual revolution they would be accused of homophobia. Gay leaders frequently made it plain to researchers that anyone who raised questions about gay sexual freedom for any reason, whether ethical or biological, would be equally accused of anti-gay bias. Few researchers were willing to venture into such a political and social hot zone, and the few who did found that they consequently lost influence within the gay male community, a bad position to be in if your research required a high level of cooperation from gay men.

The explosion of hepatitis B, however, changed everything. After a smattering of curable infections that cost no more than a course of penicillin or a few weeks of Flagyl, medical experts were sobered by what the rapid spread of hepatitis B portended. Epidemiologists who had warned about the grim possibility of something really nasty entering the gay fast lane now found themselves taken very seriously. Suddenly, people were dying. Hepatitis B woke up the research community and spurred it to action.

Since work was well advanced on a vaccine for hepatitis B, researchers decided that they needed to develop a clear picture of the rate at which the disease was spreading in the gay population, so that once a vaccine was prepared its effectiveness could be measured. And so large cohorts of gay men were recruited in New York and San Francisco in 1978 to help prepare the way for vaccine trials. Men who enrolled in the studies agreed to come in at regular intervals to have their blood tested so that researchers could measure the incidence of infection. The samples were then preserved, and they were to become invaluable measures of the rise of HIV infection once a test for HIV antibodies became available in the mid-eighties. Researchers were then able to go back, retest the blood, and obtain a stop-motion picture of HIV's deadly incursion into the gay male population.

The result is a chilling portrait of a virus that had made major inroads into that population before anybody suspected a thing. In San Francisco in 1978, 4.5 percent of the cohort was already infected with HIV when the very first blood for the hepatitis study was drawn. The next year the rate *tripled* to 12 percent. During 1980 it doubled again, so that when the first announcements of the new immune deficiency syndrome were published in 1981, HIV had already infected *24 percent* of the San Francisco cohort. Infection continued to rise thereafter at a fairly steady rate of 11 percent per year—an astounding rate of sexual transmission generally, but typical of the rates of transmission in the gay male community, where other STDs continued increasing at around 12 percent per year. Prevalence in this cohort hit 35 percent during 1981, 46 percent during 1982, and 57 percent during 1983. Figures for 1984 show 67.4 percent of the cohort infected. As saturation took hold and most of the susceptibles became infected, the number rose more slowly, peaking at 73.1 percent in 1985.

Across the continent in New York City a similar tragedy was unfolding. When New York's hepatitis B cohort was enrolled in 1978, 6.6 percent of the men were already HIV positive. This was slightly higher than the San Francisco percentage at the same time, indicating that the virus's initial incursion in the North American gay population may have occurred in New York. But from then on, HIV's progress was roughly the same. The annual incidence of infection in New York peaked from 1982 through 1984. At its highest, 10.6 percent of the entire cohort became infected in a single year. By 1984, 43.7 percent of the New York cohort was infected.

Similar numbers were seen in other cities with large gay populations. By 1984 HIV prevalence among cohorts of gay men reached as high as 41 percent in Chicago, 49 percent in Boston, and 50 percent in Los Angeles. It hit 58 percent in a gay cohort in Denver by 1985, and 58 percent in Seattle in 1986. By 1987 it had reached 60 percent in one gay cohort in San Diego and 70 percent in another in Philadelphia.

Some have questioned why it took HIV so long to begin its fateful progress. It has even been suggested that since gay core groups were firmly in place as early as the late sixties and early seventies, and HIV did not explode until the late seventies, the rise of AIDS cannot be explained by behavioral changes. But in retrospect, it's clear that HIV didn't take long to make its move. Other diseases, far older, more common, and more easily transmitted, also took several years to build into epidemics. Hepatitis B really began to explode only in the late seventies. The great herpes epidemic among heterosexuals was a product of the early eighties, even though the sexual revolution that propelled it began in the sixties. Not every pathogen will respond instantly to events. Indeed, considering how difficult it is to transmit HIV, what seems remarkable about the epidemic is not how long it took to begin, but how swift it was.

Helping the Virus

We have already seen how the change in scale of sexual activity influenced the rise of other STDS in the gay population. But were there specific factors that contributed to the rapid spread of HIV?

Experts argue that the spread of HIV among sexually active gay men in the early eighties resulted from a fatal confluence of the biology of HIV and the collective behavior of gay men. While the invention of safer sex in the form of the condom code is based on the simple idea that HIV is transmitted by infected body fluids, the reality is considerably more complex. HIV is indeed spread through body fluids, but virtually all sexually active people transmit body fluids, and very few produce rates of HIV transmission remotely approaching those of gay men. To understand why gay sexual ecology interacted with HIV in such a disastrous way, we need to look at the range of factors that influenced HIV transmission in the gay world.

Multipartner Anal Sex. Many people, including many gay men, presume that anal sex itself was the overriding factor that led to the extraordinary levels of infection in the gay population. However, it appears that the difference in risk between anal and vaginal sex is nowhere near sufficient to account for the several-thousand-fold difference in HIV prevalence between gay men and comparable heterosexuals in the developed world. True, the rectum is somewhat more susceptible to infection than the vagina or the mouth, but not by very much. So the reason that anal sex led to catastrophic levels of infection in the gay population seems to have less to do with anal sex per se, and more to do with specific ways that gay men practiced it.

The primary factor that led to increased HIV transmission was anal sex combined with multiple partners, particularly in concentrated core groups. By the seventies there is little doubt that for those in the most sexually active core groups, multipartner anal sex had become the main event. Michael Callen, both an avid practitioner and a careful observer of life in the gay fast lane, believed that this was a "historically unprecedented aspect" of the gay sexual revolution. "In the urban gay fast lane of the '70s, the expectation was that fucking would take place," he wrote. "If you didn't fuck, you were thought odd." Callen, by the way, did not believe that this was essential to homosexuality or homosexuals. "Fucking is, for most gay men, an acquired taste," he wrote, which nonetheless "became more the rule than the exception, at least in the fast lane."

A number of theories have been put forward in attempts to explain how something often considered a highly intimate activity came to be practiced with very large numbers of partners in certain core groups. One is that gay men were finally turning to each other for sex, especially in safe spaces like baths where the number of potential partners was maximal and the danger of interruption was minimal. This combination of higher self-esteem and greater safety created a powerful impetus toward greater intimacy. Another was that improved hygiene and available cures for venereal diseases made men feel safer about fucking. Still another was that the "loosen up" ethic of the sixties and seventies prompted a general move toward less self-restraint and greater sexual experimentation among both gays and straights. In addition, some have argued that as gay men came to consider their sexuality as equivalent to heterosexuality, they came to believe that anal sex ought to be as central to their sexual lives as vaginal sex is to straights'. Still others have pointed out that many gay men first developed their sexual expectations from porn films, where the most common plot is that partners meet, they have oral sex, and then they have anal sex. Some argue that this influenced many gay men to believe that anal sex was simply expected, even in anonymous encounters and one-night stands.

Probably all of these factors played a role, but whatever the case, many researchers consider the combination of anal sex with multiple partners in tightly concentrated circles of individuals to have been the single most vital element in amplifying AIDS. Some epidemiologists now speculate that if the most sexually active core of gay men had confined themselves to oral sex or mutual masturbation with large numbers of partners, and had reserved anal sex for longer-term relationships, things would have turned out very differently.

Insertive/Receptive "Versatility." In the middle of the century, and particularly in the sixties and seventies, gay men began doing something that appears rare in sexual history: They began to abandon strict role separation in sex and alternately play both the insertive and receptive roles, a practice sometimes called versatility.

In most cultures, male-to-male sexual relations were stratified and people played very defined roles. Sometimes, as David Greenberg writes in *The Construction of Homosexuality*, the stratification was based primarily on age, as when "the older partner takes a role defined as active or masculine; the younger, a role defined as passive or female." In other societies roles are not based on age as much as on outward appearances of gender—as in the macho/queen dichotomy of many Latin American societies today. In such societies anal sex is highly structured, with the "homosexual" partner always playing the feminine, bottom role and the "macho" partner being the masculine top. The same separation also applied to early-twentieth-century New York, where the "fairy" or "queer" partner virtually always fellated the (presumably) straight partner.

As modern gay sexual culture emerged in the middle of the twentieth century, however, gay men began to consider this role separation a form of self-oppression. As more and more gay men began having sex with each other rather than with trade, and as more and more adopted anal sex as part of their sexual repertoire, activists called upon men to strive for sexual equality and reject strict role separation. Carl Wittman's "A Gay Manifesto," perhaps the most influential gay lib essay from the early seventies, was explicit on this point. In the section headed "On Positions and Roles" Wittman wrote:

> Much of our sexuality has been perverted through mimicry of straights, and warped from self-hatred. These sexual perversions are basically anti-gay:
>
> *"I like to make it with straight guys."*
> *"I'm not gay but I like to be 'done.' "*
> *"I like to fuck, but I don't want to be fucked."*
> *"I don't like to be touched above the neck."*
>
> This is role playing at its worst; we must transcend these roles. We strive for democratic, mutual, reciprocal sex.

For Wittman and many others, the stratification of sex roles was a relic of an oppressive past. As the seventies progressed, this rejection of role-playing became so pronounced that in a sense versatility itself became a kind of role: Those who disliked versatility for whatever reason began to feel embarrassed to admit it, since such reticence was now perceived by some as almost an affront to homosexuality. Whether one considers this a socially liberating development or just another form of sexual conformity, it seems to have had enormous consequences for gay sexual ecology.

To achieve maximum efficiency in transmission, STDs need to circulate freely within a sexual ecosystem. But because HIV is difficult to transmit and generally needs to be injected directly into the body and bloodstream, it is much easier for the insertive partner to infect the receptive one than the other way around. This creates what some epidemiologists call the "dead-end factor" that inhibits transmission from women to men in the developed world. In the absence of mitigating factors the virus is likely to hit a dead end wherever strict role separation is practiced. As we have seen, the dead-end factor is mitigated in parts of the Third World where men frequently have venereal sores that allow the virus to enter their bloodstreams directly. It also seems mitigated among uncircumcised men, since the tissue of the foreskin seems particularly susceptible to HIV infection and since the foreskin creates a reservoir where HIV can linger for long enough to enter the body.

Nowhere was the dead-end factor canceled out more efficiently, however, than where the gay practice of insertive/receptive "versatility" was widely adopted. Now the same person into whom HIV was injected could himself switch roles and become the injector into others, who themselves could receive the microbe passively and then reverse positions and pass it along. Mathematical models of the epidemic have stressed the central importance of this factor in the dissemination of HIV among gay men.

Concurrency. Having multiple partners heightens the risk of transmission for any sexually transmitted disease, but not all forms of multiple partnering are equally risky. We have already seen how multipartnerism in core groups can amplify risk. Researchers calculate that there is also an enormous difference in risk between those who have multiple partners in a serial or a concurrent fashion.

Serial multipartnerism, which can also be called serial monogamy, means having partners one at a time. You become involved with someone, remain monogamous with that person while you're together, then break up and find a new partner with whom you are again monogamous for the duration of the relationship. *Concurrent multipartnerism* means having partners more or less interchangeably. Mathematical models have demonstrated that these two different styles create enormously different opportunities for disease transmission. Even if people in one population have an average of, say, twelve partners per year concurrently, and those in another population have the same number of partners but have them in a serial fashion, the concurrent population can suffer a rate of total disease transmission from 10 to 100 times higher than the serial population.

To illustrate how this might work with a virus like HIV, let's compare two hypothetical men who both have twelve partners per year. The man who mixes his partners concurrently—let's call him Joe—goes back and forth among his twelve partners throughout the year, while Tom has his twelve partners in a linear fashion, taking one exclusive lover each month, then breaking up with that person, taking up with a new lover for a month, and so on.

Let's say that of Joe's twelve concurrent partners, Partner Ten is infected with HIV. Partner Ten is not very infectious, so although Joe has sex with all of his partners randomly from January through December, he does not become infected by Partner Ten until October. Once Joe is infected, however, he becomes highly infectious himself, as people newly infected with HIV tend to be. Since he is still having concurrent sexual relations with all eleven of his other partners, he can now quickly and easily transmit his new infection to any of the other partners in his circle. As a result, throughout the rest of October, November, and December, several or perhaps even most of his other partners become infected.

Tom also has twelve partners that year, but has them one at a time. Tom's Partner Ten is also HIV-positive and mildly infectious, and Tom also becomes infected by this partner in October, at which point Tom becomes highly infectious. But while Tom can easily pass his new infection along to his next two lovers, Partners Eleven and Twelve, he cannot pass it along to Partners One through Nine, since he is no longer having sex with them. So even though Joe and Tom both have twelve partners that year, and even though the circumstances of their infection are the same—infection by Partner Ten in the tenth month of the year—their abilities to transmit their infection are vastly different. While that difference seems notable in individuals, imagine how it would be further magnified if all of Joe's partners are also concurrent with twelve other partners, all of whom are also concurrent with twelve other partners, and so on, while all of Tom's partners practice serial monogamy.

Among core groups of gay men, concurrency was the overwhelming rule. Indeed, the urban gay culture of the seventies and early eighties so avidly promoted and celebrated concurrency—in the baths and sex clubs, among circles of "fuck buddies," and so on—that even many men in long-term committed relationships saw little reason why they should not engage in concurrent relations with others. Men frequenting bars, bathhouses, and sex clubs and having anonymous sex with dozens or even hundreds of partners were mixing them together in what, from a virus's point of view, would be the most efficient possible way. It is impossible from today's vantage to go back and determine precisely the extent to which sexual concurrency increased transmission among gay men, but some investigators now believe that the prevalence of concurrency amplified transmission among gay men by factors of 10 to 100 times.

Viral Load. One of the reasons that concurrent partners are so much more likely to transmit HIV than serial partners has to do with a factor of HIV infection known as viremia, or viral load. Viral load varies widely in the sexual fluids of HIV-positive men. For example, some studies indicate that there is detectable HIV in the semen of less than 30 percent of all HIV-infected men. Of this group an even smaller percentage appears to have a viral load hundreds of times higher than the average infectious HIV-positive man. This very high level of viremia typically occurs at two times during the course of HIV disease: at the very beginning, in the months after infection, and again near the end, when the virus has overwhelmed the body's immune system. During the initial period, which can last up to six months, the invading HIV blooms throughout the body of its new host almost unchecked, and the newly infected person can have a viremia level many hundreds of times greater than will be typical later on. In all likelihood, this is the period when people are most able to transmit HIV.

Within several months of initial infection, however, the immune system mounts a more effective response. The body begins manufacturing millions of T cells to counterattack the virus, and eventually this counterattack dramatically lowers the level of free-floating HIV in the blood and other bodily fluids. The surviving HIV retreats into certain areas of the body, such as the lymph system, where it engages in a long battle of attrition with the immune system. During this period, which typically lasts for several years, the level of free-floating virus remains comparatively low, and the infected person is thought to be much less likely to transmit infection during sex. This is not to say that such a person *cannot* transmit infection. Indeed, transmissions during this period have been well documented. But the odds seem somewhat lower than they were during primary infection.

Eventually, however, HIV is able to mount a final assault of its own, manufacturing billions of virions a day to replace those lost in the battle with the immune system. At this point things begin to tip in favor of the virus. The level of viral replication overwhelms the ability to combat it, HIV swarms throughout the body, the level of viremia in bodily fluids rises to levels comparable to those in the first several months of infection, and the infected individual usually begins to suffer from opportunistic infections. At this stage the person again develops a heightened ability to transmit HIV, and this time that ability appears to be for keeps.

This limited period in which a person is highly infectious could have a significant impact on transmission in populations that have concurrent partners. What it implies is that for HIV to have the greatest chance of spreading, an infected person not only needs to have unsafe sex with lots of partners, but to do so within the relatively brief time that he is highly infectious. In other words, lots of concurrent partners in the briefest possible time span will equal the greatest chance of epidemic spread. Precisely those conditions were most prevalent among the core of gay men who had large numbers of partners. If, however, a person remains monogamous during the peak period of infectiousness, and especially if that person remains monogamous with the very person who infected him or her, that highly infectious period is wasted from the virus's point of view. Such would tend to be the case where people practice serial monogamy.

The Synergy of Plagues

Other STDs. Researchers have recognized that a number of other factors make gay men more susceptible to viral infection, both by lowering the body's natural immunity and by placing people in the position where they are more likely to encounter infection. High on the list of other factors facilitating HIV's spread in the gay population was the enormous increase in other STDs. We have already seen how increased STD infection raises the risk of HIV transmission by causing venereal sores that allow direct viral access to the bloodstream, and by placing a ready pool of easily infectible white blood cells at the point of entry. Most middle-class gay men who contracted lots of STDs had ready access to health care and usually did not walk around for long with untreated venereal sores. Ironically, however, their immune systems were depleted by repeated courses of antibiotics prescribed to fight other STD infections. Such continuous use of powerful antibiotics can compromise the immune system in ways that make infection by many different microbes, including HIV, far more likely. So, in this way, the very access to quality health care that helped make the gay sexual revolution possible contributed to the rapid spread of HIV.

Substance Abuse. Drinking and drug abuse also lower immunity and tend to increase risky behaviors. Alcohol had long been an important part of gay social life, partly because of the central role that bars played in fostering a gay identity, partly because those engaging in deeply stigmatized sex often needed to dull their inhibitions. In *Cherry Grove*, her wonderfully evocative history of the gay Fire Island resort, Esther Newton writes that for many homosexuals, sex was possible only under the heavy fog of drink. "It is no exaggeration to say," she writes of Cherry Grove in the 1940s, that "alcohol was the lifeblood of Grove social life and that drunkenness was not only accepted but conferred status." She quotes one Grove resident as saying, "Until you had fallen off the boardwalk you were not really a Cherry Grover." Pre-Stonewall clinical studies show extremely high rates of alcohol consumption among gay men, while later studies of gay men drawn from more representative samples in the seventies present conflicting results: Some indicate that one third of gay men had problems with alcohol and that gays were twice as likely as straights to be alcoholics. Others have found fewer differences between heterosexuals and homosexuals in alcohol consumption and abuse.

Since gay liberation coincided with a steep rise in society's use of recreational drugs generally, it is no surprise that the gay world had an active drug subculture. The most sexually active urban gay men tended to consume large amounts of recreational drugs, including cocaine, marijuana, THC, MDA, LSD, and speed. The party circuits in the gay resorts of both coasts were famous for their open use of drugs, and the literature of the era is filled with romanticized depictions of drug use as an integral part of the gay male experience.

Gay life even had its own favorite drugs, the most ubiquitous being nitrate inhalants, or "poppers." Poppers were initially manufactured as treatments for angina pectoris, a painful heart condition. But they also produce a momentarily powerful "rush" that dilutes blood vessels and, for many, enhances sexual pleasure and prolongs orgasm. They also relax muscles, including the sphincter muscle, making them an aid to both anal sex and fisting. Poppers became so popular in urban gay circles in the seventies that popper manufacturers rivaled bathhouse owners as the biggest advertisers in the gay press. A CDC study during the early eighties showed that 85 percent of gay men used poppers, compared to only 15 percent of heterosexual men, making poppers the closest thing we had to a truly gay drug. Poppers became so ubiquitous in the urban gay world that many investigators long suspected that AIDS was caused by poppers. Since poppers have been shown to have an adverse effect on the immune system, they may have played a significant role in making people more susceptible to HIV infection.

A significant subset of gay men straddled the line between the gay community and the world of injection drug users (IDUs). Since injection drugs had created a parallel HIV epidemic among IDUs, this intersection between gay men and IDUs created a viral "bridge" that linked the two epidemics. Of the first 1,000 AIDS cases, for example, 642 were gay men and 154 were injection drug users, but an additional 81 were both: gay male IDUs. (By contrast, only 1 out of the 54 Haitians and none of the 7 hemophiliacs in the original cohort of 1,000 were also IDUs). There has been much speculation on the significance of this connection, a linkage between the two most intense pools of infection that continues to this day.

Travel. Still another factor contributing to rapid dissemination was widespread travel and mobility. As we have seen, this affected the health of the whole world by making possible the rapid spread of new diseases from isolated pockets to great urban centers and from one urban center to another. As a glance at the travel ads of any major gay publication will attest, many gay men love to travel, and few populations in history have been as mobile. Sexual vacations to Third World countries with thriving sex industries, such as Haiti and Thailand, were very popular in the seventies. Within the United States a party circuit evolved—called simply the Circuit—

that found men gathering several times per year for huge, nationally known megaparties that often lasted several days. In some sense the gay meccas of L.A. and New York and San Francisco became one large, interconnected bicoastal community during the seventies, a community in which well-heeled travelers intermingled sexually as well as socially. The importance of this factor was highlighted at the very outset of the epidemic, when researchers discovered clusters of gay men in New York, San Francisco, and Los Angeles who were connected to each other through sexual relations. Patient Zero, the airline steward made notorious by Randy Shilts in *And the Band Played On* (not because he was thought first to introduce HIV to North America, as sometimes erroneously reported, but because his mobility and sexual activity placed him at the center of several important clusters of early AIDS cases), was only one among thousands of highly mobile gay men who helped transport HIV quickly and efficiently.

Increased Virulence. According to a theory advanced by Amherst biologist Paul Ewald in his 1993 book *Evolution of Infectious Disease*, the high levels of HIV transmission among gay men and IV drug users may have led to the evolution of new strains of more virulent and infectious HIV. Viral infectiousness is defined as the ability of a virus to enter and infect a cell in the target host. Virulence describes the ability of that virus to replicate within that cell, in the process disrupting the cell's natural function and causing illness. According to the theory of natural selection, which operates with the same relentless logic among viruses as among elephants, only those viral strains best suited to their environment will survive and be passed along. When people had relatively few sex partners and might spend many years with the same person, the only strains of HIV likely to survive and be passed along were those that delayed causing illness for long enough to give their relatively monogamous hosts a chance to have sexual relations with other partners and pass the strain along. In other words, only those strains so mild that they allowed their hosts decades of healthy life were likely to survive in a relatively monogamous world. More virulent strains would cause their hosts to fall ill and stop having sex relatively quickly, before they could find additional partners, and so those more virulent strains would generally die with their hosts.

When HIV entered communities characterized by large numbers of concurrent partners, however, the virus no longer had to reside in the same person for decades in order to be passed along. As a result, whenever a random mutation of a highly virulent strain arose that also had a high degree of infectiousness, it now had a distinct advantage. Since it was more aggressive, it was more likely to be passed along in any given sexual encounter. And since its more promiscuous host was likely to have many partners in the few years before becoming ill, it had ample opportunity to be passed along. Thus, the logic of natural selection ceased favoring the extremely mild strains and now increasingly favored the most aggressive ones.

The Core and the Bridge

We have already seen evidence that STD epidemics often begin in small cores of people who suffer from multiple risk factors. This phenomenon was observed among gay men from the very beginning of the epidemic. In 1983 leading AIDS doctor Joseph Sonnabend wrote in an influential article that "it appears that the disease has been occurring in a rather small subset [of gay men] characterized by having had sexual contact with large numbers of different partners in settings where the carriage of CMV [cytomegalovirus] in particular (but also of other sexually transmitted infections) is high." He attributed this to the "unprecedented level of promiscuity" within this subset. A few years later PWA activist Michael Callen would not feel any need to elaborate his statement that "unwittingly, and with the best of revolutionary intentions, a small subset of gay men managed to create disease settings equivalent to those of poor third-world nations," thereby facilitating the explosion of AIDS. Even within gay urban circles and even among activists, AIDS was thought of as a disease of the promiscuous. And, at first, it probably was.

In the late eighties Professor James Thompson, chairman of the department of statistics at Rice University, published statistical models that calculated what would happen to the incidence of HIV in gay populations with and without such core groups. His work indicated that the overall level of sexual interaction that characterized most gay men was not sufficient to push HIV over the epidemic threshold in most communities, but that the extraordinarily

high levels of activity that characterized a subset of the gay population made epidemic amplification inevitable. In perhaps his most
startling and disturbing model, Thompson created two scenarios.
In one, a theoretical gay population has a uniform sexual rate of 30
contacts per month. In the other, the total number of contacts
within the population remains the same, but most sexual activity is
shifted to the core, so that 10 percent of the population has 150
contacts per month and the other 90 percent has only a few contacts. Thompson showed that despite the fact that this second
population has the same total number of contacts as the first, the
fact that most of the contacts have been shifted to the core has the
same effect as if the entire group had doubled its number of contacts. In other words, the same number of contacts produces twice
as much new infection if those contacts are concentrated among a
small core of men. Thompson's models, which are rarely discussed
in gay prevention circles, are unambiguous. It is not anything particular about homosexuality that renders AIDS possible in the gay
population, Thompson wrote. "It is the presence of extraordinarily
sexually active individuals in the homosexual community which
causes the problem. . . . It should be pointed out to the gay community that even if most of the members of the community cut
down on their activity and/or practice 'safe sex,' even the less
promiscuous are seriously endangered by a small, highly promiscuous sub-group."

Bridging. In many societies, however, small subsets of people
can be burdened with high levels of sexually transmitted diseases
without contributing to a wider epidemic. The factor that most
often prevents a disease from bridging from a core to the rest of
the population is, quite baldly, prejudice and stigma. People in
cores tend to be members of poor, oppressed minorities who are
often marginalized and visibly ill—and therefore often shunned as
sexual partners by the majority. In the gay world, however, almost
the opposite was the case. There was no prejudice or stigma
directed against the A-list: beautiful, well-heeled men who were
both the most sexually active and the most desirable. Virtually no
one stigmatized their behavior. Indeed, many people felt the
behavior of A-list gay men represented the apex of gay liberation,
something to be envied and emulated rather than shunned. And
among the majority who did not participate in the extremes of the

gay fast lane, there was very little or no stigma against having affairs or brief encounters with those who did. The seventies and early eighties were, after all, a relaxed era in which many gay men—including many in relationships—prided themselves on being more open-minded and tolerant about the occasional tryst than heterosexuals. As a result, there appears to have been a tremendous amount of sexual mixing between the most highly active (and infected) gay men and the rest of the population. Men who had only one extracurricular partner a year mixed freely with those who had hundreds. Someone involved in a long-term relationship in which he himself chose to remain monogamous might often assume, or know for certain, that his lover had dalliances with other casual partners, sometimes lots of them. Because of this, any disease agent becoming endemic within the sexual core of gay men had ample opportunity to radiate out efficiently through the rest of the gay population.

This kind of mixing happened throughout the gay landscape and was facilitated by all sorts of institutions, but some experts believe that bathhouses played a particularly crucial role in this process. In the first place, the virus took advantage of the baths to exploit the fact that people with HIV tend to be highly infectious for a couple of months right after they become infected themselves. What likely occurred (on a massive scale) is that a regular bath-goer would become infected one night at the tubs and then, during the next couple of months when he was extremely likely to transmit infection, would return many times and have perhaps dozens of partners, infecting several. Many of those partners would also frequent bathhouses and they would repeat the process, primarily using the medium of baths and sex clubs to accumulate large numbers of partners in the limited window of maximum transmission. While those who habituated baths quickly became saturated with HIV, there were tens of thousands of additional men who went to the baths much less often—from once every few weeks to once a year or less. These men were spread out all along the behavioral continuum. Some might even be in fairly monogamous relationships, for whom the baths were simply an occasional treat. But once there, they ran a high likelihood of having sex with the very people whom, from a biological standpoint, they most needed to avoid. So it appears that the baths both created the conditions for the most sexually active core to become quickly infected, and then created the ideal conditions to bridge the resultant epidemic rapidly across the gay landscape.

Some researchers now believe that under these conditions HIV spread almost like measles or chicken pox in its original, explosive phase in the early eighties. It has been estimated that in the early eighties the average infected gay man infected an average of five additional gay men. Such a mind-boggling reproductive rate for a virus that's relatively difficult to transmit would require several conditions: that infected men had very large numbers of partners, that they engaged in the most transmitting form of fluid exchange, and that they had those partners in quick succession, during the brief initial period of high infectiousness at the outset of their own infection. Commercial sex establishments are obviously not the only ways that people can engage in such behavior, especially in urban populations where much of social life centered around cruising and bars. But bathhouses and sex clubs clearly fulfilled those conditions in extraordinarily efficient ways, causing some researchers to believe that they played the vital role that schools and movie theaters play for diseases like measles and chicken pox. A 1989 epidemiological survey of AIDS transmission in the gay world noted that "gay bath houses and sex clubs functioned for gay men in the same way that 'shooting galleries' have functioned for drug injectors in establishing the AIDS epidemic and the spread of HIV infection."

Understanding the role of core groups is hardly just an academic exercise. Because of core groups' concentration and their ability to spread infection both inside and outside the core, they make logical targets for prevention programs. In the early nineties researchers created models to examine what might happen to the future number of infections if public health officials prevented 100 new infections today within a core, as opposed to preventing 100 new infections outside the core. One study indicated that within ten years a "policy of targeting the one-time intervention at the core averts *ten times as many cases* as would have been averted by a policy directed at the non-core." If, for example, 100 cases of gonorrhea are prevented in a non-core today, that would prevent an additional 426 cases within ten years. But preventing 100 cases of gonorrhea within a core prevents an additional 4,278 cases. Approximately the same numbers apply to HIV. Preventing 100 cases in a noncore today, the study reported, prevents an additional 201 cases in ten years, while preventing 100 cases within a core prevents an additional, 2,106 cases.

All These Factors Are Central to Gay Life

"It was an historic accident that HIV disease first manifested itself in the gay populations of the east and west coasts of the United States," wrote British sociologist Jeffrey Weeks in *AIDS and Contemporary History* in 1993. His opinion has been almost universal among gay and AIDS activists even to this day. Yet there is little "accidental" about the sexual ecology described above. Multiple concurrent partners, versatile anal sex, core group behavior centered in commercial sex establishments, widespread recreational drug abuse, repeated waves of STDs and constant intake of antibiotics, sexual tourism and travel—these factors were not "accidents." Multipartner anal sex was encouraged, celebrated, considered a central component of liberation. Core group behavior in baths and sex clubs was deemed by many the quintessence of freedom. Versatility was declared a political imperative. Analingus was pronounced the champagne of gay sex, a palpable gesture of revolution. STDs were to be worn like badges of honor, antibiotics to be taken with pride.

Far from being accidents, these things characterized the very foundation of what it supposedly meant to experience gay liberation. Taken together they formed a sexual ecology of almost incalculably catastrophic dimensions, a classic feedback loop in which virtually every factor served to amplify every other. From the virus's point of view, the ecology of liberation was a royal road to adaptive triumph. From many gay men's point of view, it proved a trapdoor to hell on earth.

It would be reassuring to say that in the epidemic's second decade all of this has become common knowledge, that AIDS prevention is now grounded in a frank and full understanding of the ecological principles briefly sketched here, principles learned painfully with much death and loss. But sadly for gay men, that is not the case. As we will see in the next chapters, our collective gay response to AIDS has never included a sober evaluation of the ways the sexual culture of the seventies produced the AIDS epidemic. Quite the opposite. The enterprise of AIDS prevention in the gay world has strenuously avoided any detailed examination of these mechanisms. Their very discussion is considered offensive, homophobic, self-loathing. Instead, we have sought to minimize or even deny these factors, partly in order to preserve as much as possible the gains of the gay sexual revolution—the very "gains" that brought us AIDS.

In one sense, the behavioral changes that characterized the seventies were indeed accidental. No one at Stonewall, or for many years afterward, could have guessed the dire biological consequences of what at the time seemed like the blossoming of freedom, the logical response to years of repression and homophobia. But as we will see, once those consequences became known, innocence was lost. Or should have been.

Chapter 4

The Birth of the Condom Code

The first halting attempts to reconfigure gay sexual ecology began almost as soon as the epidemic was noticed, and within a few years culminated in the creation of what is now called safer sex. This was developed almost exclusively by gay men and disseminated through a broad network of gay institutions that had sprung up in the seventies, as well as institutions that were created specifically to cope with AIDS. Its creation was mostly unassisted by government or media, which remained embarrassed by the mention of homosexuality, indifferent to the deaths of homosexuals, and loath to contribute to discussions on how gay men could continue having sexually fulfilling lives in the midst of a sexually transmitted epidemic—or, for that matter, under any circumstances at all.

The Dual Imperative

Those who sought to create a theory of safer sex had to contend not only with the confusing and deadly dynamics of AIDS itself—even its basic cause was unclear for several years—but with two enormous social challenges. First, anti-gay forces almost immediately seized upon AIDS to argue that since liberated male homosexuality had apparently unleashed an epidemic, the "lesson of AIDS" was that gay liberation was a mistake that should be reversed. Conservative columnist Patrick Buchanan spoke for many when he wrote: "The poor homosexuals—they have declared war on Nature, and now Nature is exacting an awful retribution." In the process of crafting a social and medical response to the epidemic gay men were constantly on the defensive, and had to examine their own pronouncements and conclusions continually to make sure they did not seem to give credence to such claims.

The other challenge was perhaps more dire. The epidemic seemed to implicate two central aspects of gay sexuality: the practice of anal sex and what one gay liberationist called the "brotherhood of promiscuity" that gay men had built in cosmopolitan cities. The very behaviors that gay activists had spent years promoting seemed to have contained the seeds of disaster. But since promiscuity and anal sex were perceived by many (though certainly not all) gay men to be central to liberation, and since it was felt that most gay men would not accept any safer sex regimen that questioned their right to have multiple partners and anal sex, many gay theorists and activists considered it absolutely crucial that any response to the epidemic not stigmatize either behavior. The question then became, if anal sex and promiscuity equal liberation, and AIDS is spreading due to anal sex and promiscuity, how can gay men control the spread of AIDS without sacrificing liberation?

These two challenges created a dual imperative that has characterized gay AIDS prevention to this day: to prevent the spread of HIV, but only in a way that defends gay men against attacks from the right and preserves the multipartnerist ethic of the gay sexual revolution. In what was undoubtedly one of the tallest orders a prevention strategy ever had to fill, safer sex was to be a political and social as much as a medical or ecological construction.

The First "Crisis of Ideology"

The AIDS epidemic is usually dated from June 5, 1981, when the Centers for Disease Control published a brief item in its *Morbidity and Mortality Weekly Report* (*MMWR*) describing a strange new outbreak of pneumonia in five otherwise healthy gay men. In fact the first mention in the media was not in the *MMWR*, but in the May 18 issue of the *New York Native*, a gay newspaper. Written by pioneering gay journalist and physician Dr. Lawrence D. Mass, whose early coverage was the most incisive and extensive of the epidemic, this brief report displayed the twin approaches that would define much of gay men's subsequent reaction to the growing tragedy: acknowledgment and denial. The initial headline the editors placed above the article, DISEASE RUMORS LARGELY UNFOUNDED, seems to encapsulate that early reaction, acknowledging a problem and trying to minimize it at the same time. This attitude, by the way, is hardly confined to gay men and AIDS, but seems a staple initial response to epidemics throughout history. During a serious outbreak of cholera in New York City in 1832, the *New York Evening Post* snorted, "We have some cholera in the city, and a great deal of humbug."

It quickly became clear, particularly in Mass's subsequent coverage, that the rumors were very well founded and that something terrible was stalking homosexual men in America. As the months went by and gay men and public health experts slowly began to discern the outlines of a major epidemic, they naturally became anxious to find out what, if anything, unafflicted men could do to protect themselves. Since AIDS was initially associated almost exclusively with homosexual men, suspicion naturally focused on behaviors that gay men shared in common. Some theorized that repeated rectal exposure to the semen of different partners might be leading to an immune breakdown. Others believed that the cumulative effects of multiple sex partners, which led to increased bouts of STDs, which in turn led to prodigious consumption of antibiotics, had devastated gay men's immunity. Still others suspected that the recreational use of poppers were to blame. And some suspected that a new sexually transmitted pathogen, probably a virus, had entered the gay population and was spreading in the conditions created by gay sexual ecology, a suspicion that slowly solidified as the epidemiology of AIDS was found to resemble closely that of hepatitis B. But whatever one's theory of choice, virtually all of these theories implicated basic aspects of gay sexual freedom in one form or another. And for many gay men, that posed a problem almost as threatening as the epidemic itself.

So before the cause of AIDS was nailed down, even before many people had become sick, prescient gay men suspected they were faced with an issue that might strike at the heart of the political and sexual culture they had so carefully constructed in the face of such opposition from homophobes and moralists. Within the gay community a "crisis of ideology is threatening to explode," wrote Mass in the *New York Native* as early as March of 1982. "With much confusion on all sides, advocates of sexual fulfillment are being opposed to critics of promiscuity." In a sense, they still are.

The First Safe Sex: Partner Reduction

The root of the crisis was an unambiguous connection. The very first group of gay men with the syndrome were found to have had twice as many partners as those without it, and their partners were in turn found to have more than average numbers of partners as well. So it appeared obvious that in the absence of a known cause, any rational prevention strategy must involve partner reduction. Accordingly, the very earliest literature produced by gay and AIDS groups, long before HIV was discovered, urged gay men to "reduce" their partners.

The first explicit advice about AIDS prevention appeared in 1982 in the form of pamphlets and newsletters by the San Francisco gay and lesbian doctors' group Bay Area Physicians for Human Rights, by Houston's Citizens for Human Equality, and by New York's Gay Men's Health Crisis. This material emphasized partner reduction as the primary strategy for avoiding the syndrome. The newsletter distributed by Gay Men's Health Crisis put it simply: "The fewer different partners, the less your risk of acquiring a disease." In addition to partner reduction, gay men were urged to "know" their partners and to examine each other's bodies before sex for evidence of lesions and swollen glands, under the assumption that infection ought to produce visible signs. Some early material also recommended that partners avoid exchanging "bodily fluids," and some advised men to consider wearing condoms, but this was rarely emphasized at first. An early *Advocate* article on safer sex advised men to "know" and "reduce" their partners first and foremost. It relegated advice on condoms to seventh on the list, and seemed skeptical even then. "Wearing a condom may reduce the risk," it tepidly suggested.

Government health experts also focused primarily on partner reduction. The first guidelines for gay men issued by the Public Health Service in March 1983 consisted of these two sentences: "Sexual contact should be avoided with persons known or suspected to have AIDS. Members of high risk groups should be aware that multiple sexual partners increase the probability of developing AIDS." Other mainstream groups concurred. "Sex with multiple partners . . . increases your chance of exposure," said the United Way of Los Angeles, while the American Red Cross advised, "Don't have sex with multiple partners. . . . The more partners you have, the greater your risk."

Although in retrospect the message to reduce partners did not go anywhere near far enough, even this tepid advice was seen by many as going too far—a direct attack on gay sexuality. Openly gay anthropologist Ralph Bolton, who has strongly defended gay male promiscuity in scientific papers and articles, cited one reason he believed the partner reduction strategy was ill advised—it would be seen as anti-gay:

> Resistance to limiting the number of partners was sure to arise because the sexual liberation for which gay men had fought so hard included the right to be promiscuous. Promiscuity was a key feature of gay culture as it evolved, and attempts to extirpate promiscuity could be interpreted as an attack on gay culture and gay liberation, much more so than an emphasis on eradicating risky practices could be. . . . It was sex, after all, that gay men had in common; it was their sexuality that differentiated them from the larger society. Cruising was the favorite pastime for many, and sexual adventures were conversational center-pieces. . . . Calling for a reduction in the number of sexual partners implied a radical restructuring of all of gay social life. . . .

Nonetheless, many gay men followed the advice to reduce partners. Long-term cohort studies show declines beginning in 1982 and continuing steadily through the late 1980s. Unfortunately, partner reduction proved woefully inadequate by itself. For one thing, reduction was an ambiguous concept. Reduce to what, from what? Many gay men in the most sexually active core groups were having dozens or even hundreds of partners a year. Would reducing from 500 partners to 100 make a difference? What about reducing from 50 to 10? No one knew, and no one got specific. As a result, many gay men reduced their number of partners to two thirds, or half, or one third, of their former level, and discovered too late that such reductions made little difference.

One reason, according to mathematical models of the epidemic, is that for partner reduction to work by itself, the overall prevalence of disease in your population—in other words, the percentage of your potential sex partners who are already infected—must be quite low. Harvard statistician Victor de Gruttola, for example, has demonstrated that in a hypothetical population where just 2 percent of potential new partners are infected, a person who has only two partners a year faces about one tenth the risk of one who has thirty partners a year—a very significant decrease in risk. But in a population where 40 percent of potential partners are infected, then the risk facing the person with two partners rises to about two thirds of the risk facing the person with thirty partners. In a population like that, reducing to two partners provides very little benefit.

In retrospect, many experts believe that the only reduction likely to have slowed the epidemic at this early point would have been widespread adoption of monogamy—one partner at a time, for fairly long periods of months or years. Some epidemiologists now believe that given the prevalence rates that confronted gay men when the partner reduction message first went out in 1982 and 1983—rates ranging from well below 10 percent in most small cities, towns, and rural areas to 20 percent in some of the largest cities—if most men had reduced to a single partner and stayed with that partner for extended periods, this might have significantly slowed the epidemic or even halted it entirely. But virtually no one suggested that at the time, and those who did were ridiculed and sometimes vilified. If mere "reduction" was controversial, monogamy was quite out of the question, considered neither desirable nor practical, or, for that matter, even possible, by those constructing the new ethic of safer sex. Instead, the gay population as a whole continued engaging in a level of partner change far higher than HIV required to maintain its exponential spread. Even many gay men who followed the vague advice to reduce partners still tended to have many more partners than the heterosexual norm. On the face of it, such reductions often amounted to major behavioral change, but they proved woefully unable to halt the rising tide of infection. And the additional advice to "know one's partner" and examine each other for lesions and sores seems, in retrospect, pathetically misguided. Since HIV is most transmissible in the first few months after a person's initial infection, when symptoms are wholly invisible, knowing or examining each other means nothing.

The Early Prevention Dissidents

Some voices cried out for a more radical approach. Dr. Alvin Friedman-Kien urged gay men to stop having sex altogether, or at least to use condoms consistently until the cause of the new malady was found. Larry Kramer, who had cofounded Gay Men's Health Crisis, urged its board to take this position, but the board refused, and Kramer was accused of sex negativity, a serious charge among those for whom sexual freedom was a central point of gay liberation. "Read anything by Kramer closely," wrote playwright Robert Chesley in a now-famous letter to the *Native* in December of 1981. "I think that you'll find that the subtext is always: the wages of gay sin are death. . . . I am not downplaying the seriousness of Kaposi's sarcoma. But something else is happening here, which is also serious: gay homophobia and anti-eroticism."

Braving this kind of vilification, AIDS physician Joseph Sonnabend not only criticized the culture of multipartnerism but extended his critique to physicians who countenanced it. "A desire to appear nonjudgmental, a desire to remain untinged by moralism, fear of provoking ire, have all fostered a conspiracy of silence," he wrote in September 1982. "For years no clear message about the danger of promiscuity has emanated from those in whom gay men have entrusted their well-being."

The Lost Window of Opportunity

It is tempting to wonder what might have happened if such advice had been more widely given or more universally accepted in those crucial years, or if the advice to reduce partners had been coupled with insistent advice to wear condoms every time with every partner. In retrospect these were the very years—1981 through 1984—that infections rose from modest to catastrophic levels among gay men in most American cities (with the possible exception of San Francisco, where over 25 percent of the gay male population was already infected as early as 1981). This now looks like a lost window of opportunity, a period between the time the medical establishment and gay leaders first became aware of the epidemic and the time the virus eventually saturated the community, in which it was at least biologically possible to have prevented the extraordinarily high levels of prevalence that now confound prevention efforts and will bedevil gay men well into the next century. In most cities there was a crucial period between the time that most gay men became aware of AIDS (more than half of the gay men in one New York study, for example, had heard about AIDS by the end of 1981), and the time that saturation set in, generally around 1985.

In later years it became common in gay circles to blame the failure almost entirely on the media and the government, and it is undeniable that both were seriously derelict in reporting and publicizing the epidemic and providing resources to assist in prevention. But focusing exclusively on them begs the question of what gay leaders and the community as a whole were actually prepared to do, and the record argues that they were neither prepared nor probably able to do what was necessary. Right from the beginning voices were raised in well-informed gay circles that proposed the very solutions that might have worked, and those voices were by and large shouted down—not by the mainstream media and government, but by the gay media and gay men ourselves. People demanded absolute proof before they were willing to advise gay men to wear condoms every time, to reduce partners to one monogamous partner at a time, to close commercial sex institutions, and such proof was impossible to provide in that early period. What if abstinence, monogamy, the shutting down of institutions like sex clubs and baths were encouraged, it was argued, and then it turned out that AIDS wasn't sexually transmitted? Or was only sexually transmitted under very specific circumstances?

Some today also plausibly argue that even if such advice had been given, it would not and could not have been followed by more than a small fraction of the gay male population, particularly in the major urban areas where AIDS spread first and fastest. There was no social support network for the kinds of changes that might have made a difference, no cultural consensus on what those changes might be, certainly no support for such changes from outside the gay community. While it can be argued that all societies can and do change, it is more difficult to argue that they can turn on a dime, and more difficult still to argue that they can turn on a dime without any wider network of support, rewards, and encouragements, virtually all of which were lacking in this case.

All this is certainly true. And so, while the larger society did its best to ignore the tragedy unfolding in the gay world, the gay community itself was almost intrinsically unable to do what was necessary to contain the tragedy unfolding within its ranks. With the inevitability of a Greek disaster, gay men dithered and argued among themselves about appearing to be "sex-negative," and gay leaders, including medical leaders and heads of the new AIDS organizations, worked to "avoid causing panic." The farthest most were willing to go was the advice to reduce partners. It was advice that very large numbers of gay men, desperate for leadership, willingly followed. But at each step of the way, their reduction was too little, too late, and during the explosive phase of the early epidemic tens of thousands of men who followed such advice nonetheless became infected.

Some might consider it pointless or even mean-spirited to raise this issue today, arguing that whether one accepts this analysis or not, it's all ancient history. However, while it is certainly true that the events of this period are history, that history deeply colors how we view and cope with the epidemic today. Perhaps the most fundamental complaint of AIDS activism has centered on what everyone else did, or rather failed to do, during the precise period in question, when the epidemic first exploded. How the government failed to warn, the media failed to report, the scientific establishment failed to investigate, the drug industry failed to produce remedies or vaccines. Within the gay and AIDS movements an entire analysis of how AIDS happened to gay men is centered on the idea that others, "they," the mainstream world, could have saved us during this crucial period and did not. If it is so important to constantly raise awareness about that massive failing—and I believe it is—how can it be unimportant for gay men to examine our own actions and failures during this same period?

On the contrary. Our failure then may have been inevitable, but it remains at the root of today's crisis. Despite the invention of the condom code, despite our huge increase in sophistication about AIDS, and health and disease, we continue to shy away from analyzing how our own ecology, including our desire to preserve what appear to be toxic aspects of our hard-won sexual freedoms, contributed to the tragedy of AIDS. I suppose we continue to shy away from such an analysis precisely because it is so painful, and because many will be quick to call anyone who attempts it mean-spirited. But in this case the classic admonition that those who forget history are condemned to repeat it could hardly be more true. And in this case the consequence of such a repetition could hardly be more grim.

The Rise of the Condom Code

Almost from the beginning there was another message that, subtly at first and then more directly, seemed to contradict or even negate the advice to limit partners. This message held that since HIV is probably transmitted in bodily fluids, the way to prevent transmission is not to limit the number of partners but to limit fluid exchange by using condoms. The first activists to advocate this strategy forcefully were Michael Callen and Richard Berkowitz, two patients of Joseph Sonnabend's, who believed that AIDS was caused by multiple factors, especially repeated exposures to CMV in semen and to semen itself. Their May 1983 pamphlet, "How to Have Sex in an Epidemic," stated their solution in forthright terms. "The key," they wrote, "is modifying what you do—not how often you do it nor with how many different partners. . . . Sex doesn't make you sick—diseases do. . . . Once you understand how diseases are transmitted, you can begin to explore medically safe sex."

At first this advice was not widely echoed by most AIDS groups. Uncertain about what caused AIDS, few were willing to say with confidence that condoms would prevent transmission. Guidelines spoke of "possible germs" that might be transmitted in "fluids." Gay publications and pamphlets advised that "wearing a condom *may* reduce the risk." But once it became widely accepted that HIV was the viral cause of the new syndrome, and once it was demonstrated that HIV could indeed be blocked with latex condoms, the advice to reduce partners was slowly abandoned and the advice to use condoms became the central tenet of the new gay sexual ecology. Indeed, so central did condom use become that David L. Chambers, in an insightful article in the *Harvard Civil Rights Civil Liberties Law Review*, dubbed the entire safer sex regime the "Code of the Condom." According to the code, risk lies almost exclusively in the exchange of fluids during anal sex, and therefore the use of a condom is a biological necessity.

Chambers points out that the adoption of this code was not inevitable. At least two other safer sex messages might have taken root in the gay world. According to Chambers, "One message would simply have provided accurate information about the risks of anal sex" with and without condoms, and let individuals decide what level of risk they were willing to accept. That approach was favored by some who felt that, like partner reduction, the condom code was too judgmental and implicitly devalued a central aspect of gay sex—namely, unprotected anal sex. But while this "here are the facts—you decide" approach was sometimes adopted for oral sex, it rarely appears in advice about anal sex.

The other approach, writes Chambers, "would have urged men to refrain from anal sex altogether," in favor of things like oral sex and noninsertive activities such as masturbation. Such a policy was followed in Holland until 1991. Men were encouraged to give up anal sex completely, and many apparently did. Cohort studies of Dutch gay men reported that the practice of anal sex declined dramatically from 1984 to 1985. Since the level of HIV prevalence in these cohorts remained lower than in most American cities—the rate of new infections actually reached zero in one cohort in 1987—this advice may have been quite effective. Nonetheless, this approach was never seriously entertained by gay AIDS groups in the United States. Anal sex had come to be seen as an essential—possibly *the* essential—expression of homosexual intimacy by the 1980s. Perhaps the most famous articulation of this view appeared in a 1985 *New York Native* interview with Joseph Sonnabend. "The rectum," Sonnabend said, "is a sexual organ, and it deserves the respect a penis gets and a vagina gets. Anal intercourse has been the central activity for gay men and for some women for all of history. . . . We have to recognize what is hazardous, but at the same time, we shouldn't undermine an act that's important to celebrate."

Michael Callen was openly scornful of any attempt to discourage gay men from practicing anal sex. In his 1989 article "In Defense of Anal Sex" in the *PWA Coalition Newsline*, Callen listed three basic reasons. First, he considered such a message an equivocation. If, Callen wrote, the premise is that condoms aren't fully safe, then the message should be that everyone should "stop having anal sex entirely." This seems a rather muddled objection, since the message Callen was objecting to was precisely that: to stop having anal sex entirely. His second objection was that this avoids more difficult and complex messages, such as advising men to perform coitus interruptus, demanding better condoms from manufacturers, educating gay men about proper condom use, and demanding a "national AIDS education campaign which speaks bluntly in non-clinical language that people can understand." His third (and, I suspect, core) objection was that any message advising abandonment of anal sex was homophobic, since similar messages about giving up vaginal sex were not being directed toward heterosexuals.

Callen was hardly alone. Chambers reports what happened when he asked the associate director of education at a large AIDS service organization whether the best advice to a young gay man was to avoid anal intercourse altogether. "His response was abrupt and unequivocal. His organization, he said, would never recommend avoiding anal intercourse. To him, a gay man who told another gay man to avoid anal intercourse had probably absorbed the larger society's hatred of gay sexuality or was himself ashamed of the allure of anal sex. At a minimum, he said, advice of this sort would be ineffective because it would be seen as coming from such a person."

There was, of course, a third possibility that Chambers does not raise. AIDS advocates could have followed the partner reduction theory to its logical conclusion and endorsed monogamy as a form of prevention, working to create and shore up institutions that supported long-term, monogamous gay relationships and attacking the ethic of multipartnerism. This was never seriously considered by any gay AIDS organization.

Instead, the code of the condom became virtually the entire message of prevention. "Condom distribution" became a rallying cry in gay bars, "condom availability" a major goal of public education programs. The condom became a symbol of safety, prevention's magic bullet. All this was carried out, however, in knowledge of the fact that the condom code contained certain inherent risks.

Condom Failures

One risk concerned condoms themselves. Studies have repeatedly reported major problems with condom efficacy. Condom failure rates of approximately 10 percent have long been a fact of life for heterosexuals attempting to use them to prevent pregnancy. In anal sex virtually every study of condom efficacy has found that condoms sometimes break, fall off during or after, or are otherwise misused. A survey published in the *American Journal of Public Health*, for example, reported failures of 4.7 percent to 8 percent. Factors that led to failure included condoms being "too small or too thin, the use of oil as opposed to water-based lubricants, breakage due to fingernails or jewelry, inexperience in condom use, physical stress on condoms inherent to anal intercourse, and the use of condoms not designed for anal intercourse." In addition to mechanical failure, condoms often fail to provide protection because people fail to use them consistently, which is hardly surprising given the lack of rational thinking that often precedes sex.

These levels of failure in both vaginal and anal sex have resulted in HIV infections even among consistent condom users. An August 1992 update in *MMWR* reported that among serodiscordant heterosexual couples, the rate of HIV transmission was 9.7 percent among those who used condoms "inconsistently," and 1.1 percent among those who used them "consistently." A 1990 study in the *Journal of AIDS* estimated that for heterosexual serodiscordant couples, the overall failure rates for HIV "may approach those for pregnancy," which the study cited as 10 percent. Among gay men, the Multicenter AIDS Cohort Study (MACS) reported the infection of seven gay male participants despite reporting that they used condoms every time with every partner. Other studies have found similar results.

As the condom code became solidified, however, these considerations tended to be minimized by prevention activists. Since the primary message of safer sex came to revolve around getting men to use condoms every time they had anal sex, anything that might undermine confidence in condoms was felt to undermine confidence in safer sex itself. It was hard enough to get gay men to use condoms in the first place, hard enough to convince governments to promote them, hard enough to get schools to make them available to sexually active teens. If in addition it were admitted that condoms failed on a low but fairly regular basis, the job of condom promotion might become impossible. As became depressingly customary with AIDS, the struggle for prevention became a struggle not only against the virus, but also against efforts by right-wingers to use the virus to delegitimize all sex that was not procreative, including all gay sex. Anti-gay conservatives seized upon and often exaggerated negative data about condoms to proclaim that safer sex was a total lie, that the proper heterosexual response to the epidemic was lifelong monogamy, the proper gay reaction abstinence or conversion to heterosexuality. Prevention activists were thus forced into a defensive posture, and as such were very reluctant to give any ground at all on the issue of condom effectiveness. It became a matter of faith among gay AIDS activists that condoms were unquestionably effective. As the massive incursion of HIV into the gay community became clear and a similar incursion into straight America seemed imminent, many came to feel that undermining confidence in condoms was tantamount to undermining the very concept that there could be something called safer sex.

Isolating HIV

A second major flaw of the condom code was that it focused solely on anal sex and ignored the larger behavioral and ecological picture. From the beginning gay men tended to isolate the HIV epidemic from the syphilis and gonorrhea epidemics, from the hepatitis epidemic and the herpes epidemic and the CMV epidemic and the Epstein-Barr epidemic and the intestinal parasite epidemic and the myriad of other sexually transmitted epidemics that were part of the bigger picture in which AIDS was embedded. Gay men taught ourselves to think about HIV as a separate entity, a loose bug that had somehow tragically entered an otherwise sound system.

Perhaps because HIV is primarily transmitted via anal sex among gay men, or perhaps because of residual moralistic beliefs about the practice, many gay men also came to think that anal sex was somehow uniquely capable of transmitting disease in general. People who were convinced that anal sex with multiple partners was inherently dangerous remained skeptical that oral sex with multiple partners was particularly risky for certain diseases, and outright scoffed at the idea that deep kissing with multiple partners could spread certain infections. Such beliefs, however, reflect more about social and sexual attitudes toward anal sex than biological realities. Anal sex is indeed the easiest mode of transmission for HIV among gay men, but oral-anal contact is the easiest mode of transmitting many other diseases, and oral-genital sex and even deep kissing, when practiced with large numbers of partners in high-prevalence core groups, can become vectors for the amplification of a number of infections from hepatitis and herpes to mononucleosis.

When looking at the long list of diseases that swept the gay male world in the years leading up to AIDS, one sees that quite a few were primarily spread by oral-anal sex and many others were spread just as readily orally as anally. The list includes all forms of hepatitis, most forms of oral and genital herpes, oral gonorrhea, cytomegalovirus, Epstein-Barr virus, and all of the major intestinal parasites. The common wisdom then and now has been that these diseases are insignificant, mild, and easy to cure, and that they didn't have much to do with AIDS. But the common wisdom is largely wrong. Herpes remains incurable in all its forms, as do Epstein-Barr virus and CMV. Gonorrhea has mutated into deadly and incurable antibiotic-resistant strains. Hepatitis remains a killer, and although a highly effective vaccine is now available, very few gay men have taken it. The gastrointestinal parasites are cured only with great difficulty, and the large doses of drugs needed to cure them place a major strain on the immune system. Throughout the period leading up to AIDS scientists were discovering a succession of new STDs in the gay population that they had never considered sexually transmitted before, and several of these were primarily transmitted orally. Clearly the practice of anal sex with many partners was not the only problem, although it was the first to produce such a catastrophic result. Yet the condom code focused almost exclusively on anal sex, preferring to ignore this wider web of ecological and behavioral cause and effect.

Oral Sex. Other diseases aside, there is also evidence that receptive oral sex—sucking—while significantly less risky than receptive anal sex, nonetheless carries a risk of HIV infection, but this, too, was largely glossed over by the condom code.

Oral sex has been a contentious subject in AIDS prevention from the start, for good reason. Many studies indicate that oral sex is the most popular sexual practice among gay men. Most studies also indicate that people find condoms extremely intrusive during oral sex, quite literally ruining the experience for many. As a result, prevention workers are understandably loath to advise using condoms unless the evidence of risk seems clear and present. And it has not been clear. Epidemiological evidence about oral risk has always been murky. Many studies show little or no statistical risk, while others indicate that risk is real but much lower than in anal sex. Those epidemiologists who have studied the issue most closely tend to concur that the risk of infection during receptive oral sex is probably from one fifth to one tenth of the risk during receptive anal sex, perhaps even less. The reason even this degree of risk is not seen more often in studies, they argue, is that whenever a newly infected man indicates that he has had any anal sex whatsoever, the infection is automatically assigned to that practice, producing a masking effect that makes the precise delineation of oral risk impossible.

The tendency of anal sex to "mask" the risk of oral sex has had a psychological effect on the gay community as well, reinforcing the popular conception that oral risk is minuscule. A common opinion among gay men is that if oral sex were really risky we'd be seeing new AIDS cases everywhere. This seems questionable logic, since we are indeed seeing new cases everywhere. But it has been bolstered by the fact that the condom code is essentially agnostic about oral sex, defining no obligation to use condoms when sucking or getting sucked. Most AIDS groups and safer sex brochures traditionally have left it up to individual choice: You might want to use a condom during oral sex, but many people choose not to. It's up to you. More recently, some have begun promoting unprotected oral sex, sometimes even to ejaculation, as a form of "harm reduction." One slogan: "Oral Sex *Is* Safer Sex."

Consequences of the Condom Code

By the mid eighties the use of condoms during anal sex was declared virtually the entire message of safer sex in the gay world. One small concession to its imperfections was contained in a new nomenclature that declared sex with condoms *safer*, not necessarily safe, since a remote possibility of transmission remains. But the limits and problems of the code were otherwise glossed over and sometimes simply denied. Gay men were told that using condoms fulfilled the entire obligation to oneself and others in the age of AIDS.

As the code gained widespread acceptance, certain logical consequences followed in its wake. Chambers points out that one concerned the issue of whether sexually active gay men have an obligation to get tested. HIV antibody testing became widely available in 1985, but initially most gay AIDS groups advised gay men to avoid the test. Lack of effective therapies, they argued, meant that knowledge of HIV infection could not lead to useful therapies but would almost certainly lead to despair. In addition, there was the very real danger that the confidentiality of test results might be breached, and since there was often serious discrimination directed against people with HIV, that was not to be taken lightly.

In the late 1980s, however, prophylactic drugs and antiretrovirals became available that prevented or delayed common opportunistic infections like pneumocystis, and it became clear that infected people could benefit from early interventions provided they could afford them. At that point most gay AIDS groups reversed course and advised gay men to take the test. But none of these groups propounded an ethical *obligation* to get tested. "On the contrary," writes Chambers, "the condom rule fully answers the obligations to others. So far as others are concerned, if we use condoms, then it does not matter whether we have the virus." So when AIDS groups advised gay men to get tested, the advice was almost always couched in terms of self-interest, not altruism.

A second question answered by the condom code was what, if any, obligation a person who knows he is HIV infected has to *inform* his partners of his serostatus. "The case for a moral obligation to inform the partner is even easier to state than the case for testing," Chambers points out, since "providing information gives the partner a chance to make more fully informed decisions about sex." The fact is that, whether rational or not, many uninfected people who might have sex with someone whose serostatus they do not know would refuse to have sex—even safer sex—with someone they know to be HIV positive. Nonetheless, in the opinion of most AIDS groups, the condom code fulfills any obligation an HIV-positive person might have to inform his or her partner. GMHC's pamphlet "Safer Sex for HIV Positives" was typical:

"If you follow [the guideline to use condoms], you don't need to worry about whether your partners know that you're positive. You've already protected them from infection and yourself from reinfection. . . . Just use your judgment about who to tell—there's still discrimination out there." Implicit in this advice (aside from the assumption that HIV-positive men will continue to have multiple partners) is the idea that the risk of discrimination to the infected person is as serious, or even more serious, than the risk of infecting one's partners. Therefore the right to remain silent and protect oneself from possible discrimination trumps the obligation to disclose and allow one's partners to make more informed decisions about the level of risk they are willing to take.

Self-Defense

But this is not necessarily as callous as it sounds. The reason is that an even more central tenet of the condom code is the need of all people to adopt a position of self-defense in sexual matters. This was first promulgated in the days before HIV was discovered. Back then no one could possibly know their HIV status (aside from those who had full-blown AIDS), so it was imperative for everybody to proceed from the assumption that every potential partner was infected. Once widespread testing became available and thousands of asymptomatic men discovered their serostatus, however, a new situation developed. Now many men knew that they were HIV-positive, and a great gulf opened up in the gay male world between HIV positives and HIV negatives. Many who were positive saw little incentive to practice safer sex for their own protection. True, health experts warned of the possibility of re-infection with different strains of HIV, but many men considered that possibility less than fully proved. Experts also warned about the danger of other opportunistic infections, but many positive men were not particularly impressed with admonitions that they ought to forgo unprotected anal sex out of fear of contracting infections they might just as easily get from oral sex or, for that matter, kissing.

Given that, it might have made sense to amend the condom code, adding an absolute obligation to get tested and know your serostatus, and adding, for those who find out they are HIV-positive, an absolute obligation to protect others from infection, even if those others are momentarily willing to take a risk. No such amendment, however, was made. HIV-positive men continued to be told to practice safer sex for their own benefit, not out of any altruistic obligation to protect others. This had the unfortunate effect of implying to many HIV-positive men that they were off the ethical hook when engaging in unsafe sex, particularly with anonymous partners. The condom code's ethic of self-defense allowed them to reason justly that if they found a partner who was willing to engage in risky sex, that partner must be doing so out of informed choice. And if that partner became infected, it was his own fault. A catch-22 thus arose in many sexual situations. An HIV-positive person could assume that if his partner was willing to engage in risky activities, that partner must also be positive ("After all, he'd never risk letting me infect him"), while the HIV-negative person could assume that since his partner was willing to engage in unsafe sex, that partner must also be negative ("After all, he'd never knowingly risk infecting me").

But perhaps the most significant result of the condom code was the belief that since condoms provide ample protection from infection, there was no reason why anything else about gay sexual ecology needed to be addressed. If everyone simply used a condom with every partner, every time, the problem was solved. Gay men could return to the golden age of the sexual revolution that had started to fade into memory during the dark early years of the epidemic.

Avoiding "Transformative" Change

It is sometimes said that the adoption of the condom code was the "least transformative" change that gay men could have made in the face of the epidemic. Other possible approaches might have looked at the interlocking reasons for the epidemic, seen a series of ecological connections, and then attempted to address them collectively, advocating a transformation of gay sexual culture. But this approach was not merely avoided, it was deliberately shunned. Indeed, the desire to avoid a "transformative" change in gay sexual culture was a cornerstone of prevention. Author Edward King speaks for many gay AIDS prevention workers and organizations when he writes, "AIDS educators have a responsibility to aim only for the minimum necessary changes in individuals' lives which are needed to reduce the risk of giving or getting HIV." King applies this principle directly to the condom code and anal sex:

> The known effectiveness of condoms in preventing HIV transmission during anal sex means that the appropriate intervention for gay men who enjoy fucking is to encourage condom use, rather than attempt to persuade them to abandon anal intercourse in favor of non-penetrative forms of sex. Likewise, it is relatively commonplace to read accounts of the ways in which the impact of AIDS has changed the way gay men

related to each other, with more emphasis now being placed on friend-ship and relationships, and less on sex. While this may or may not be the case, and may or may not be a desirable outcome, it is important to recognize that such changes cannot in themselves be considered legiti-mate aims of HIV education.

This approach, common to most gay AIDS organizations, is often extended to the issues of multipartnerism and the whole complex of behaviors that characterized gay sexual life in the seventies and led to AIDS. Do not interrupt the cultural and behavioral context of AIDS transmission, it argues. Just interrupt the virus.

Harm Reduction

Among a number of reasons this least transformative idea has been so readily embraced, a primary one is "harm reduction." Harm reduction has been described as "a philosophy wherein the professional health care provider sets aside all judgments in order to meet clients at their own level regarding a problem or crisis." It is considered particularly effective in dealing with certain drug abusers. If, for example, an IV drug user comes to health workers and asks for help in avoiding HIV infection, health workers should not insist that the user give up injecting drugs in order to receive help. Instead, they should provide the user with clean needles and information to help avoid infection. Help in quitting drugs may also be provided, but only if asked for. The reasoning is that many IV drug users don't want to quit using drugs; they just want to avoid HIV. So if health workers demand that they quit using drugs in order to get help, many users will be driven away from HIV preven-tion programs and needlessly become infected.

In a sense, the almost exclusive focus on the condom code rep-resents an effort by gay AIDS organizations to apply harm reduction to the gay community as a whole. Gay men, this reasoning goes, don't want to change most aspects of their sexual culture, and they will resist and dismiss anyone who suggests they should. They simply want to avoid HIV. If AIDS groups suggest that gay men need to transform their sexual culture, they will be lumped together with moralists and homophobes and their advice will simply drive many men away from prevention. This nontransformative approach is reinforced by the widespread belief that gay men cannot change their sexual culture even if they want to. Many activists openly express what the late journalist Randy Shilts called the "sex fiend" argument: that many gay men are insatiable satyrs who would respond to admonitions to change their basic patterns of behavior by hiding and perhaps even increasing that behavior rather than actually attempting to change it.

This reasoning is also buttressed by the dual ideological imperative to fight AIDS but only in ways that support what is sometimes called "sex-positive" gay male culture. Gay author Frank Browning, in his book *The Culture of Desire*, relates that some of his straight friends were incredulous at the behavior of gay AIDS activists and prevention workers at the Fifth International AIDS Conference in Montreal:

> For five days the discos were packed with gay doctors, nurses, activists, and researchers shamelessly cruising each other. A nearby bathhouse was doing land-office business. A JO (jack-off) club posted promotional fliers in the conference exhibit hall.... Most of my straight friends have told me that they cannot fathom how an AIDS conference can also be a sex carnival. My standard flip response has frequently been "But what else could it be?" The lust of men for other men has not evaporated just because funerals and memorial services have become nearly as ordinary as an evening at the theater. To a considerable degree, those gay men who have committed themselves to trench duty in the battle against AIDS have done so exactly because they would not and, perhaps, could not relinquish passion to death. Simple survival as whole human beings forced them to face AIDS squarely and to determine how much they would permit it to control them.

One can go further and say that psychological survival has impelled many gay men to resist, sometimes bitterly, any analysis of the ecological implications of AIDS. Instead, many believe that a proper goal of AIDS prevention should be the opposite—to defend the gay sexual revolution and to fight off any analysis that might tend to call it into question. Many were uncomfortable with the original (and certainly unsuccessful) emphasis on partner reduction not because they assumed it would fail, but because they felt it undermined the whole point of gay liberation. As Michael Lynch wrote in the gay Canadian publication *Body Politic* during the heyday of the partner reduction message in the early 1980s, "Gays are once again allowing the medical profession to define, restrict, pathologize us." Gay liberation was founded, he said, on a "sexual brotherhood of promiscuity," and any abandonment of that promiscuity would amount to a "communal betrayal of gargantuan proportions." The condom code eliminated such concerns. By declaring that condoms fulfilled all obligations to prevention, the culture of multipartnerism could be justified and celebrated anew. In the minds of many, the code has the added benefit of seeming to absolve multipartner sex from any role in the epidemic whatsoever, since it was now explained that multipartner sex is, in fact, perfectly compatible with a healthy sexual ecology. Because of the condom code we could continue to look at AIDS as an "accident" that simply happened to strike gay men first.

Hail the Conquering Code

As the eighties progressed, this view seemed eminently justified. Researchers assured gay men that even though many continued to have large numbers of partners, they had done an astonishingly successful job in bringing the rates of HIV infection down to very low levels. The most widely quoted statement to this effect was contained in a study of a cohort of gay men in San Francisco by researchers Maria Elkstrand and Thomas Coates. The changes this cohort had made in reducing its previous levels of risky sex, they write, "may represent the most profound changes ever observed in the literature on health change behavior." Other studies seemed to offer confirmation. Researcher Warren Winkelstein and his colleagues reported in 1988 that the annual HIV infection rates in previously uninfected members of a San Francisco cohort had declined by 88 percent in just two years, "from 5.9 percent during the first six months of 1985 to 0.7 percent during the last six months of 1987." Winkelstein also reported "declines of approximately 80 percent in the prevalence of sexual behaviors associated with HIV transmission" in the sample.

Research in New York in the late 1980s painted a similar picture. In 1987 the number of men in a New York cohort who reported always using condoms for receptive anal sex had risen from virtually zero to

62 percent. There, and in similar cohorts across the nation, the rate of new HIV infection appeared to be dropping dramatically among gay men, as did the rates of other sexually transmitted diseases. One cohort that had been decimated in the early eighties reported zero transmissions in 1987. Gay prevention organizations were so certain of their success that San Francisco's Stop AIDS Project, a model gay-run group that had aggressively promoted a community standard of safer sex and condom use beginning in 1985, disbanded in 1989, convinced that its job was done (it would soon be back).

The idea that gay men had largely solved the problem of transmission had a tremendous impact on gay people's analysis, or lack of analysis, of their sexual ecology. As the reports began to pour in during 1986 and 1987, we felt fully justified in congratulating ourselves that our invention of the condom code was an unqualified success. Whatever prevention work remained to be done was in the form of reinforcing "education" and condom distribution, of explaining to those in the gay world who had not yet heard, and to those millions in the straight world who did not want to hear, the triumphant message of the code. We were now in the driver's seat of AIDS prevention. We had discovered and successfully promulgated the answer. Now it was time for the rest of the world to listen to us, the experts.

The Degaying of AIDS

All this contributed to a complementary idea that began to take on the force of dogma in the late 1980s: the idea that AIDS is not a "gay and junkie disease" and that heterosexuals are equally at risk. The propagation of this idea produced a phenomenon often described as the "degaying" of AIDS, and it, like the supposed "success" of prevention, has had a dramatic effect on how gay men have come to view themselves and their sexual ecology.

Degaying began in 1985 amid the flurry of publicity surrounding the illness and death of actor Rock Hudson. His illness was a great turning point in the epidemic, the moment when AIDS first became a burning national issue. And one reason, ironically, was that many people presumed that the quintessentially masculine Hudson was heterosexual, and that his illness proved that AIDS was spreading into the heterosexual mainstream. "I thought AIDS was a gay disease," one man told *USA Today* in a typical reaction, "but if Rock Hudson can get it, anyone can." A thousand headlines concurred. Now, the public was suddenly told, everyone is at risk.

The fact that Hudson's illness sparked this reaction may seem odd in retrospect, since Hudson was a sexually active gay man, and one who apparently didn't practice safer sex even after he knew he was infected. But in another sense the reaction seemed long overdue, since evidence had been accumulating from the start that AIDS was not limited to gays even in the United States. First IDUs, then people from Haiti, then the recipients of blood products and blood transfusions, then the heterosexual partners and infants of the above, were all found to have the disease. By the end of the first year the full outlines of these "non-gay" types of transmission were well known to medicine. Nonetheless the vast majority of heterosexual Americans still considered themselves immune. Even many who engaged in multipartner heterosexual sex did not consider themselves at risk since they were not members of "risk groups." This logic went, and still goes, to the illogical extreme that some men who have frequent homosexual relations presume they are safe because they don't consider themselves gay in a social sense, while at the same time some young gay men who have not yet had sex believe they may be infected simply because their psychological orientation is homosexual. In an attempt to fight these dangerous ideas about risk groups, many health educators used Rock Hudson's illness (ironically, as it turned out) to emphasize that AIDS was no longer just a gay disease. In the process, they contributed to the degaying campaign.

Meanwhile, AIDS activists also promoted degaying. One reason was purely altruistic: We believed, with considerable justification at the time, that the terrible experience of AIDS in the Third World was a harbinger of what was to come in developed countries, and that HIV's widespread dissemination among heterosexuals in Africa and Asia was simply a result of those continents' "head start." In this view, heterosexuals around the world are pretty much all alike, so that what happens among heterosexuals in Uganda is bound to happen to their counterparts in Utah given enough time. Unless heterosexuals in industrialized nations quickly took steps to adopt the condom code, the African disaster would repeat itself here.

Aside from these biological concerns, which were shared by many health experts, the degaying campaign was strongly pushed by AIDS activists for a pragmatic reason. Activists were painfully aware that the epidemic had been ignored in its early days largely because of a perception that it affected only stigmatized groups. Thanks to that perception there had been a virtual news blackout, which many believed had contributed to the spread of HIV in the gay population. Thanks to it as well, very little money was being spent to fight the disease or find a cure. If, however, the public began to fear that AIDS might spread to the mainstream, then perhaps media organizations and governments and drug companies might begin to take the disease seriously.

Degaying as a political strategy was also eagerly embraced by many conservatives, who believed that AIDS had the potential to reverse the sexual revolution and corral heterosexuals back into monogamy. It's hardly a new idea. In the early 1700s a preacher named Edmund Masses wrote that "the fear of disease is a great restraint to men. If men were more healthy, 'tis a great chance they would be less righteous." In the middle of this century sociologists argued that fear of both pregnancy and STDs played a major role in restraining sexual activity in many cultures. Conservatives' chagrin at the loss of that role is illustrated by the title of a 1948 lecture by prominent bacteriologist Thomas B. Turner. He called his talk "Penicillin: Help or Hindrance?" The hindrance he referred to was the loss of fear as a restraining factor in extramarital relations, and the possibility that as a result humankind would see multiple reinfections with dangerous STDs in the future. (He was right: It did.) In the 1980s and 1990s, what better way for moralists and "family values" conservatives to inculcate fear than to emphasize that incurable, fatal AIDS lay in wait for those who partook of sex merely for pleasure? Conservatives also understood (in ways that many gay AIDS activists did not) that degaying actually *added* to the stigma of homosexuality, since a disease that first erupted in that marginal population was now seen as a threat to everyone. The spread of AIDS to those outside the gay demimonde implied that gay men were, in the uncharitable phrase of author Michael Fumento, "the rats and fleas of the new plague."

And so through the genuine concerns of activists and health workers and the highly politicized motivations of those on both the right and the left, by the end of the eighties the degaying agenda had come to seem an unqualified success. Countless articles proclaimed that AIDS was no longer a "gay and junkie disease," that it could strike anybody, and indeed was already doing so. The press was full of reports that "heterosexual AIDS" was the fastest-growing form of transmission, that women were the fastest-growing demographic segment of the epidemic. When author Fumento challenged these ideas in his book *The Myth of Heterosexual AIDS* in 1989, he was savaged virtually everywhere.

Degaying as a Positive Feedback Loop

The widespread acceptance of degaying had a profound impact on gay men's vision of their own sexual ecology. If AIDS was not a "gay disease," why should gay men examine the ecological reasons their community was so devastated? Clearly it was just an accident of history, a fluke, a momentary incursion of an otherwise universal pandemic. Degaying had the opposite effect that many AIDS activists hoped. It caused governments to shift vital resources away from prevention programs for gay men, IDUs, and their sexual partners (where the overwhelming need was situated) and spread those resources across the entire population. But it also had an unexpected psychological impact on the gay world itself. Gay men's focus naturally shifted away from ourselves and our gay sexual culture. There was nothing particularly amiss in the gay sexual arrangement that needed rethinking, since whatever we were doing, everybody else was doing too. Indeed, the original stigmatizing, "anti-gay analysis" of AIDS could be reversed. Gay men had solved the ecological problem of AIDS through the condom code, but straight people had not. It was our turn to gloat.

In the late eighties a sort of gay triumphalism appeared, an attitude that if anything, the gay male culture of sexual frankness had given us an edge in HIV prevention, an edge that would be unavailable to uptight heterosexuals. As the condom code appeared to solve the problem of transmission, as the idea that AIDS would soon be striking millions of heterosexuals sank in, the obvious ecological implications of the epidemic for gay men could now be not only ignored but indignantly denied. Gay sexual culture came to be viewed by many AIDS activists not as an inadvertent culprit that underlay the astonishing spread of HIV among gay men, but as a tool to *prevent* HIV transmission. We would be saved by our sexual sophistication, by our willingness to explore nonpenetrative forms of sex, by our frankness. Cindy Patton, in her book *Inventing AIDS,* remarked that while gay men "knew a lot about sex," heterosexuals "had little sense of themselves as 'heterosexual' and functioned under an implied ethical code in which vaginal intercourse was the paradigmatic practice and in which women negotiated from a position of lesser power. Given these different sexual ethics, it is no surprise that it is heterosexuals—the amorphous general public—who have such profound difficulty accepting safer sex." Gay theorist Douglas Crimp spoke for many when he castigated the prudishness of gay critics of multipartnerism like Randy Shilts and Larry Kramer. Their attitudes, he wrote, were perversely distorted. "[T]hey insist that our promiscuity will destroy us when in fact it is our promiscuity that will save us."

In light of the triumph of the condom code, the unprecedented success of gay HIV prevention, and the coming avalanche of heterosexual AIDS, who could disagree?

CHAPTER 5

The "Second Wave"

On December 11, 1993, more than twelve years after the first reports of a new disease syndrome in gay men, readers of the *New York Times* awoke to a startling front-page article. Beneath the headline SECOND WAVE OF AIDS FEARED BY OFFICIALS IN SAN FRANCISCO ran a story by *Times* reporter Jane Gross that seemed to confound eight years of hopes and efforts by AIDS educators and prevention workers. Gay men in San Francisco, Gross reported, were practicing unsafe sex in significant numbers and were becoming infected with HIV at "worrisome" rates. The article presented a number of explanations by experts and Bay Area psychologists for this apparent "relapse," among them depression, a sense of fatality or inevitability, lack of motivation to remain healthy, survivor's guilt, grief, and trauma. Oddly, however, the article quoted demographic surveys in which the men themselves mentioned none of these reasons. Instead, they indicated that they often did not use condoms because they "wanted to enhance their pleasure, or they were under the influence of alcohol or drugs, or they were swept away by passion." And the youngest gay men, those who had suffered comparatively little loss and grief due to AIDS or even none at all, had the highest levels of unsafe sex and the worst levels of new infections. They mostly reported a "sense of youthful invulnerability, a belief that AIDS is the plague of an older generation, and a dread of growing old in a culture that prizes youth and beauty."

The article sent shock waves through gay and AIDS activists, but in a sense it shouldn't have. The phenomenon Gross was describing had already been described by researchers in scientific journals for several years. Gross's article shocked many because the troubling information it contained had, with certain notable exceptions, been almost completely ignored or overlooked by AIDS activists and gay community leaders. Now, with the morning *Times* on breakfast tables across the nation, the news was out. Safer sex was in serious trouble, and the problem could no longer be ignored.

The Early Signs of Trouble

In retrospect, it's surprising the news took so long to surface, since the fact that gay men were not using condoms consistently had been clear to researchers for some time. As early as November of 1989 the CDC's *Morbidity and Mortality Weekly Report* reported that gonorrhea cases among gay men attending STD clinics in King County, Washington, which had peaked at 720 cases in 1982 and dropped to a mere 27 cases in 1988, had risen to an alarming 71 cases in the first nine months of 1989. Within months, similar trends among gay men were being reported from STD clinics around the nation and from locations as far-flung as England, Australia, and the Netherlands. Since transmission of gonorrhea is effectively blocked by condoms and can spread rapidly only when people are engaging in unprotected intercourse with multiple partners, the obvious inference was that this was what was happening.

Increased occurrences of unsafe sex with multiple partners soon showed up in direct studies of HIV transmission itself. Medical journals began publishing reports based on data that had been collected in the late eighties, and most of it looked grim. A groundbreaking 1990 study in *Journal of AIDS* by epidemiologist Ron Stall and associates in San Francisco reported that a significant minority of gay men who had initially adopted safer sex had, in the researchers' term, "relapsed." This finding was culled in San Francisco in 1988, during the height of what novelist Andrew Holleran has called the Fear, that period when the terror of AIDS in the gay world was so strong that the fast lane seemed practically to disappear from the public landscape. The study's authors themselves said this period had produced "the most profound community wide health-related behavioral risk reductions ever measured." But now relapse into unsafe behavior, they wrote, had become "the predominant kind of high risk sex, accounting for approximately two thirds of all prevalent high risk sex" in their cohort in 1988.

Data from the Chicago Multicenter AIDS Cohort (MACS) confirmed that the problem was as serious in Chicago. Analyzing data collected from 1986 through 1988, Chicago MACS researchers reported that only 45 percent of gay men consistently maintained safer practices, while 47 percent had "relapsed" into unsafe behavior at least once, and 3 percent consistently had unsafe sex. And the problem was noted in other countries. In 1989, for example, the level of anal sex among gay men in England's Project SIGMA slowly began to rise after years of decline, as did the men's average number of partners and their rate of HIV infection. By 1991, only one third of the men in Project SIGMA reported using condoms every time they had anal sex, and a significant minority said they never used them at all.

Reports of high levels of unsafe sex were not confined to urban gay men. A 1992 study of gay American men in small cities in upstate New York, West Virginia, northern Wisconsin, Montana, and other locations reported that about one third of the subjects said that they had engaged in unprotected anal intercourse in the preceding two months. The mean frequency of this behavior was 8.4 occasions over two months, and only a quarter of those occasions were with partners the men described as monogamous. The researchers concluded that a new "front line" of HIV prevention had shifted to smaller cities, and that "prevention efforts in these areas are urgently needed to avert sharp increases in future [HIV] infections in this population."

In study after study—in gay populations in the United States and other industrialized countries, in large urban centers and small cities, among young men new to gay life (and the epidemic) and older men—the same pattern was repeated. The condom code did not seem to be working nearly as well as originally hoped, or hyped. The problem seemed particularly acute among young gay men and gay men of color. In one 1993 San Francisco study, 2.9 percent of gay men aged 18 to 29 were becoming infected per year. Another report estimated that 20 percent of all AIDS cases in the United States occurred among men of color who had sex with men.

Perhaps the most disturbing piece of news came in 1991 when researcher Donald R. Hoover and his associates set out to predict the future course of AIDS infection among gay men. Using combined data collected from cohorts in Baltimore, Chicago, Los Angeles, and Pittsburgh who had been originally uninfected in 1984, the researchers reported that about 46 percent of these men had become infected by January 1990. In other words, almost half of the gay men who were uninfected at a time in which AIDS had already become the central news story in the gay world were now infected. Even worse, Hoover then attempted to estimate future trends based on the hazards observed between 1986 and 1990. Assuming that those trends would remain stable into the future, his team predicted the prospects of a twenty-year-old gay man remaining uninfected over subsequent years:

> Such a man [Hoover's team wrote] has a 20.2 percent chance of sero-converting before reaching the age of twenty-five years (a 4.4 percent yearly hazard). The annual hazard drops to 2.5 percent between twenty-five and thirty years, to about 1.5 percent between thirty and forty-five years, and to 1.0 percent between forty and fifty-five years. The overall probability of seroconversion prior to age fifty-five years is about 50 percent, with seroconversion still continuing at and after age fifty-five. Given that this cohort consists of volunteers receiving extensive anti-HIV-1 transmission education, the future seroconversion rates of the general homosexual population may be even higher than those observed here.

The significance of this result, whose outlines have been generally confirmed since, can hardly be overestimated. The population Hoover was studying consisted of volunteers who trekked to the researchers' offices every six months, provided detailed summaries of their sexual activity, were tested for HIV, and were given extensive counseling to help them avoid infection. Researchers consider such men the most educated and motivated portion of the gay male population, and therefore among the least likely to become infected. (Indeed, it is partly for that reason that many similar cohorts were disbanded in the early 1990s; researchers and government funders felt that the men's high level of AIDS awareness rendered them

unrepresentative of the gay population as a whole.) Hoover's estimates were based on the assumption that levels of unsafe activity
among such men would remain "stabilized" at their relatively low
1986–1990 levels, when in fact many reports indicate that levels of
unsafe activity have risen substantially since then.

"Relapse"

By the mid 1990s this problem was being widely reported and
had acquired a name: relapse. The word first appeared in a single
research paper presented at the 1989 International AIDS Conference in Montreal, but by the next year's conference in San Francisco it had become prevention's hot new term. Relapse
originally had a very specific meaning: It described the behavior
of men who had once consistently used condoms but who had
then given them up on at least some occasions. The term quickly
grew more encompassing, however, to the point where it sometimes came to describe a general breakdown in condom use
among gay men.

The term has been criticized by some researchers and activists
who consider it judgmental and complain that it smacks of anti-
gay bias. "Outside medicine," writes British researchers, "the term
relapse is more clearly pejorative, and refers to backsliding, or
slinking back to an unacceptable position. Relapse, then, is concerned with bad behavior or state of being." He objects that
"when applied to gay men, it reinforces their otherness as out-
siders." And he criticizes its accuracy, since quite a few men who
return to unprotected anal sex are in steady relationships with
partners of the same serostatus, and their behavior should not be
considered relapse because it's not really unsafe. Edward King
agrees, arguing that a "particularly misleading" suggestion implicit
in the term is the idea that "making the choice to practice unprotected anal sex is necessarily always wrong and to be actively discouraged by AIDS educators, or worse still, that anal sex is
unhealthy *per se.*"

Controversy over the term has tended to overshadow an even
more significant fact, which is that a substantial number of gay
men never consistently adopted condoms in the first place. One
study of gay New Yorkers' sexual practices at the height of the

Fear in 1987 found that the percentage who said they always used condoms during receptive anal sex had risen to around 60 percent (up from 2 percent in 1981), but that the remaining 40 percent did not use condoms consistently, and some never used them at all. Other studies showed similar levels of condom use during the late eighties, while a slew of studies reported that significant numbers of gay men continuously cycled in and out of protected sex and had from the beginning, using condoms for a while, returning to unprotected sex for a while, then adopting condoms again, in much the same way that dieters lose weight and gain it back. Some researchers plausibly argue that this cycling phenomenon accounts for most unsafe sex among gay men, and always has.

All in all, in comparing studies published from the mid eighties to the mid nineties, it is reasonably accurate to say that no more than about half of all gay men have ever used condoms consistently as a response to AIDS. Given that, the sudden shift from self-congratulations about safer sex to panic about relapse looks more like a shift in perspective than reality. In the late eighties the glass of prevention seemed half full as activists, researchers, and journalists focused on the impressive percentage of the gay population who used condoms consistently. Then, when it became apparent that transmissions were continuing at high levels into the nineties, the glass began to look half empty and they began to focus on the percentage that did not.

Nonetheless, for those committed to the condom code the idea of "relapse" remains alluring, since it helps to avoid facing the stark possibility that the condom code is unworkable even under the most compelling of circumstances. After all, if we can convince ourselves that the condom code was successful once upon a time, there's a reasonable chance it could work again. But if we are forced to admit that it never really worked, we're in much more serious trouble. Such an acknowledgment would tend to lead to either of two equally unpalatable conclusions. Either safer sex can never really work, or safer sex is going to have to go much further than the condom code, perhaps by attacking the ecological and multifactorial roots of HIV transmission in the gay population, roots that are tied up in many people's very definition of gay identity and community.

Measuring Success

At this point it's worthwhile to define precisely what we mean by success or failure as applied to the condom code and safer sex generally. AIDS prevention experts argue that there are two fundamental goals of prevention, and the success or failure of any strategy ought to be measured against both. You might say that one is personal and concerns the individual, the other ecological and concerns the population as a whole.

The personal goal is simple: Did this strategy prevent me from becoming HIV infected if I am seronegative, or prevent me from infecting my partner if I am seropositive? In that sense, the question of whether the condom code has "worked" can only be answered individually by each of the millions of people who employ it in their lives. Since we can safely say that when used consistently and correctly condoms provide considerable protection from HIV infection, the strategy has undoubtedly been a success for lots of people.

But the second, larger goal of prevention is just as crucial for the gay community. That goal is to reduce HIV transmission below the epidemic threshold. In other words, to reduce r to less than one. By that measure, if r is less than one and transmission is declining, prevention is working. And if it is rising, prevention is failing. Success does not require that *all* new infections be prevented, a state sometimes called "risk elimination." No prevention strategy in an epidemic as large and complex as AIDS can be expected to do that. But prevention can be expected to produce a shift in the right direction, and if it is not doing that it is failing in its larger, ecological goal. So to determine whether the condom code ever worked, we need to ask at least two questions. First, did HIV transmission ever drop below the epidemic's tipping point in the gay world? And second, if it did, was it due to the condom code by itself, a combination of the condom code and other behavior changes, or some other phenomenon altogether?

There is no question that HIV transmission dropped substantially in the late eighties among American gay men. Levels of transmission that had risen to as high as 12 percent per year in the early eighties dropped to a mere 1 or 2 percent per year by the end of the decade. But as successful as that sounds, the more important question is, Is that 1 or 2 percent low enough to extinguish the epidemic eventually?

One attempt to answer this question is contained in an epidemiological study called "Effect of Sexual Behavior Change on Long-Term HIV Prevalence among Homosexual Men." Its authors, Martina Morris and Laura Dean, are researchers at Columbia University's School of Public Health and have spent years tracking the AIDS epidemic among gay men in New York City. It's worthwhile examining their study in some detail because their methods and assumptions help illuminate the dynamics of HIV transmission among gay men.

Morris and Dean begin by asking whether the changes in gay men's behavior have been sufficient to reduce the rate of HIV transmission below the epidemic threshold. They note that "current analyses suggest that the answer is no." Standard epidemiological formulas (called Kaplan-Meier-based projections) like those by Hoover suggest that seroconversion rates of 1 to 2 percent per year will lead to a 50 percent infection rate eventually, which is hardly successful by anybody's lights. But they point out that such analyses are based on static seroconversion rates, and that real rates are actually quite fluid, depending on three variables: "the rate of sexual contact (new partner acquisition rate), the prevalence of infection (the likelihood of selecting an infected partner), and the infectivity of the disease (the probability of disease transmission per partnership)." What would happen, they ask, if two of those variables, contact rates and infectivity, remained steady for several years but the third, prevalence, declined? This might happen if the large group of men who were infected early in the epidemic died. "With other things being equal," they note, "this should eventually lower seroconversion." They also note that future infection rates are highly dependent on the sexual ecology of younger gay men, since the future of epidemic growth is contingent on the infection of the young. So rather than using a static model, they employed a dynamic model, one that had proven remarkably accurate in predicting the actual course of the epidemic up to the point of their study.

Into that dynamic model went their basic data about gay men's behavior during the height of the Fear from 1985 to 1991, data collected from a large cohort of gay men in New York City that was enrolled in 1985 but that continued to add young gay men as time went on. According to this data, gay male New Yorkers had originally averaged about eleven "unsafe contacts" per year in the years before the epidemic, an unsafe contact being defined as a person with whom one has anal sex without condoms at least once. By 1991, gay New Yorkers had reduced that number to just one per year, a signal of how greatly behavior modification had altered gay men's sexual practices in New York City.

Using their dynamic model, Morris and Dean then attempted to determine if that level of condom use was enough to lower HIV transmission below threshold. Spinning out the next thirty-five years based on the 1991 average of one unsafe contact per year, they found that that level lies "very close to the level necessary to reduce transmission below the epidemic reproductive threshold." If that level of condom use is "maintained in the future, then the transmission of HIV in the population could eventually die out." Morris and Dean published a chart that vividly showed that as the years go by, the percentage of gay men infected with HIV could slowly drop from around 40 percent in 1991 to a mere 5 percent in 2030.

The researchers couched this first part of their finding as good news, but even this was worrisome because even at the extremely high level of condom use in 1991, the transmission rate of gay New Yorkers was teetering right on the brink of the epidemic's tipping point. The researchers then created a second model to predict what would happen if gay men returned to a level of two "unsafe contacts" per year. That small difference—between one unsafe partner and two per year—produced disaster. Transmission rose well above the epidemic threshold in every age category, so that instead of a 5 percent prevalence level in thirty-five years, it rose to more than 50 percent, and among those age forty-five to fifty-four more than 60 percent. In other words, the seemingly negligible difference between one unsafe contact and two per year marks the difference between teetering right on the brink of disaster and tumbling into the abyss. "The implications of even temporary returns to unsafe practices are not simply an increase in individual risk," the researchers wrote, "but also the persistence of HIV transmission at epidemic levels in the [gay] population."

Unfortunately, 1991 was the last year that Morris and Dean received funding to follow their cohort, so we cannot determine what this group's number of "unsafe contacts" were in later years. But most surveys indicate that gay men are having more unsafe sex with more partners than they were in 1991. In New York itself, sub-sequent surveys revealed an increase in gay men's total number of partners, an increase in the number of unsafe partners, and rises in the amount of unprotected sex. The same has been true for San Francisco, Chicago, Boston, Denver, and most other cities with ongoing epidemiological surveys. Of course, this does not prove that Morris and Dean's second scenario is the current reality for the gay world. In fact, in a very real sense there is no single current reality, since even among gay Americans there are many different ecosystems and many different epidemics, each with its own dynamic. But the probable answer to our first question—did HIV transmission ever drop below threshold in the gay world—is maybe, but not by much, and not for long.

Farr's Law and the Theory of "Saturation"

If the condom code at its best barely got us to the brink of epi-demic threshold, why did new infections drop so dramatically among gay men in the late eighties? There's no question they did drop. One of the main reasons AIDS educators were once so opti-mistic was the decline in the rate of HIV transmission to just 1 or 2 percent per year by the end of the decade. Doesn't that alone indi-cate that new infections had dropped far below the replacement level?

Over a century ago epidemiologists discovered that infectious epidemics develop in a predictable way: They start slowly, enter a phase of explosive growth, then level off and finally experience a rapid decline in new infections. The reasons are fairly simple. At the beginning of an epidemic only a few individuals are infected, so the disease spreads fairly slowly. But as anyone can easily demonstrate by doubling the number 2, then doubling 4, then doubling 8, and so reaching over 1,000,000 in only nineteen steps, the process of doubling quickly produces astronomical numbers. So once an epi-demic gets a firm foothold and begins the implacable doubling process, it doesn't take long for it to begin racing through the sus-ceptible population in an exponential way. However, any popula-tion of susceptibles constitutes a finite number of people, and once this population approaches saturation, the remaining uninfected population will necessarily be dominated by people who, for various reasons, are less susceptible or not susceptible at all. As this happens, the rate of new infections has to slow. Eventually, if nothing halts the natural progress of the epidemic, prevalence hits what is sometimes called the "saturation point," at which most of those who are susceptible have been infected. Now the rate of new infections drops dramatically along a mathematical curve almost the opposite of the one it initially rose upon. Finally, when virtually no susceptibles are left to infect, new cases can sputter out and almost cease altogether—that is, until a new generation of susceptibles enters the population. At that point new infections can begin to rise again. This classic rise and fall of an epidemic is sometimes called Farr's Law after a nineteenth-century British physician and pioneer epidemiologist who correctly predicted the rise, duration, and termination of a cattle plague based merely on reports of early infections. Since the rapid rise and rapid decline of new HIV infections among gay men in the eighties followed the basic curve of Farr's Law, it is possible that what we witnessed when new infections dropped was not the triumph of prevention, but the tragedy of saturation.

The concept of Farr's Law applied to the spread of HIV in a population of sexually active gay men might work like this: In the beginning, as HIV entered gay ecosystems through just a few individuals, it took several years of slow doubling before it really took hold. But eventually its doubling time decreased and people engaging in the riskiest behaviors with the most partners began experiencing very high rates of infection and very brief doubling times. The incidence curve rose dramatically, and within just a few years this initial core quickly became saturated. Eventually, as the men in the core were removed from the pool of susceptibles, the rate slowed for two basic reasons. One is that much of the unsafe sex was now being conducted among pairs in which both partners were already infected, and this activity was "wasted" from the virus's point of view. The other was that a large percentage of those who remained uninfected did so precisely because they did not engage in risky behavior, or engaged in it less often and with fewer partners than the original core, and were therefore less susceptible. As a result, members of this less susceptible group became infected at increasingly slower rates. Still, as those among them had unsafe sex they too became infected and were removed from the ranks of susceptibles, and the rate of infection slowed even more. Eventually, HIV had infected most people who engage in risky behaviors, and the so-called saturation point was reached. Now new infections had to drop to extremely low levels or even temporarily cease altogether. There was virtually nobody left to infect. And that's where things would have to remain until a group of new susceptibles entered the population (young gay men coming of age, or older gay men coming out of the closet) and began engaging in risk behaviors. At that point, new infections ought to begin a slow but steady rise, leading to a Second Wave of the epidemic.

Success or Saturation?

The dramatic rise of HIV prevalence in gay male cohorts from 1978 to 1985, and the equally dramatic cresting of new infections and subsequent drop once prevalence levels reached around 50 percent, appears to follow closely the classic curve predicted by Farr's Law and observed in epidemics throughout the world. The all-time high-water mark of HIV prevalence in the gay population was measured in a San Francisco cohort in 1985 that suffered a cumulative total infection level of 73.1 percent. No other cohort of gay men attained such astronomic levels, but many saw cumulative prevalence rise to between 40 and 60 percent by the mid eighties, at which point new infections slowed dramatically.

Some have argued that a 40 to 60 percent prevalence level cannot amount to saturation, since a large percentage of gay men remained uninfected. But saturation is a misnomer in epidemiology in much the way that "full employment" is a misnomer in economics—it does not mean that every single person in a social community has been infected. Some who engage in high-risk behavior will remain infection-free thanks to plain luck. A few others will likely be naturally immune to HIV. Such natural immunity is still a poorly understood phenomenon, but it has nonetheless been plausibly demonstrated by studies of prostitutes in high-prevalence areas. Most importantly, a significant percentage of sexually active gay men will remain uninfected because they never, or virtually never, engage in sexual acts that put them at risk (such as receptive anal sex), or do so only within mutually monogamous partnerships where both members are uninfected. Even in the pre-AIDS era when fear of HIV was not an issue, studies indicated that up to 40 percent of gay men did not engage in receptive anal sex, or did so very rarely, or with very few partners. So it seems reasonable to assume that only between 40 to 60 percent of gay men fall into the susceptible category, and once prevalence hits that level, that's about as saturated as you're likely to get. After that, the rate of new infections has no place to go but down.

This model of saturation does not in any way diminish the importance of behavior change for individuals. For those who practiced anal sex and who avoided infection by using condoms consistently, behavior change played the decisive role. But from a population-wide perspective, the sudden drop in new infections seems not the result of the success of prevention, but of its tragic failure.

Small Cities, Towns, and Rural Areas

But what about the gay communities in towns and smaller American cities, where studies show that HIV prevalence often peaked at only 20 or 30 percent? Surely, some argue, the condom code worked in these places. And since it did, the argument goes, doesn't that prove that it *can* work, and that we just have to try harder?

While prevalence plateaued at lower levels in small cities than in larger ones, there are several factors that raise doubt over whether this had much to do with the condom code. First of all, study after study indicates that gay men in smaller cities and towns used condoms *less* consistently than gay men in bigger cities. Part of the reason is less proximity to education and support: Most AIDS education programs were created in big cities and directed at the populations there. Another reason is that until quite recently gay men in small-town America tended to be more closeted, and were therefore harder to reach with supportive prevention messages. Even when such men receive AIDS education, some studies indicate that they may be less amenable to putting that education into practice. Safer sex, after all, requires a fairly high level of sexual self-confidence and negotiation skills, not things that are frequently associated with people who live in the closet or confine their sexual activity to brief, sometimes shame-ridden encounters. Probably for that reason some early studies have shown that being closeted or deeply ashamed of one's sexual orientation was itself a risk factor for HIV infection. Finally, adoption of safer sex is closely associated with perception of risk, and such a perception most often stems from personal knowledge of friends or acquaintances who have become infected. Since AIDS was far less prevalent in outlying gay populations in the eighties, men in such places naturally tended to have a lower perception of risk.

For all of these reasons, gay men's use of condoms lagged in small cities and towns. Yet paradoxically, so did the prevalence of HIV infection. So before we credit the condom code with saving middle-American gays from saturation, we need to look for other factors in the sexual ecology of middle-American gay life that might account for the lower level of infection. Such factors are not hard to find.

As we have seen, the great engines of infection in gay America were the high levels of sexual multipartnerism in urban gay core groups, particularly multipartnerism combined with anal sex; a lot of mixing between cores and everybody else; and a synergy of additional factors from high levels of other STDs and repeated use of antibiotics to substance abuse and versatility. Individuals in big cities could easily have hundreds of partners per year within large core groups where most of their partners also had hundreds of partners per year. Bathhouses and sex clubs provided highly efficient venues for this activity, as did bars and cruising areas. One could easily go out cruising every night for years in Houston, Chicago, Atlanta, New York, Boston, San Francisco, and many other cities, have sex with a different man each night, and never have sex with the same person twice. Yet even gay cohorts in large American cities had dramatically different rates of partner change in the late seventies, ranging from a mean of 18.1 partners in a four-month period in a cohort in St. Louis, to 36.1 partners in a four-month period in a San Francisco cohort.

Obviously some gay men in small American cities and towns and rural areas also have multiple partners, but a comparison of studies of both big-city and small-town gay men tends to show that those in smaller towns on average have fewer partners than those in the largest cities. Reasons include the fewer potential partners in small-town America, fewer venues like bathhouses and sex clubs and public cruising grounds, and less anonymity. Another possible reason is that gay men who place a premium on sexual adventure often migrate to cities where such adventures are more easily attainable. In general the opportunity for sex with hundreds or thousands of partners in smaller cities and towns is greatly reduced for all but a small minority of the most determined.

Another difference that may have affected rates of transmission is that gay men in middle America often have less geographic proximity to the great centers of AIDS infection. Many epidemiologists complain that the role of geography in sexual ecology is still underrated. The geographical peaks and valleys of HIV infection indicate that HIV spreads not only in time but in space. The epidemic began in certain physical epicenters—primarily New York, San Francisco, Los Angeles, Miami, and Houston—spread out from there, and is still spreading. Those who engage in risky behavior in areas near these epicenters are at far greater risk than those farther afield.

Certainly saturation can still occur within smaller ecosystems. Saturation is, after all, a relative concept. It does not mean that most people in a given *social community* have been infected, but simply that most of those engaging in certain behaviors within certain ecosystems have been infected. So it is entirely possible that a prevalence level of only 25 percent of the gay population of some small American city or town represents saturation for that community.

Without taking these factors into account, it's easy to assume that the peak level of infection ought to be the same in every gay community, and that since AIDS peaked in one San Francisco cohort at over 70 percent, that marks its natural high-water mark in any gay population, so that whenever it falls short of that mark, prevention has scored a success. It seems more likely, however, that every gay community has its own continuously shifting level of saturation, and that the levels in smaller cities and towns are almost certainly lower than those of the biggest cities.

None of this is meant to imply that the condom code had no impact on prevalence. A small city's 20 percent prevalence might easily rise to 30 percent if nobody used condoms. But the message of the late eighties—that the condom code was the first and foremost reason why new infections dropped—seems unsubstantiated by either the facts of the epidemic or the theory behind them.

Discrepancies

Some have dismissed these arguments entirely by maintaining that the Second Wave is a statistical mirage that isn't happening at all. The primary piece of evidence used to bolster this contention is that cases of rectal gonorrhea remain extremely low in most gay populations, at least compared to their levels in the late seventies. Since rectal gonorrhea is spread through the same activity that spreads HIV, why, they ask, isn't the Second Wave producing a major epidemic of rectal gonorrhea as well?

To understand why, remember that STD transmission relies on three factors: infectivity per sexual act, the rate of partner change, and *prevalence of the disease among potential partners*. Let us, for the sake of illustration, say that to maintain rectal gonorrhea transmission in a hypothetical gay community at a rate of 1,000 cases per year, there needs to be a 10 percent prevalence of the disease in that population, and the average person has to have 10 partners a year. (These are not the actual figures, which would vary from population to population.) Those two things together—10 percent prevalence times 10 partners per year—will produce 1,000 new cases annually. If either of those factors is reduced, you would have to have a proportional increase in one of the other factors to maintain 1,000 annual cases.

Now let's suppose that this population becomes comparatively safe for one year, and that during this "safe year" virtually everybody who had rectal gonorrhea goes to the doctor and gets cured. By the end of our safe year gonorrhea prevalence has accordingly dropped from 10 percent to 0.1 percent, virtually eliminating the disease from this population. Then let's suppose that at the end of the safe year many people return to unprotected anal sex with an average of 5 partners per year. What happens to the rectal gonorrhea rates? Well, remember that to have 1,000 new cases a year requires a 10 percent prevalence multiplied by an average of 10 partners a year. This population has only a 0.1 prevalence and an average of 5 partners a year. If this is below the tipping point for rectal gonorrhea, the disease will continue to disappear slowly. Even if it is above the tipping point, it will take many years before a noticeable epidemic got under way with such low prevalence.

Unlike rectal gonorrhea, however, HIV is not curable and is therefore not banished from our hypothetical population during their "safe year." In fact, because HIV is slow moving and incurable, the prevalence of HIV infection has hardly declined at all. So if this population stops using condoms and begins to average five partners per year, the rate of new HIV infections has the potential to rise dramatically, while the rate of rectal gonorrhea will remain vanishingly low. The fact that we can take little comfort in comparing notes of HIV transmission with other diseases illustrates a basic fact: that each STD has its own ecology and responds to its own factors.

Beyond Nontransformative Change

The condom code was never adopted more than partially by gay men, even during the tremendous wave of fear that swept gay America in the mid eighties. As a result, while the code undoubtedly succeeded in keeping many individuals uninfected, it does not appear to have succeeded for the overall gay population. It seems reasonable to conclude that if it didn't work when fear ruled the day, it is even less likely to succeed in the future as AIDS evolves into a more manageable disease and becomes an accepted part of life.

This would strongly suggest that the basic "nontransformative" strategy of containing HIV exclusively through the condom code is destined to continue to fail. If gay men want to avoid continued saturation with HIV, or avoid a repeat of the AIDS disaster with new strains of HIV or new diseases altogether, a larger transformation seems required. Yet the reaction to date does not suggest that this idea has been widely accepted. There was clear evidence that the condom code was failing as far back as the late eighties. There was fairly straightforward evidence that saturation was more responsible for the decline in new infections than safer sex. And there was practical and theoretical evidence that new waves of infection were inevitable once new groups of susceptible young gay men entered the gay life. Yet the mechanisms of denial were tremendous. Brave individual researchers and prevention workers sounded alarms, but as we will see in the next chapter, even today the long-term implications of this problem are widely obscured in denial, false optimism, and politics as usual, straight and gay.

CHAPTER 6

Surfing the Second Wave

As news of the Second Wave washed over the gay community in the mid nineties, it provoked a complex series of responses. One, of course, was denial. Some community activists argued that the statistics emanating from HIV studies simply had to be wrong, and often pointed to the low rates of rectal gonorrhea as proof. Most, however, reluctantly accepted the HIV data and struggled to do two basic things. One was to figure out what exactly was happening in the psychological lives of individual gay men that caused them to fail to use condoms consistently. The other was to try to devise new approaches, programs, and strategies that might increase condom use. In both cases, the debate remained focused entirely on the condom code, accepting as a given that all approaches to prevention in the gay community must implicitly validate a casual attitude toward sex with lots of partners. In this view, the proper response to the grim new situation was not to question the condom code, but to question why gay men seemed unable to comply with it more effectively, and then to use that information to devise new ways to get them to comply.

Almost immediately after researchers began exploring this question, however, they hit a series of snags. Many of the reasons given early in the epidemic for not always using condoms—lack of education, lack of AIDS awareness, lack of access to condoms—no longer seemed valid. Many of the additional reasons put forth by the new prevention activists—low self-esteem, survivor's guilt, fatalism, self-hatred—did not seem supported by actual studies of gay men. And many of the reasons that did show up in controlled studies seemed part of normal human behavior, the kind of all-too-human failures that interventions can't do much about.

The Usual Suspects

Education. Some initially argued, and a few still argue, that the shortcomings of the condom code are largely failures of education: People don't use condoms because they don't know about them, often because governmental indifference and right-wing hostility have prevented lifesaving information from getting to those who need it. However, convincing evidence shows that lack of education has faded as a major factor. There are undoubtedly some men, particularly the young, who become infected because they simply don't know about condoms or how to use them properly. But study after study indicates that AIDS awareness is nearly universal among those homosexual men of all races and classes who are becoming infected in the Second Wave. Some prevention workers even report that when they do outreach among men in what are usually considered the hardest to reach groups—namely, men who have sex with men but do not necessarily consider themselves gay—they often end up being given helpful and accurate tips about using condoms by the very men they are trying to reach.

The inability of education to lead automatically to consistent safer sex was underscored in 1995 when a number of prominent gay and AIDS activists began publicly confessing that they had recently been unsafe. Not only did all of these men know about condoms, many were also experienced AIDS educators who taught others about condoms. Basic education remains a necessary precursor to behavior change, especially for the young and those just becoming sexually active. But it is increasingly clear that education and AIDS awareness, while necessary foundations of behavior change, are not sufficient by themselves to produce consistent behavior change. This should be no surprise in a world where the public is well educated about the dangers of smoking, obesity, substance abuse, drunk driving, and so on, yet significant numbers of people engage in all these behaviors. Some AIDS educators and activists may have felt that the horrors of AIDS were sufficiently more horrible than those other things to act as a deterrent, and anti-gay sentiments may have led others to believe that gay sexual intimacy was easily expendable. The evidence argues that neither is the case.

Condom Availability. Others initially argued that the problems of the condom code were largely problems of availability: People don't use condoms because they don't have access to them. Since the early years of AIDS, a great battle has been waged to make sure condoms are available to those at high risk. This battle has been fought particularly bitterly in school districts where AIDS educators try to ensure that teenage students have ready access to condoms and some parents resist, arguing that condom availability condones teenage sexual activity. So some have naturally suggested that lack of condoms is a prime reason for unsafe sex among gay men. But this, too, no longer appears to be the case.

Lack of condoms occasionally appears in studies as a reason for not having safer sex, but it does not generally show up as a major factor. Almost the opposite is true. Studies indicating that condoms are widely available have prompted major gay-run AIDS organizations to discontinue the free distribution of condoms to bars, discos, and community centers, assuming it is no longer needed and the money can be better spent elsewhere. That move could backfire, of course, since it may be that one reason that condom availability has receded as an issue is the success of such programs. But at any rate it's difficult to argue at present that lack of condoms is a major contributor to unsafe sex in urban gay America.

The Closet. As we noted, in the early years of the epidemic there was some evidence that openly gay men were more likely to have safe sex than those who were closeted or bisexual or conflicted about their homosexuality. The main explanations were that openly gay men lived in communities where peer norms supported safe sex, that they had more access to education and condoms than closeted men, more firsthand experience of friends with the disease, and higher sexual and personal self-esteem, which led to greater assertiveness and better communication skills. As a result, many activists and educators believed that AIDS prevention efforts should try to assist closeted men in coming out and becoming less conflicted about their sexual orientation.

In the nineties, however, this equation seemed reversed, particularly among young men. In study after study, openly gay men reported being less safe than those who are closeted, conflicted, or bisexual. The Young Men's Study in San Francisco, for example, reported that "high-risk-taking men were found to be well integrated into the gay community; they reported more gay friends, more comfort being gay, less loneliness and were more likely to have a lover. However, they also reported less social support for safe sex, more interpersonal and communication barriers to safe sex, greater enjoyment of unsafe sex, and more often engaging in sex while high on drugs/alcohol and in public cruising areas." The report's conclusions were that "social norms and interpersonal pressures within the young gay men's subculture promote engaging in unsafe sex." These findings were replicated across the nation. One 1991 Chicago study found that "AIDS-risk behavior is lower [among closeted bisexuals] than among gay men," although the authors noted that it was "still significant" among the closeted group. A 1990 Mississippi study found that "self-rating of outness" was positively associated with unsafe sex. A 1991 Milwaukee study reported that "homosexual outness" was associated with heightened risk. Experts cautioned that they were finding little evidence that closeted or conflicted men were becoming safer than they once were. What they were finding instead was that openly gay men were becoming less safe. Some argued that the primary reason was that peer norms in the gay community that had once vigorously supported safer sex had relaxed. Whatever the reason or reasons, one thing seemed clear: The closet could no longer be considered a major cause of unsafe sex, and encouraging young gay men to come out into urban gay communities that did not seem to really support safety, or that actually seemed to encourage unsafety in some cases, no longer ranked as an effective AIDS-prevention strategy.

Substance Abuse. If education, condom availability, and the closet were no longer showing up in studies as major reasons why many gay men were unsafe, one factor that continued to show up again and again was substance abuse. Research consistently indicates that up to 60 percent of those who have unsafe sex are either drunk or high at the time. Alcohol itself is quite capable of inducing people to take risks, but of particular concern has been the resurgence of drugs like D-methamphetamine (crystal meth), special K, and Ecstasy, powerful intoxicants that often cause users to disregard norms of safer sex completely. Crystal meth in particular, which in the nineties became the drug of choice on the gay party circuit in many major cities, contributes to unsafety in many ways. "Far cheaper and longer lasting than cocaine," writes Doug Sadownick, "and more available on the streets than Ecstasy, crystal meth raised sexual cravings to superhuman levels." Some men say it prolongs erection but delays ejaculation, allowing them to engage in longer bouts of intercourse that lead to abrasions and bleeding. Others report that prolonged use makes them unable to achieve erections at all, at which point they may allow themselves to be penetrated, sometimes by multiple partners without a care as to whether or not those partners are wearing condoms. A Seattle King County Department of Public Health study in 1993 showed that 60 percent of gay and bisexual crystal meth users were HIV-positive, the highest prevalence levels in the state.

Researchers have at least two ways of looking at the connection between substance abuse and unsafe sex. One is that the phenomenon is essentially an outgrowth of preexisting substance abuse problems among gay men, and the best way to deal with it is to help men stay sober or better control their intake of drugs or alcohol in situations where they are likely to have sex. As a result, the gay community has made a genuine and serious effort to deal with substance abuse, both through twelve-step programs and through AIDS-specific efforts like GMHC's Substance Use Counseling & Education program, a project that draws direct connections between substance abuse issues and safer sex.

But there is another side to the substance abuse equation that may make it less amenable to interventions. Some men report that they get intoxicated precisely because they want to have unsafe sex and are unable to have it when sober. Only when they are drunk or stoned are they able to lose their inhibitions, forget about AIDS, and have the sex they dream of. In these cases, attacking an underlying addiction may not be effective at all, since it is not a chronic addiction but the conscious or unconscious use of drugs to achieve a specific, desired result that motivates men to get high.

In both cases substance abuse is clearly a serious contributing factor to the failure of many gay men to adhere to the condom code. But it is also clear that substance abuse is one of society's most intractable problems, and will continue to affect vast numbers of people despite the best efforts of social workers and educators. If we have learned anything about substance abuse in the decades since the invention of twelve-step programs, it is that people will not successfully address such problems until they are personally ready to do so. Society can make sure that programs are in place to help people when they decide they want help, but it cannot make them want help. If many gay men are alcoholics or chronic abusers, and many more find the condom code untenable and see intoxication as the only way they can have the sex they desire, it is doubtful that even the best-designed programs can make more than a modest dent in this problem. If the success of the condom code requires solving the issue of substance abuse, its prospects look exceedingly dim.

The New Prevention

Since lack of AIDS education and awareness or lack of condoms are clearly not the main reasons for the breakdown in safer sex, and since the critical problem of substance abuse is unlikely to be solved anytime soon, one might expect us to begin questioning the underlying precept of the condom code—namely, that it is possible to contain AIDS among gay men simply by getting everybody to use condoms all the time. If evidence strongly argues that it is not possible, then logic ought to dictate that prevention leaders explore entirely new approaches to prevention. And I believe those approaches ought to take the logic of ecology into account, particularly ecology's critique of technological fixes that often don't go far enough to address fundamental problems.

However, a new generation of prevention activists has moved in the opposite direction. These "new prevention" leaders essentially argue that the condom code is failing not because it doesn't go far enough, but because it goes too far: that it's too strict, too restrictive, too "homophobic." That if anything, gay men need to loosen up.

A major figure to emerge in this debate is California psychologist Walt Odets, whose speeches and writings have made him a leader of the "new prevention" activism. Odets is probably best known for his cogent argument that AIDS prevention programs ought to direct different messages to those who are HIV infected and uninfected. He argues that positives and negatives naturally have different motivations for having, or not having, safer sex, and that effective prevention must acknowledge that its main targets are HIV-negative men and craft its messages accordingly. Odets maintains that these differences have often been papered over by prevention leaders determined not to exacerbate a split in the gay world.

There is strong logic to this argument, and in the mid nineties several large prevention organizations began moving toward this approach, tailoring their messages toward HIV-negative men. But many new prevention leaders carry their critique much further. A central charge is that much of AIDS prevention lacks psychological sophistication and fails to recognize that uninfected gay men are suffering from a massive psychological epidemic of loss, survivor's guilt, and anxiety, much of it exacerbated by what Odets calls the "profound and destructive effects of denial and repression that we are erecting against fear, grief and depression." New prevention leaders argue that instead of employing psychological insight to combat these problems, safer sex tries to shame and coerce gay men into changing their behavior, a strategy Odets believes is often based on AIDS educators' own internalized homophobia and moralism. He argues that prevention educators have attempted to cover up the difficulty that gay men have with condoms, and have manipulated gay men's self-loathing to get them to make sexual changes that would be unthinkable for straights. "Had the epidemic first occurred among heterosexuals," he writes, "it seems very likely that unprotected vaginal sex would have come to be considered a calculated risk necessary to live an ordinary human life as we expect to lead it, very much like driving an automobile." The reason that this is not the case for unprotected anal sex is homophobia. "Our education has been laden with homophobic assumptions," he writes, "and has exploited the 'internal' homophobia of gay men in an attempt to accomplish behavioral change." The very idea that gay men would adopt readily to condoms is, he argues, rooted in homophobia.

Odets argues that society has "projected this horrific disease onto a reviled minority—in order for it to be *other*." "Society's assignment of AIDS to gay men," he writes, "is intelligible—it is another example of the projection of self-hatred and fear onto others. Through socialization and other learning, gay men have always internalized such projections, and in internalizing society's homosexualization of the epidemic, gay men have thoroughly 'AIDSified' homosexuality."

Odets argues that educators need to remove homophobia from their programs, especially the homophobic assumption that men ought to use condoms every time. "The male heterosexual population would . . . not have accepted it," he argues, and neither should gay men. He urges prevention workers to stop "withholding information and lying" to gay men that safer sex can be satisfying and rewarding, to stop moralizing, to acknowledge the social realities of the epidemic, and to pay real attention to the psychological devastation that AIDS has wrought among gay men.

Justifications and Excuses: The Work of Levine and Siegel

Odets bases much of his theory on the conditions he finds among the gay men who are his patients in Berkeley, California. His attitude toward qualitative research into the lives of gay men is upfront. "I write as a clinical psychologist and an observer of people in everyday life," he informs us. "I am not interested in 'scientific' psychology that 'objectifies' and quantifies data, and I have found little of such work useful in understanding the epidemic, our feelings about it, or what to do about it." However, some of the most illuminating explanations of unsafe sex in the gay world have come from researchers who have applied basic rules of research to the field. Such researchers often come up with very different conclusions from those of the new prevention thinkers.

Perhaps the most interesting investigation into what is actually happening among gay men who have unsafe sex was published by researchers Martin P. Levine and Karolynn Siegel. Titled "Unprotected Sex: Understanding Gay Men's Participation," Levine and Siegel's study undertook to discover the actual motives of a large group of New York City gay men who engage in unsafe sex. They found little to substantiate the idea that gay men are having unsafe sex because they are suffering from broad mental-health problems compounded by the homophobia of prevention workers. What they found instead was that gay men who had unsafe sex were acting much like other people in similar circumstances, and their motives could be divided roughly into two categories: justifications and excuses.

Those who cited "justifications" were men who intentionally and routinely engaged in unsafe sex, but justified it by arguing that their behavior was not actually risky. They either openly doubted the validity of a practice's classification as risky (this was limited primarily to unprotected oral sex) or believed they could eliminate, or at least minimize, the risk of HIV transmission during unprotected intercourse through strategies that prevented the transmission of infected body fluids into the bloodstream. Researchers found that these justifiers could be grouped into four basic categories.

No Signs of Infectivity. Some men had unprotected sex because they assumed their partners were uninfected. Many reasons were given for this assumption, among them that the partner said he had tested negative or had high T-cell counts, that he claimed a history of monogamy or said he rarely took the receptive role in anal sex, or that he came from a geographical area with a low number of AIDS cases. One thirty-eight-year-old, for example, reported that he didn't bother using condoms with "imports," men from countries with few AIDS cases.

No Fluid Transmission. A second group who routinely had unprotected sex justified it by arguing that there was no fluid exchange. These men were roughly divided into two groups: those who believed that preseminal fluid does not contain HIV and those who believed that both semen and preseminal fluid carry HIV, and who therefore opted for only "dry" intercourse.

No Lacerations. Men in this group believed that for HIV to enter the bloodstream there must be a visible cut or laceration, and that if such lacerations are not visible, it's safe to have unprotected sex. Most of these men avoided receptive anal sex, but were willing to engage in insertive anal sex and receptive oral sex.

Saliva, Gastric Juices, and Urethral Acids Kill HIV. This group felt safe in engaging in a number of behaviors because they believed that the defensive properties of certain body fluids kill HIV.

Many of the men giving justifications were articulate and well educated, and had elaborate rationalizations that allowed them to have the kind of unprotected sex they wanted without worrying too much that they might be contracting, or spreading, infection. They did not seem to fit the psychological profile of men having unsafe sex for reasons of low self-esteem, survivor's guilt, and so on. While it could be argued that their behavior and beliefs indicate low AIDS awareness, the opposite could also be argued. Many actually knew a great deal about AIDS and HIV, and had configured that knowledge in a way that allowed them to do what they wanted.

The other major group was those who also had sex that put them at high risk for HIV infection, but who recognized the danger they had placed themselves in, were sorry about it, and offered "excuses" for these lapses, excuses that invariably attributed their behavior to forces beyond their control. "They regarded instances of unprotected sex as an unintentional relapse from their normal pattern of protection, which emerged from either 'extenuating circumstances' or 'external forces' beyond their control." Levine and Siegel grouped these excuses into four categories.

Drugs and Alcohol. The most common excuse came from men who maintained that "drugs or alcohol impaired their judgment, lowered their inhibitions, or reduced their ability to resist a partner's urging or pressure" to engage in unprotected sex. Many of these men expressed regret at what they had done as soon as they were sober.

Sexual Passion. This was the second most commonly cited reason, and "nearly all the men offering this excuse felt their behavior was uncharacteristic of them and attributable to uncontrollable urges, which overwhelmed their intent to use protection. These men typically described these urges as powerful biological needs and drives."

Emotional Needs. Men in this group explained their unsafe sex as "an expression of love, affection, or acceptance. Typically these men participated in unprotected intercourse to demonstrate their emotional feelings for their partners who were usually their lovers or boyfriends. Many described their behavior as a sacrifice made for their partners."

Partner Coercion. Finally, there was a group of men who claimed they had been coerced into having unsafe sex. Some reported that they had been pressured by their partners to forgo condoms, and thus had the unsafe sex knowingly but essentially unwillingly. Others claimed they were deceived, saying that they thought their partners were using condoms but discovered too late that they were not.

In evaluating these various justifications and excuses, Levine and Siegel noted that two very different models of HIV risk behavior were circulating in the gay world. The first, which they call the *public health construction*, is the one that's been widely publicized by health authorities and AIDS prevention groups. According to this model, there are different risk levels between receptive and insertive anal sex and between oral and anal sex, but all forms of intercourse are essentially risky unless both partners know beyond a reasonable doubt that they are uninfected. The second model is what the researchers call the *gay folk construction* of risk. According to this view, a lot of things the health authorities consider unsafe really are safe, or almost completely safe. This includes oral sex, or at least oral sex without ejaculation, and also sometimes includes the belief that HIV must directly enter the bloodstream through visible lacerations on the penis or the lining of the anus or mouth in order to cause infection.

The Heterosexual Equation

In what was perhaps their most significant finding, Levine and Siegel reported that gay men who have unsafe sex are acting in much the same way as most heterosexuals who engage in "problematic erotic conduct," such as adultery or sex that might result in unwanted pregnancy or STD transmission. "Within the broader culture, there are a set of socially legitimate reasons for engaging in improper sexual behavior," they wrote:

Typically these explanations affirm the validity of normative expectations but attempt to neutralize reputational damage by denying the risk of discovery, pregnancy, or disease as well as individual responsibility for participating in the act. That is, they assert that the act was wrong but maintain that there was almost no chance of either being found out or becoming pregnant or sick, and attribute responsibility for this behavior to situations and forces out of the individual's control, such as insobriety, lust, affection, pleasure or duress.

The crucial point here is that gay men who have unsafe sex seem to act very much like their straight counterparts. This flies in the face of the new prevention thinkers' increasingly elaborate theories that attribute unsafe sex to gay dysfunction, survivor's guilt, fatalism, neuroses, and low self-esteem, and argue that if AIDS educators and gay men had less internalized homophobia, compliance would be much better. Studies like Levine and Siegel's paint a different picture, implying that significant condom noncompliance stems from natural human failings that exist among gays and straights, the psychologically devastated and the relatively healthy.

As if in conformation, data emerged in the nineties concerning heterosexual couples where one partner—usually the male member of the couple—had been infected with HIV from a blood transfusion or clotting factor. In such cases the couple was duly advised that the man was infected and that they must always use condoms. But studies showed that among such couples, consistent use of condoms was nowhere near the rule. One typical study showed that only 48 percent of such couples "consistently" used condoms, and other studies showed similar rates. Since many of the uninfected partners in these couples subsequently became infected, the rate of new infection bore out the fact that they were indeed taking serious risks. Yet obviously none of these heterosexual couples could suffer from homosexual self-loathing and the other self-esteem and behavioral problems said to afflict gay men.

These results were no surprise to family planning experts. It is generally considered well established that while some couples who rely on condoms for birth control manage to use them absolutely properly every time they have sex throughout their reproductive lives, this seems to be the exception. Most people employing condoms for birth control use them most of the time, and hope for the best the rest of the time. In decades past there were even names for the results of such imperfect compliance, such as "bottle babies," a term that described the children born to parents who intended to practice birth control but who "forgot" once they got a bit tipsy. Today's abortion rates attest to how often heterosexuals fail to use birth control even when the penalty is an unwanted birth or a costly, physically painful, and emotionally traumatic operation. The same was true in the past when abortions were illegal and often fatal for the mother.

Sex aside, people have traditionally had major problems maintaining a perfect commitment to any difficult behavior change. We seem to be good at crafting well-intentioned resolutions to deal with knotty problems, and some people seem fairly adept at sticking to those resolutions most of the time. But few of us seem capable of sticking to them all the time, in every situation, forever. Dieters slip off their diets. Alcoholics fall off the wagon. Former smokers impulsively light up. Responsible drivers sometimes drive drunk, or fail to buckle up. Couples desperate not to have a child sometimes fail to use birth control. Failure at compliance is not a specifically "gay" problem, and although failure to be perfect can be exacerbated by contributing factors like lack of education, substance abuse, self-hatred, or survivor's guilt, such failure is not in its deepest sense *caused* by those factors, at least not for most people. It seems part of many of our natures to be occasionally impulsive creatures who do not always act in our own genuine long-term best interests. In fact, from the perspective of behavior change, the amazing thing about gay men's rate of condom use is not that it is so low, but that it is so high. Compared to campaigns that attempt to encourage people to quit smoking, or to diet and exercise, or to quit using addictive drugs, campaigns that often measure success in single percentage points, the consistent adoption of condoms by approximately half of all gay men is a remarkable success by almost any behavioral scale.

Many heterosexuals and even many gay men who read accounts of gay unsafe sex and the Second Wave of the AIDS epidemic express surprise that anyone, under any circumstances, could be foolhardy enough not to use a condom when having sex in a high-risk population. Yet many of those expressing such wonderment are themselves overweight, or smoke cigarettes, or fail to get enough exercise, or drive too fast, or eat junk food, or drink too much, or don't get regular checkups even though they may be at risk for breast cancer or prostate cancer or high blood pressure. And those who argue that such risks are simply not comparable to

AIDS are not being very realistic. Smoking kills over 400,000 Americans a year, well over a thousand people a day. Obesity leads to dramatically high rates of morbidity and mortality. Experts estimate that about half of the annual deaths in the United States are caused by factors relating to people's behavior. It's more or less accepted that there will always be people with reasons for doing such things, no matter how perfect we make our society.

Occasional Unsafe Sex and the Human Condition

Since less-than-perfect compliance seems to be the human condition, it may seem odd that gay men and gay-run AIDS organizations spend so much energy arguing that unsafe sex is a result of a specific gay male dysfunction. The idea seems more consistent with the philosophy of anti-gay conservatives, who have a vested interest in the belief that gay men are compulsive sexual neurotics incapable of exercising self-control. To such homophobes and moral conservatives the Second Wave seems welcome proof not of universal human frailty, but of their contention that gay liberation was a mistake that needs to be reversed.

In the face of that, one might expect gay liberationists to be eager to point out that far from having a death wish, gay men actually seem to be using condoms at least as consistently as heterosexuals facing similar risk. But increasingly as the news of the Second Wave sank into gay consciousness in the nineties, one heard the opposite argument: that the failure always to use condoms indicates that something has gone terribly wrong with gay men. Why would gay advocates advance this argument, especially when it doesn't find much support in the more objective scientific literature on relapse like Levine and Siegel's study? One possible explanation is that there exists a collective unwillingness to believe that the condom code might be inherently unworkable, a hesitation to accept that truly effective safer sex might involve going beyond the condom code and questioning some cherished ideas about the compatibility of promiscuity and safety. For many, the code is the only possible approach to AIDS prevention because it is the only possible response that allows the so-called sex-positive aspects of gay male ideology to go essentially unchallenged. In a community whose practice of sex-positivity helped produce a bona fide ecological catastrophe, the condom code is the only strategy that allows many gay men to pretend that sex without consequences is still a possibility. As such, it simply *has* to work.

Yet the occasional failure to use condoms seems to result far more from human imperfection than gay dysfunction. Gay men are selling themselves short by confusing the two, and by continuing to focus on why they are not good enough for the condom code, rather than on why the condom code is not good enough for them.

Tinkering with Hopelessness

In a sense, prevention boxed itself into a corner in the nineties, and as it did it was enveloped by a feeling of irrelevance and doom. A lack of realistic solutions within the context of the condom code created a sense of purposelessness and even hopelessness among many rank-and-file gay men and, perhaps more ominously, among prevention workers and AIDS educators. Much of the prevention discussion revolved around mere tinkering with the condom code to finesse a bit more compliance here and there. As people became demoralized, many came to accept that prevention could never really contain AIDS.

This attitude seemed to come to the fore in the summer of 1994 when the American Association of Physicians for Human Rights (now the Gay and Lesbian Medical Association), a gay doctors' group, hosted a summit conference in Dallas that brought together 150 of the most influential "opinion shapers" in the nation working on the AIDS problem among gay men and lesbians. The purpose was to exchange new ideas, propose bold new strategies, and send gay prevention workers off in brave new directions.

Dallas was a defining moment in the demise of the condom code, but it hardly seemed recognized as such by most of its participants. No one at any of the seminars and forums and encounter groups I attended questioned the ultimate viability of the code, nor was it questioned in the thick published report that was sent to summit participants a few months later. In that report, organizers listed the five big issues that dominated discussions. First and foremost was the issue of "how and whether HIV-negative and HIV-positive men should be separately targeted," essentially endorsing the commonsense idea of pitching the condom code differently to

HIV-negative and HIV-positive men. The second concerned the empowerment of affected communities, with many attendees expressing "strongly held beliefs that gay and bisexual men of color and youth should have the resources to design and carry out their own prevention strategies" to promote the condom code to their communities. The third was "building community" and "reducing both internalized and societal homophobia." One could hardly argue with these goals, perhaps the most basic goals of gay liberation, yet in the context of AIDS prevention they tended to gloss over studies presented at the conference indicating that new infections were raging in the most cohesive gay communities, and among men with the strongest gay identity. The fourth was challenging "the pervasive perception that HIV is not a lesbian issue." And finally the conference endorsed the idea of actually evaluating prevention programs to see what works and what doesn't, something that had almost never been done in the past, and that has remained rare ever since.

Published along with this evaluation were dozens of specific one-sentence recommendations for action by individual summit participants. There was much written about identity and identity politics. "Combat bi and transphobia in lesbian and gay organizations." "Remember that substance abuse treatment must address queerness." And there were lots of process suggestions: "Move the focus of HIV prevention from a disease model to a health promotion model." "Establish a national mailing list of services for HIV negative people." And finally, as if this meeting were not discouraging enough, there were recommendations to repeat it across the nation.

What is striking about these undoubtedly well-meaning suggestions is how irrelevant most are to the actual crisis of transmission. Absent from the summit were discussions of the role of multiple partners in HIV transmission, or the role of core groups, or versatile anal sex, or almost any substantive discussions of gay sexual ecology. No one raised the question of why the epidemic was not spreading randomly throughout the heterosexual population. Few had the bad taste to mention the resurgence of sex clubs or bathhouses. Virtually no one questioned the feasibility of the condom code at all. A couple of speakers briefly mentioned the possibility that gay culture subtly encourages unsafe sex even as it purportedly tries not to, but little was made of this. The condom code was a given; the problem was how to get more people to comply more often. And this despite the fact that several of the most educated, informed men at the conference admitted to having recently failed to use condoms during anal sex.

AIDS Groups and Sexual Libertarians

What could explain this myopia? How is it possible that at a forum of the most influential thinkers on AIDS prevention in the gay world, virtually no one was willing to discuss what any college-level instructor in epidemiology would consider the most basic biological reasons for the epidemic's continuation? The answer, it seems, is political rather than medical.

Under different political circumstances, one might expect that prevention advocates would focus almost exclusively on the kinds of changes needed to contain the epidemic, leaving no subject off the table. That kind of freewheeling discussion is the norm in other realms where public health is the issue, such as highway safety. Car safety advocates and consumer groups are generally quite fearless in exposing the reasons why automobiles and highways are unsafe, and quite adamant in proposing measures— lower speed limits, helmet laws, seat belt laws, the improvement of car safety—even when those measures involve some restrictions on the individual's absolute right to drive fast and free, or car manufacturers' rights to earn a maximum profit. Since many of these proposals conflict with the political or financial aspirations of others, opposition arises to them from car makers and "anti-helmet" and "anti–speed limit" libertarians whose primary concerns are, respectively, profits and absolute personal freedom, and for whom safety is secondary when it conflicts with those concerns. From the inevitable tension and debate between these two forces, compromises in strategies are hammered out.

If the world of AIDS prevention worked that way, the process might look like this. Gay AIDS prevention advocates at forums like the Dallas meeting would fight tenaciously to develop strategies designed to contain new infections, even to the point of advocating unpopular things such as bathhouse regulation, provided a strong case could be made that such sacrifices might lower HIV transmission below the epidemic threshold. Meanwhile, bathhouse owners and sexual libertarians would fight for profits and absolute sexual freedom first, and put concern about AIDS second. These two sides would slug it out, and a practical solution would emerge somewhere between the two positions.

This has not occurred in the field of gay AIDS prevention, however. The prevention movement, like the gay world generally, is intensely focused on sexual liberty and privacy concerns, and practically everyone working in AIDS prevention, from staffers in community-based organizations to more radical AIDS activists in groups like ACT UP, generally come from the ranks of sexual libertarians. Many have retained their primary allegiance to the principle of almost absolute sexual liberty even as they have risen to responsible positions in the prevention movement. Indeed, many say that the primary reason they got involved in AIDS prevention in the first place was to fight from the inside to keep prevention from being used to challenge sexual liberty. Most of these folks are well intentioned, and many sincerely believe they are being practical, since they argue that any safer sex message that does not explicitly validate the principles of gay male sexual freedom would be rejected by the very people it most needs to reach.

In any event, the traditional balance between those who would put prevention first and those who would put profits and/or absolute freedom first is almost completely absent from the equation. There are powerful voices arguing for absolute sexual freedom, filling prevention agencies, health departments, and civil liberties groups with staffers committed to resisting any impingement on sexual freedom for any reason whatsoever. And there are powerful forces fighting to turn the maximum profit from gay sex, filling the pages of gay magazines and newspapers with sexy ads enticing gay men to, as one ad for a Miami disco party put it, "go ahead and cross the line." But there are virtually no powerful forces within the gay AIDS prevention movement arguing for prevention first. Indeed, among the "new approaches" to AIDS, the most heralded ones actually seem likely to increase transmission, not lessen it.

Openness

One of those approaches is based on the idea that a major way to address unsafe sex is for gay men to begin publicly talking about the unsafe sex they personally have. According to this idea, safer sex has become a moral posture among gay men, which has rendered the whole subject of occasional unsafe sex a sort of taboo. As a result, those who are trying but failing to stay safe have a difficult time talking about their lapses, since they are ashamed to admit them. Unsafe behavior has become the loony aunt in the attic of gay life, unspoken and, because of its silence, beyond help. The advocates of openness argue that we need to erase the taboo against unsafe sex to make it possible for people to talk honestly about the unsafe sex they are having.

However, this leaves a nagging contradiction unaddressed. If gay men begin making a virtue of confessing that they don't always have safer sex, and are applauded when they do, won't that create a new community norm in which unsafe sex is acceptable? After all, urging people within a community to admit openly to a certain behavior and insisting that no stigma be attached to it when they do seems like a very effective way of creating a new community norm validating that behavior. And if community norms are among the most powerful motivators of behavior, won't that lead to more unsafe sex, not less?

In a sense, the widely touted "openness" policy seeks to do for unsafe sex what gay liberation does for homosexuality: bring it out of the closet and normalize it. As such it finds deep resonance among gay leaders and prevention workers accustomed to the idea that all stigma is inherently bad, all openness and honesty good. But there's a big difference between AIDS prevention and gay liberation. We attack anti-gay stigma in order to encourage homosexuality to flourish. But if we attack the stigma against unsafe behavior, we might just do the same for that. If strong community norms against unsafe sex are the bedrock upon which individual behavior change is built, a new community norm of openness and acceptance of unsafe sex might crack that foundation beyond repair.

Yet as the debate heated up in the mid nineties, gay men witnessed a major national trend in this direction. At the Dallas summit a number of top prevention leaders stood up and admitted to having had unsafe anal sex in the preceding months. Afterward similar accounts began appearing in newspapers and magazines and community forums around the nation, as writers and activists electrified the prevention movement by openly admitting to having unsafe sex. This certainly opened up the subject and dragged it out of the closet. But it is questionable whether it made gay men, particularly younger gay men, feel there was much that anyone could do about it. After all, if the leaders of AIDS prevention have unsafe sex, what hope was there for the average Joe?

Responsibility

As we have seen, another new idea in prevention is the idea of targeting positives and negatives with different messages. Many proponents of this idea argue that a major flaw of AIDS prevention has been its failure to acknowledge that infected and uninfected men have fundamentally different reasons for having safe sex. The motivation of the uninfected is clearly to save themselves. The motivation of the already infected is altruism, the desire not to infect others. It is plausibly argued that these two basic motivations are so different that they deserve separate educational campaigns, one for negatives and one for positives.

This idea makes a lot of sense, and has received the endorsement of many professionals, behavior change experts, psychologists, and others involved in prevention. The problem is that while everyone seems comfortable with the half of the message telling HIV-negative men why it is in their best interests to stay uninfected, almost no prevention group has been comfortable with the other half, the part directed at telling positive men why they have a moral responsibility not to risk infecting others, even if those others are momentarily willing to assume risk. Such a message is considered judgmental and stigmatizing by some and useless by others, who argue that positive men are so volatile that they are beyond appeals to conscience.

Indeed, the very idea that HIV-positive men have a responsibility not to infect others is seen by some as judgmental and stigmatizing. In a 1996 essay in the *New England Journal of Medicine*, ethicist Ronald Bayer described how, in the early years of the epidemic, "the very idea of responsibility . . . was viewed as alien and threatening. It was a concept more common to the moral and religious right, which had shown a profound indifference to the plight of those with AIDS." Many prevention experts argued that emphasizing HIV-positive responsibility could increase risk by lulling the uninfected into a false sense of security, and that it might lead us down a slippery slope toward criminalization of infected people. In seeking to maintain solidarity with the infected, they emphasized that if everyone simply protects themselves, no one can be harmed without their own consent.

This attitude has remained so entrenched into the nineties that when New York City was preparing to mark its fifty-thousandth AIDS case in 1993 by launching a campaign that urged the HIV positive to protect others as well as themselves, it had to be canceled when forces within the city health bureaucracy objected that this was a dangerous form of blaming the victim. As a result, the enlightened concept that different strategies need to be addressed with the infected and the uninfected has in most cases only been half instituted. Those who are uninfected continue to be told to protect themselves. Those who are positive are essentially told the same thing, or nothing at all.

Oral Substitution

Another major new approach in prevention is the idea that gay men should be encouraged to have unprotected oral sex. The theory behind this strategy is that a prime reason gay men are having so much unsafe anal sex is that they have been led to believe, falsely, that unprotected oral sex is risky. As a result, they develop a feeling of hopelessness about ever being able to survive the epidemic, and just give up, returning to unprotected anal sex. To combat this trend, the theory goes, gay men should be encouraged to believe that unprotected oral sex is safe, or in the parlance of prevention, "low risk."

Walt Odets puts it this way:

> Were we to support gay and bisexual men in the practice of ordinary oral sex—with or without ejaculation in the mouth—it is likely that we would see an overall reduction in HIV transmission. This probability rests on the probabilities that we would see a reduction in the incidence of anal sex; an even greater reduction in the incidence of semen exchange through anal sex; and would help place the task of protected-sex-for-a-lifetime back in the realm of possibility.

Former Shanti Project director Eric Rofes goes even further. The gay male community, he writes, needs to shape "a major, long-term commitment to stop scaring men away from oral sex and to allow the elevation of cocksucking, including the swallowing of semen, as the central act of gay identity. A wide variety of strategies should be encouraged which, over the long haul, shift giving head into the position currently occupied by getting fucked."

While this purports to be a new and revolutionary strategy that challenges traditional skittishness about oral sex among American AIDS prevention groups, it actually dovetails with the advice most gay-run AIDS prevention programs have been giving for years. These programs have long relegated oral sex to a fairly low position in the hierarchy of risk. The wording of a 1991 brochure by New York's GMHC is typical of this approach: "Sucking and getting sucked without coming are considered low risk for HIV transmission," it advises. "You're the only one who can decide how risky you want to get." This is followed by several explicit tips on how to reduce risk when having unprotected oral sex.

Many of those supporting this "oral substitution" strategy seem to be calling for two distinct but related approaches. The first is that AIDS educators and activists need to "stop scaring" people about oral sex. The second urges gay men to elevate oral sex to the place currently occupied by anal sex. Neither promotes an ecological message or makes any attempt to discourage people from having multiple or concurrent partners, but rather both assume that they will. In that sense, both are consonant with a basic impetus behind the condom code—keep the multipartner gay sexual ethic alive. But both seem extremely problematic and poorly thought out, and if implemented might just result in an increase in infections.

At first glance it might seem that a call to "stop scaring" people about oral sex merely requires us to refrain from *overestimating* its risk. That, of course, is reasonable. After all, AIDS education is supposed to rest on a bedrock of truth, and educators should never overestimate the risk of anything. But it's difficult to square any imperative to "stop scaring" people about oral sex with truth telling. After all, if the imperative is to stop scaring, what do we do with evidence that oral sex does carry some risk? Unfortunately, there is a great deal of such evidence—anecdotal, bench, epidemiological, and theoretical. It has been trickling in for years and will continue to do so. If AIDS education is about truth telling, and oral substitution is about not scaring people, what happens when the truth is scary?

Some advocates of oral substitution maintain that this question is moot: The risk of oral sex is "low," they say, and any evidence to the contrary is simply wrong. But what is low? Sadly, whether we like it or not, many scientists, researchers, and doctors, not to mention individual gay men who believe they were orally infected, maintain that oral sex holds a risk that is significantly higher than many gay men would feel comfortable with. Researchers working on this question are unsure of the relative risk, but some have placed the comparative odds of infection between oral and anal sex at from 1 in 5 to around 1 in 10. Certainly anyone committed to informed consent should not object to giving people all the data to make an informed decision, even data that might scare them. Which brings up another major problem with oral substitution: its apparent elitism. Instead of full disclosure, it seeks to put a "spin" on the way gay men receive information, a spin designed to manipulate gay men into a sense of security about oral sex, a sense they might not have if they were simply given the facts.

Many prevention activists committed to spin-doctoring oral risk are unabashed in their criticism of those who simply present the facts. After I published a lengthy article in *Out* magazine about the current state of knowledge about oral risk, I was chastised by one prominent educator who told me that although the article seemed both balanced and accurate, it was "misguided for the simple reason that if we're going to steer men toward sucking, any discussion of the risks of oral sex amounts to overemphasis." And of course that is correct. A campaign to "stop scaring" people requires AIDS educators and journalists to "stop reporting" anything that might scare them. Including the truth.

The worst excesses of those who champion oral substitution, however, are their attempts to discredit individuals who claim to have been infected through oral sex. This usually involves calling such people liars and arguing that they *cannot* have gotten infected in the way they say they did, and that they should therefore shut up about it. This flies in the face of every message of self-empowerment that animates the PWA activist movement. So in the end, the "don't scare" strategy does not merely ask us to refrain from scaring. It actively requires us to minimize potentially scary studies, criticize those who refuse to play along, and, worst of all, silence with shame those who believe they were infected through oral sex.

The second part of the strategy purports to be boldly transformative. It calls for a cultural commitment to promote oral sex as the "central act" of gay sexuality under the assumption that if men become more comfortable about sucking, they will stop fucking. This is a very tempting idea. After all, if every gay man who currently has unprotected anal sex switched to oral sex, it is virtually certain that new infections would decline dramatically. The more germane question is, if men become convinced that oral sex is very low risk or even risk free, will they stop having anal sex, which after all is the strategy's entire point?

Unfortunately, there is no need to turn to experts in psychological forecasting for an answer. That future utopia in which most gay men believe oral sex is relatively safe is the world we have been living in since the late eighties. Since that time the vast majority of gay men have been told by their peers, their AIDS institutions, and their culture, and have constantly reaffirmed to themselves, that sucking is, if not absolutely safe, at least reasonably so. And major studies have shown that the vast majority have believed it, and have acted on that belief.

Take, for example, the 1987 Communication Technologies study in which self-identified gay men were asked to rank the risk of HIV transmission on a 10-point scale, with 10 being the most risky activity and 1 being completely safe. These men rated unprotected receptive anal sex at 9.8 on this scale, about as risky as you can get. Anal sex with condoms was rated at 3.5, about as safe as anything is likely to be during a fatal STD epidemic. And unprotected oral sex without ejaculation was rated at 3.7. In other worlds, even at the height of the Fear, gay men believed that unprotected oral sex was about as safe as the safer anal sex they were being encouraged to practice by most AIDS organizations. And they acted on that belief. In most studies, between 80 and 90 percent of all gay men report engaging in unprotected oral sex.

The same was still true in the mid nineties, when I wrote the article mentioned above. "I have always considered receptive oral sex without ejaculation to be safe, and the information in your [article] shocked me," began a letter to the editor. A second published letter was much the same. "As a twenty-two-year-old, I have been told all my short sex life that oral sex without a condom is safe." Those letters were typical of countless comments I received. Many men were aware of some vague risk associated with ingesting semen, but had always assumed that such risk was extremely low, and that the risk without swallowing was essentially zero.

If there is any difference between the late eighties and mid nineties in this regard, it is the openness and confidence with which men in the nineties are having unprotected oral sex with multiple partners. Back in the mid and late eighties oral sex had largely retreated behind closed doors. Men continued to engage in it, but somewhat more carefully and seemingly with fewer partners. Sex clubs in New York and other major cities absolutely forbade oral sex, enforcing a strict "lips above the hips" rule that was meekly accepted by virtually everybody. When the first generation of new sex clubs that allowed oral sex appeared in the late eighties, many gay men and lesbians were scandalized. In 1989 New York's chapter of ACT UP debated whether to picket a well-known disco that had recently opened a back room in which sucking was allowed, and pressured the promoter to hire monitors to prevent the activity. But by the mid nineties oral sex had become the primary activity in many commercial establishments, and nobody was batting an eye.

Yet this increased relaxation about oral sex has not resulted in a decline in unprotected anal sex. Quite the opposite. Rates of unprotected anal sex have increased during the same period that gay men have become more open about unprotected sucking. So instead of providing evidence that a belief in the safety of oral sex leads to a reduction in anal sex, current experience indicates that if anything, the opposite may be true. It seems possible that gay male sexual practices do not operate like a seesaw, where if one practice goes up the other invariably goes down, but operate instead more like a wave, where practices rise and fall together. While this is obviously speculation, the least that can be said is that the burden of proof clearly falls to anyone who argues that increased confidence in and practice of unprotected oral sex will necessarily result in a shift away from anal sex. The only thing we can say with any measure of confidence is that this has not happened so far, and that encouraging unprotected oral sex, especially with multiple partners, will surely result in a rise in oral transmissions of many serious

STDs, since many people who otherwise might have practiced oral sex with caution, or with fewer partners, will have been led to believe there is no need.

Still, this has not stopped the "new prevention" juggernaut from endorsing the concept of oral substitution. About a year after the Dallas summit, posters headed ORAL SEX *IS* SAFER SEX were published by the innovative AIDS Action Committee of Massachusetts, and similar messages began to be disseminated by other groups. In 1996 the highly respected Gay and Lesbian Medical Association, after what it called "exhaustive and deliberate study," adopted the position that unprotected male-to-male oral sex should be classified as "low risk for HIV," and urged prevention groups that characterize it as "high risk" or even "somewhat risky" to "revise their materials accordingly."

Just weeks later gay men were frightened by a widely reported study in *Science* that six out of seven rhesus monkeys had been infected by the simian AIDS virus, or SIV, after researchers dabbed it on the backs of their mouths.

Fear Elimination

Another strain of thought prominent at "new prevention" venues is the idea that fear of AIDS is not, and ought not to be, a motivating factor in prevention. In a sense, the use of fear has become politically incorrect in many gay prevention circles, and attempts to bolster gay men's fear of AIDS are often seen as homophobic, counterproductive, and ineffective.

Part of the reason is that throughout the AIDS epidemic the public has harbored intense prejudice against HIV-infected people, leading to discrimination, stigma, even violence. Partly as a result, the HIV self-empowerment movement has struggled to destigmatize AIDS. One way is to emphasize the inherent innocence of all people with the disease. Another is to portray HIV infection as not such a terrible thing. People are said to live with AIDS, not die from it. The gay press in particular is filled with accounts of sexy, healthy-looking men living normal lives with HIV infection. Yet this strategy, too, runs the risk of increasing rather than decreasing new infections. Fear, after all, is the central motivating factor in prevention. Simply put, people seek to prevent what they fear. If they don't fear the consequences of a particular behavior, why should they bother struggling to avoid those consequences? Especially when the struggle is so difficult, and the behavior so enticing, pleasurable, and meaningful. So when prevention pundits argue that gay men cannot base a prevention strategy on fear, they appear to misread the very core motivating factor of prevention.

Defining Survival Down

As prevention workers concluded that absolute adherence to the condom code is unlikely, a frightening trend emerged in AIDS prevention in the mid nineties, a trend one might call "defining survival down." Many prevention workers came to believe that there was virtually no chance that prevention could contain the epidemic. Therefore, they said, we must hope for a technological rescue and in the meantime stop focusing excessively on "biological survival" and recognize that other kinds of survival are equally, or even more, important.

Again, perhaps the most eloquent proponent of this idea is California psychologist Walt Odets. "In a lifetime event of this destructiveness," he writes, "we are not addressing the human needs of the gay community by offering—or insisting on—biological survival as an exclusive and adequate purpose for human life. *Survival* must include the idea of meaningful human survival for a community that has traditionally been scorned or punished for the way it makes love, communicates intimacy, and creates human bonds. New approaches to education must take as their *primary* task such purposes. The reduction of HIV can only be a *secondary* task because it must be built on the foundation of lives experienced as worth the trouble [his italics]."

Odets is critical of those who insist on equating survival with longevity. "Has the 80-year-old man, unrealized, disheartened and disappointed with his life, survived in any important way?" he asks. "Has the 30-year-old who has contributed much to family, friends, lover, and society, but is now dying of AIDS, failed to survive in a human sense? This far into the AIDS epidemic, many find it self-evident that merely surviving the epidemic biologically is not an adequate goal, but that we must insist on lives as human beings who, above all, develop or regain our capacities to live fully and passionately."

Apparently in some cases that life of passion will include, even demand, doing things that put one at risk of HIV infection. "If some gay men feel that the fullest, richest possible life demands behaviors that may also expose them to HIV," Odets asks, "who are educators to tell them they are wrong?" He states unequivocally that "we cannot stop HIV transmission or end the epidemic through behavioral approaches without exacting catastrophic psychological and human costs. And we cannot burden every single gay with that implied task." He concludes his book *In the Shadow of the Epidemic* with what sounds like an appeal to throw off the shackles of the condom code and embrace our doom:

> [S]tingy, lonely, ruined lives will be hatched out of the fear that now tempts many of us to circle guard, in unconscious hopes of immortality, around our own living corpses—ferociously protecting lives not worth living, because they are sacrificed to nothing but their own extension. . . . We must come out as a people who refuse to live in denial or fear, who refuse to be separated from each other in life by the prospect of death, and who value life too much to spend it on nothing but its own preservation.

In the absence of a sound approach to curbing the epidemic within the crumbling edifice of the condom code, such Strangelovian "How I Learned to Stop Worrying and Love HIV" pronouncements began fast gaining ground in the nineties. And indeed, for those having genuine difficulty maintaining the condom code and incapable or unwilling to look beyond it, what other choice was there but to embrace a culture of disease?

CHAPTER 7

The Ecology of "Heterosexual AIDS"

Perhaps nothing better illustrates the fact that the condom code is fraught with serious limitations than the fact that entire populations that hardly ever use condoms remain almost completely free of AIDS, while others that use condoms with fairly high levels of consistency remain saturated with the disease. The highly selective spread of AIDS through heterosexual populations vividly illustrates the fact that overall sexual ecology is the chief determinant of whether or not AIDS will gain or maintain a foothold.

Early in the epidemic many people believed that, as Dr. Mathilde Krim remarked in 1988, it was "a fluke of fate that AIDS landed in the gay community," and that the syndrome would soon spread randomly and relentlessly throughout the entire world. Yet by the mid nineties this has clearly not occurred. AIDS has spread in an epidemic fashion among certain heterosexual populations, but its pattern is far from random. In the Third World it has grown exponentially, but only in some regions and even in those regions, only among some groups. Among most it has barely made a dent. Here in the West it has not exploded at all, but rather remained concentrated among the same groups of heterosexuals in whom it was first noticed in the mid eighties—primarily injection drug users (IDUs) and their sexual partners. This extreme selectivity underscores a basic fact: that AIDS is neither a gay nor a straight disease, but rather one that spreads under certain ecological conditions. Where it finds those conditions, either among heterosexuals or homosexuals, it thrives. Where it does not, its incidence is occasional and sporadic.

Panic in Hetero Park

In the mid eighties, the predictions that heterosexual AIDS would lead to general catastrophe could hardly have been more alarming. Perhaps the single greatest turning point in the public's perception was the announcement of Rock Hudson's illness. But the public was already well primed for hysteria: The cover of the *Life* magazine that happened to be sitting on the newsstands the week *before* Hudson's illness was announced in July of 1985 proclaimed NOW NO ONE IS SAFE FROM AIDS. For many people, Hudson's case only reinforced that warning, which in a few years appeared not only prescient, but mild.

"Research studies now project," Oprah Winfrey told her TV audience in February 1987, "that one in five—listen to me, hard to believe—one in five heterosexuals could be dead from AIDS at the end of the next three years. That's by 1990. One in five. It's no longer just a gay disease. Believe me." That same year a number of states began sponsoring campaigns with the catchphrase "AIDS Doesn't Discriminate." The next year a four-page brochure was mailed by the surgeon general's office to 107 million households across the nation warning that everyone was at risk. Thousands of panicked heterosexuals flooded the switchboards of AIDS hotlines and swamped public HIV testing sites demanding to be tested. Those tests ended up costing those services millions of dollars at a time when money for prevention was critically short.

Not all of those raising the alarm limited themselves to warning about sex. Some proclaimed that HIV was a sort of doomsday bug that could spread through casual contact. British venerealogist John Seale informed the California Senate Health and Human Services Committee in 1986 that "the genetic information contained in [HIV's] tiny strip of RNA has all that is needed to render the human race extinct within fifty years." Author Gene Antonio's sensationalistic best-selling 1986 book *The AIDS Cover-up*, which sold over

300,000 copies, predicted that 64 million Americans would be HIV infected by 1991.

Although many people dismissed the doomsday theorists as kooks, it was harder to dismiss those who argued that AIDS was rapidly expanding through heterosexual transmission. There were, of course, the stark examples of Central Africa, Thailand, and the Caribbean, where heterosexual intercourse was the primary route of transmission. And plenty of experts warned that what was happening there would soon happen here. In 1988 respected sex therapists William Masters, Virginia Johnson, and Robert Kolodny published *Crisis: Heterosexual Behavior in the Age of AIDS*, in which they theorized that "AIDS is now running rampant in the heterosexual community." Robert Redfield, a specialist in infectious disease at Walter Reed Army Hospital in Washington, warned pointedly that the experience of gay men was about to be repeated by heterosexuals. "As AIDS enters the heterosexual population," he said, "I think it will repeat the rate of spread that occurred in the homosexual population during the last four years." These warnings were widely echoed in the mainstream press and by government spokespeople, until it became virtually an article of faith that soon HIV would cut a vast swath across the middle-class heterosexual population—that is, unless middle-class heterosexuals started adhering to the condom code.

Fumento and the "Myth of Heterosexual AIDS"

The first person to attempt to pierce this solid wall of fear was Michael Fumento, a conservative science writer and former AIDS analyst for the U.S. Commission on Civil Rights. His book *The Myth of Heterosexual AIDS* caused a storm of controversy when it was published in 1990. Fumento reviewed the epidemiology of AIDS in the United States and Western countries and came to a stunning and, at the time, highly inflammatory conclusion: HIV was not spreading widely among heterosexuals and it was not going to. Fumento went further, proposing that powerful social and cultural forces from the conservative Christian right to the gay left were in effect collaborating on the giant hoax of "heterosexual AIDS," each for its own purposes. Conservatives, he wrote, believed that AIDS had the potential to be "a shiny weapon with which to recapture their vision of a better world—one where homosexuality is pushed back into the closet (or further); where chastity, monogamy, and sexual morality are revered; and where sexual behavior is once again within the domain of law." To utilize AIDS as a weapon successfully, conservatives had to scare heterosexuals into believing they were at risk, since fear was the only force strong enough to launch a sexual counterrevolution.

Gays and progressives also pushed the same degaying agenda, Fumento charged, but for opposite reasons. They believed that if the public continued to perceive AIDS as a gay disease this would prove disastrous because "the heterosexual majority, feeling unthreatened, would not support massive funding for research into the prevention and cure of AIDS." Gays also feared, Fumento wrote, that the relentless connection of gay men to AIDS "would increase the stigma attached to homosexuality."

Fumento's book was hostile to gay people and marred by a sensationalistic tabloid style. Its very title *The Myth of Heterosexual AIDS* was grabby but misleading since, as Fumento pointed out in the text, people certainly get HIV from heterosexual intercourse. (A more accurate title might have been something like *The Myth of a Universal AIDS Pandemic*.) In particular, Fumento's credibility was undermined in the gay community by his pervasive anti-gay bias, a bias that made many gay activists feel that his anti-degaying agenda was essentially anti-gay. As British AIDS educator Edward King points out, "Fumento views practicing homosexuality as disgusting and unnatural. For example, he opines that the act of rimming is 'vile,' and maintains that 'certain bodily orifices seem to be two-way and others one-way, and if it were questionable where the rectum falls, AIDS has helped decide the issue.' "

Yet King, one of England's most prominent AIDS authors and educators, admits that while it is "unpopular" to say it in gay circles, "Fumento's book is an important and convincing one. When read as a whole, his case—and particularly his analysis of epidemiology—is very strong indeed. It is therefore all the more unfortunate that Fumento's agenda in publishing *The Myth of Heterosexual AIDS* appears to be highly questionable and, some would say, pernicious."

Unfortunate indeed. Fumento's predictions were not only scorned in the gay world, they were deemed part of an anti-gay conspiracy, a lie, a deliberate downplaying of the seriousness of the coming universal pandemic. In gay and AIDS activist circles Fumento's name became synonymous with attempts to twist or distort epidemiology. A writer at my own magazine, *OutWeek*, launched a scathing attack on *New York Newsday* (my future employer) for having the temerity to employ Fumento as a book reviewer. The idea that Fumento was perpetrating a homophobic hoax became so entrenched in gay and AIDS prevention circles that it has been difficult ever since to acknowledge that his epidemiological predictions have come true.

Perhaps the largest single piece of evidence backing him up came in a stunning 1993 report issued by the National Academy of Sciences. The report, a 320-page book written by the National Research Council and titled *The Social Impact of AIDS in the United States*, contained a bombshell. AIDS, the council wrote, was about to "disappear" in America. Not because the disease itself was abating—in that sense things were worse than ever. But, the researchers wrote, the AIDS epidemic "is settling into spatially and socially isolated groups and possibly becoming endemic within them." Instead of spreading out to the broad population, as was once feared, "HIV is concentrating in pools of persons who are also caught in the 'synergism of plagues.' "

Calling it their "major conclusion," the researchers said they believed that "many geographical areas and strata of the population are virtually untouched by the epidemic and probably never will be," while "certain confined areas and populations have been devastated and are likely to continue to be." AIDS would soon disappear, they concluded, "because those who continue to be affected by it are socially invisible, beyond the sight and attention of the majority population."

Primary, Secondary, and Tertiary Transmission

To begin any discussion of why heterosexual AIDS remains largely confined to certain populations, it's important to define our terms, starting with *heterosexual AIDS* itself. (The following paragraphs refer only to AIDS in the developed world. I will discuss the Third World experience, which is quite different, later in the chapter.)

Any sexual transmission between a man and a woman can be

called heterosexual transmission, and the resulting disease, heterosexual AIDS. But researchers sometimes find it useful to divide transmission into three categories: primary, secondary, and tertiary, since these categories illustrate major and important differences in the way we conceptualize transmission.

Primary transmission is any HIV transmission that results from the primary risk behaviors that were identified in the early years of the epidemic, behaviors that still lead to the majority of new infections in the United States and other developed countries. These are anal sex between men, needle sharing, and also, to a much lesser extent, the transfusion or injection of infected blood products.

Secondary transmission occurs when a person who was infected through one of these primary routes then infects someone through heterosexual sex. Most heterosexual AIDS in the United States and other developed nations results from secondary transmission, mainly from male IDUs to their female sex partners.

Tertiary transmission occurs when a person who was infected through heterosexual sex then infects another person through heterosexual sex. By definition, a self-sustaining heterosexual epidemic would consist of a level of tertiary transmission above the epidemic threshold, or "tipping point." This is naturally what most people tend to imagine when they think of a heterosexual AIDS epidemic, namely, AIDS that is spreading rapidly through the population via heterosexual sex. But while this is happening in certain societies in the developing world, it is clearly not occurring in the developed world. There is sporadic tertiary transmission, since it is certainly possible for a person infected through heterosexual sex to infect someone else that way. But two decades after HIV began its relentless exponential spread through gay and IDU populations, tertiary transmission still does not appear to have risen to epidemic levels among heterosexuals in the developed world. Most heterosexual transmission remains secondary, a result of IDUs infecting their female sexual partners. In effect, IDUs form the critical core group that sustains infection in the heterosexual population. If transmissions among injection drug users are brought under control, perhaps through a combination of clean needle availability and better access to drug rehabilitation, many experts contend that the problem of heterosexual AIDS in the developed world will largely subside.

Factors Affecting Heterosexual Transmission

Why has HIV transmission failed to rise above the epidemic threshold among heterosexuals in most developed countries? Part of the answer is biological, part behavioral. If we consider diseases in an ascending order of transmission, from most easily spread to most difficult, a simple fact emerges. The more difficult a disease is to transmit, the more important specific behaviors are in transmitting it. If, for example, you have an STD that's very easy for anyone to catch in just a single sexual episode with a single partner, practically anybody who is not monogamous is at risk. But with a disease whose transmission does not become statistically likely until you've had ten sexual episodes with ten different partners, a much smaller group will be at risk. And with a disease that requires an average of 100 episodes with 100 partners, only a tiny group will be in danger. Put simply, differences of behavior become increasingly significant the more difficult the disease agent is to spread.

For all people, gay and straight, male and female, the strain of HIV that has so far predominated in the Western world appears to be the most difficult to transmit of all known venereal pathogens. As a result, differences in group sexual behavior become more significant for AIDS than for any other STD. Risk for individual heterosexuals is a function of the same three variables we've already discussed: the infectivity of the disease in any given instance of sex, the rate of partner change, and the prevalence of the disease in one's pool of potential partners. In all three cases, the biology of HIV, the physiology of heterosexual intercourse, and the basic behavior of most heterosexuals in the developed world combine to keep the level of transmission below the epidemic's tipping point.

Infectivity. Men can transmit HIV efficiently to women, but women are nowhere near as efficient in transmitting it back to men. According to the World Health Organization, the likelihood of an infected woman passing her infection to a man in a single instance of unprotected intercourse is approximately 1 in 1,000, whereas the likelihood of a man infecting a woman is 1 in 100. One reason is that the vagina has exposed internal mucous membranes through which the virus can be transmitted directly to the bloodstream, and infected fluids often remain in the vagina for hours, giving HIV plenty of time to find an entry. The corresponding surface in the penis is the urethra, which has far less exposed area than the interior of the vagina. When the uninfected man has an untreated venereal sore, as is often the case in the developing world, his risk of becoming infected rises to 1 in 250, but this is a fairly rare circumstance in areas where people have good access to health care. As a result, a viral dead end factor in the developed world impedes one of the main requirements of epidemic amplification, which is an efficient flow in both directions.

Partner Change. Gathering accurate information about rates of heterosexual partner change can be tricky, since survey results can differ depending on who conducted them, on the survey techniques used, and on the group surveyed. However, surveys throughout the Western world show essentially the same themes: Heterosexuals today have more partners than they did in earlier generations, mainly because they're having intercourse earlier in life, marrying later, and divorcing more often. But they are also overwhelmingly likely to have most of their partners when they are in their late teens and early twenties, before they settle down with a single partner. Afterward they tend to have relatively few lifetime partners compared to gay men or even to heterosexuals in many other cultures.

The largest single study of Americans' sexual behavior, the *Sex in America* survey published in 1994, found that 67 percent of men and 75 percent of women said they had only one partner in the previous year, and that throughout their lifetimes, 66 percent of men and 90 percent of women had ten or fewer partners. Only 9 percent of the entire sample of Americans (17 percent of men and 3 percent of women) said they had more than twenty-one lifetime partners. This study was criticized because investigators interviewed people face-to-face in their homes, a factor that probably resulted in undercounting numbers of partners. But what is so striking about its results is how well they correlate with surveys that have been criticized for the opposite reason, because their self-selected respondents might overestimate their number of partners. The *Janus Report*, for instance, has been criticized for this reason, and indeed people in its sample claimed to have more partners than those in the *Sex in America* sample. Yet almost three quarters of the Janus respondents had fewer than thirty lifetime partners, and only 15 percent of divorcees, 9 percent of singles, and 5 percent of married people reported over a hundred lifetime partners. And among virtually all segments of the heterosexual population the vast majority of partners were racked up early in adulthood, roughly from ages sixteen to twenty-six.

Not only do heterosexuals have relatively few partners, but many report being faithful to their partners once they are either married or involved in a serious relationship. Various studies, from the *Kinsey Report* to the *Redbook Report on Female Sexuality* to the *Almanac of the American People*, indicate that about one third to slightly more than one half of heterosexuals in American couples have been unfaithful to their partners at least once during marriage. Kinsey, for example, found that 50 percent of married men and 26 percent of women engaged in extramarital sex at least once, and other studies found similar results. What is perhaps more important for sexual ecology than the percentage of people who commit adultery is how often they do it and the number of partners they do it with. If the average adulterer in a given population has sex with only one or two people over the course of a marriage, that will have a dramatically different effect on population-wide transmission of disease than if the average adulterer has relations with 50 people, or 500. And it appears that the aggregate number of partners in heterosexual adultery is quite low. One study of middle-class white respondents, for example, found that 11 percent of husbands had between two and five adulterous partners, 6 percent had between six and twenty, and 2 percent had more than twenty. Among wives, 8 percent had two to five extra partners, 3 percent had six to twenty, and only 1 percent had more than twenty. In addition, many of those who are unfaithful tend to be faithful much of the time. Only a very small proportion of heterosexuals in long-term marriages are regular adulterers, and the percentage who regularly patronize prostitutes is in the low single digits for men and virtually zero for women. As a result, the magnifying effects of concurrency (lots of partners in the same time period, which can increase disease transmission manyfold) are not likely to occur in most American heterosexual populations.

Comparing these figures with those of gay men in the pre-AIDS era is like viewing two different worlds. Bell and Weinberg's highly regarded 1978 book *Homosexualities*, written at the time when HIV was beginning its spread into the gay population, reported that 75 percent of white gay men had more than a hundred lifetime partners, 43 percent had more than five hundred, and close to one third had more than a thousand. They also reported that 39 percent of gay men were in a major relationship with a significant other, but that only 14 percent were in what the researchers termed a "closed," or monogamous, relationship. Researchers found that 66 percent of gay male couples were not monogamous within the first two years of the relationship, 89 percent were not monogamous in the period from two to ten years, and 94 percent were not monogamous in relationships older than ten years.

The difference is so pronounced that in discussing the data with both straight and gay friends, I have found a general reluctance on either side to believe what they were hearing about the other. Many heterosexuals find it hard to believe that a third of gay men in the seventies had over a thousand lifetime partners. Michael Callen wrote that "by the age of twenty-six I'd had an estimated three thousand different men up my butt," and that when he mentioned this fact, people gasped. "My sense is that . . . most people who are not familiar with the fast lane simply can't fathom how such sexual feats were logistically possible." Meanwhile, men in gay communities often cannot believe that many heterosexuals pass through life with so few partners, and remain sexually faithful to the same partner long after the initial attraction has mellowed. Within the course of one day I was told by a straight colleague that "any gay man who says he's had a thousand partners has to be a liar," and told by a gay friend that "any straight man who says he's faithful to his wife is probably lying." Most people tend to believe their own experience. Yet STD transmission does not discriminate. Throughout the sexual revolution of the seventies, STD rates rose by an annual 1 percent in the heterosexual population and 12 percent among gay men, mirroring these reported differences between gay and straight behavior.

Heterosexual Risk Groups

Despite this apparent lack of a self-sustaining heterosexual epidemic, women are now the fastest-growing proportion of people with AIDS. This fact is often highlighted in the media, and leads to the impression that there is a self-sustaining heterosexual epidemic.

In fact, most women are infected not by men who were themselves infected heterosexually by another woman (tertiary infection), but by men who were infected through injection drug use (secondary infection). Injection drug users can create highly efficient core groups that in some circumstances have amplified HIV to saturation levels. It all depends on how much needle sharing is going on. In areas of the West Coast where users tend to buy drugs individually and inject them alone at home, infection rates among IDUs have remained fairly low. But in cities where shooting galleries are common, rates are catastrophically high. This is largely the case among inner-city neighborhoods on the East Coast and in the South, and in such areas HIV infection is so high that adult female residents—the potential sex partners of these men—are at serious risk. That is one reason why heterosexual AIDS is no "myth." Since the risks are faced disproportionately by African-American and Latina women, the idea that it is can amount to a dangerous form of racism.

But although core groups of drug users have spread infection to many women, those women have tended not to spread infection beyond themselves and their children. The apparent reason is that such women do not themselves constitute the kind of sexual core group that's likely to radiate infection outward. Remember, people in cores need to play two basic roles: place themselves at heightened risk of infection and, once infected, place others at heightened risk. Most female partners of IDUs satisfy half of that equation—they put themselves at risk by having unprotected sex with male IDUs or former IDUs. But in general they do not tend to have the very large numbers of partners that a woman needs to have in order to infect an average of more than one other person. As a result, the real engine of epidemic transmission in these communities is not heterosexual intercourse but needle sharing, which helps explain why AIDS in the inner city has adhered so closely to its original epicenter except in sporadic cases. It is not resulting in a heterosexual epidemic because sex is not its primary engine.

Crack Cocaine

There is, however, one population that has created a self-sustaining epidemic transmitted primarily through heterosexual sex. That is the population of crack cocaine users. Crack cocaine is smoked, not injected, so except in cases where crack users are also injection drug users, most infections among them occur through sex rather than from the direct ingestion of this powerfully addictive drug. Yet crack users form one of the most HIV-infected core populations in the United States. One study of crack-using female prostitutes in the New York metropolitan area found an HIV prevalence rate of 84 percent, perhaps the highest prevalence point ever reported in the United States. The reasons are thoroughly ecological: Crack users form a relatively closed core group characterized by a complex of behaviors that make them highly susceptible to HIV infection, and make them highly likely to pass their infections on to others.

Crack seems to increase susceptibility for several reasons. Constant crack use itself is thought to damage the immune system, both chemically and because addicts often take extremely poor care of themselves, forgo adequate nutrition and medical attention, and harbor untreated diseases of many kinds, including other STDs. Crack addiction often leads to sexually compulsive behavior, often by users who do not use condoms and who are willing to sell their bodies to maintain their access to drugs. Prostitution is endemic among female users, since it's a primary source of obtaining money for the drug during the "binge cycles" of use. One study of female crack users in the Midwest found that 80 percent had exchanged sex for crack and 86 percent had engaged in prostitution to get money to buy the drug in the previous three months. Many crack users have dozens or even hundreds of unsafe partners per year, often within circles where those partners also have similarly high rates of partner change, creating a concentrated sexual ecosystem ideal for the spread of STDs.

The self-sustaining heterosexual HIV epidemic among crack users presents a stark example of how the transmissibility of sexual acts themselves can be altered by ecological factors. For one thing, couples having sex while on crack often engage in prolonged oral or vaginal intercourse that can lead to penile abrasions, which in turn make it easier for men to become infected. So the viral roadblock that inhibits transmission from women to men is often greatly reduced among crack users. In addition, one New York City study of female crack users showed that those who engaged predominantly in fellatio "were significantly more likely to be HIV seropositive than those who performed predominantly other sex practices." The researchers discussed three interrelated reasons why oral sex was more risky among crack users. The first was that "due to crack-induced hypersexual behavior and crack-specific prostitution" women often perform oral sex for very extended periods, and do so with large numbers of partners. The second was that many of these women have poor oral hygiene, and are particularly likely to have burns and cracks on their lips, tongues, and the inside of their mouths from smoking hot crack pipes. Finally, they rarely use condoms for fellatio, even though their partners are highly likely to be HIV infected. One study even found that crack users virtually never used condoms for fellatio because of "a common folk belief . . . that HIV cannot be transmitted through oral sex."

Crack users present a case study of how heterosexual activity can become extremely unsafe by combining several risk factors—unprotected sex with large numbers of partners, chronic drug use, multiple STD and other infections, poor hygiene—within a concentrated population. Crack users have created core groups biologically similar to those that subgroups of gay men created in the seventies and early eighties, with almost identical results as far as HIV is concerned. Their plight clearly illustrates that AIDS is not a gay or a straight epidemic, but one that thrives on specific ecological conditions.

The Shrinking Pie

The American news media remain filled with stories about rising cases of heterosexual AIDS. We frequently hear that AIDS is increasing fastest among heterosexuals, that it is now the major killer of young women. How could heterosexual AIDS be increasing as a percentage of all AIDS cases here in the developed world if there is no self-sustaining heterosexual AIDS epidemic?

Briefly put, the number of people infected via heterosexual sex in the early days of the epidemic was so small, and the number of gay men infected so large, that once the initial gay epidemic reached its saturation point, it became inevitable that thereafter the rate of increase would favor heterosexuals—even if that rate of increase among heterosexuals was quite modest. In addition, the overall profile of the epidemic has become a shrinking "pie," due largely to the fact that hundreds of thousands of people who were infected early in the epidemic, most of whom were gay men, have died. In such a shrinking pie, even a decline in heterosexual transmission would look like a comparative increase.

Deliberate Exaggeration

In May 1996 the front page of the *Wall Street Journal* led with a story headlined: AIDS FIGHT IS SKEWED BY FEDERAL CAMPAIGN EXAGGERATING RISKS. Typical of that paper's excellent AIDS coverage, the article explained another reason why much of the public still believes in an imminent heterosexual epidemic.

> In the summer of 1987, federal health officials made the fateful decision to bombard the public with a terrifying message: Anyone could get AIDS. While the message was technically true, it was also highly misleading. Everyone certainly faced some danger, but for most heterosexuals, the risk from a single act of sex was smaller than the risk of ever getting hit by lightning. In the U.S., the disease was, and remains, largely the scourge of gay men, intravenous drug users, their sex partners and their new-born children.
>
> [A]s CDC officials well knew, many of the images presented by the anti-AIDS campaign created a misleading impression about who was likely to get the disease. The blonde, middle-aged woman in the CDC's brochure was an intravenous drug user who had shared AIDS-tainted needles, although she wasn't identified as such in the brochure. The Baptist minister's son who said, "If I can get AIDS, anyone can," was gay, although the public service announcement featuring him didn't say so.

Nonetheless, for "people devoted to public health," the everybody-gets-AIDS message "seemed the best course to take." As long as AIDS was seen as a problem of marginal communities, funding was under constant threat. In addition, "many credited rampant fear with achieving pro-family goals that no amount of moralizing alone could have accomplished." And even for low-risk heterosexuals, "greater caution would reduce their already low rate of infection."

However, the *Journal* reported that this policy had had "a perverse, potentially deadly effect on funding for AIDS prevention" since it prevented targeting those groups at greatest risk. Worse, the "same forces that shaped public policy in 1987 are making it difficult for the government to change directions, even now" in 1996. The CDC continues to target a broad spectrum of young people and emphasize "that women constitute a growing proportion of AIDS cases [when] close analyses of the data indicate that the vast majority of these victims are drug users or sex partners of drug users."

Virtually all news organizations get their information about AIDS from the CDC. In light of the already complex dynamics of heterosexual AIDS detailed above, it has been relatively easy for CDC officials to slant the release of AIDS data to support a policy of overemphasizing heterosexual risk in the United States. It was interesting that just weeks after the *Journal* article appeared, the CDC issued a news release reporting that intravenous drug users are responsible for the vast majority of new infections among women and heterosexual men.

The Uneven Course of AIDS in the World

Those who still support the agenda of degaying AIDS make much of the fact that AIDS is spreading rapidly in some developing countries through heterosexual behavior, and is a bona fide catastrophe in many nations. If AIDS is not a threat to heterosexuals, they ask, how can we explain Thailand or Uganda or India, where the epidemic is racing through the population?

To begin to answer the question, it's important to note that two decades after the epidemic began HIV has so far made little headway in most of the world. Measured at the rate of cumulative HIV infection per million people, for example, the sub-Saharan region has 32,433 infections per million, the Caribbean 17,840, the Arab world 196, and northeast Asia (Korea, Japan, and parts of China) only 51. Some argue that this difference is based on the time that HIV first entered the population, and that all populations will eventually catch up, but statistics from the World Health Organization indicate that HIV began spreading in much of the world at about the same time, becoming statistically noticeable in the early eighties in regions as varied as Japan, the Caribbean, and Central Africa. But while it then spread in some societies at breakneck speed, doubling the number of cases seemingly overnight, in many other societies it has hardly spread at all. After perhaps the most extensive overview of AIDS epidemiology ever undertaken, the Global AIDS Policy Coalition wrote in 1992 that "it is clear that so-called explosive HIV epidemics may not occur in many—even most—populations." The argument that such epidemics are inevitable has begun to sound as unconvincing as the argument that AIDS will eventually saturate American heterosexual populations the way it saturated American gay men. It just isn't happening that way. Instead, HIV is spreading around the world in a fairly predictable way, becoming epidemic only in those populations where sexual ecology provides it with a niche.

A stark example is Thailand, a country whose sexual ecology is ideally suited to epidemic amplification. For centuries the male aristocracy of Thai society considered it their prerogative to have large numbers of wives and concubines. Most ordinary men were far too poor for such arrangements, but during the Vietnam War Thailand developed a large, prosperous mercantile class that adopted the aristocracy's belief that men of wealth and power were entitled to plenty of concubines and "pleasure women." At the same time the war itself created a huge market for prostitutes to service the American military. As a result, Thailand developed perhaps the world's largest sex industry, employing approximately 500,000 to 800,000 female prostitutes out of a population of 57 million, or about 10 percent of all women ages fifteen to twenty-four. Patronizing prostitutes became a casual pleasure for Thai males in a way almost unknown in most other societies. Some studies report that almost 90 percent of Thai boys have visited their first prostitute by the age of sixteen, and an estimated 450,000 Thai men visit a brothel every day.

Just as Thailand's sex industry was expanding, so was heroin addiction. Again the Vietnam War played a crucial role, introducing widespread heroin use to a population that lived in a poppy-growing region and had relatively easy access to the drug. When inexpensive disposable syringes were introduced in the seventies, the practice of injecting heroin exploded. By the mid eighties there were 200,000 IDUs in Thailand, most of whom shared needles.

Both IDUs and commercial sex workers and their clients formed huge and efficient core groups in Thai society. As a result, the rate of HIV transmission was dramatic, and prevalence rose alarmingly in the late eighties. In some provinces, up to 50 percent of IDUs, 90 percent of the female sex workers, and 15 percent of all

21-year-old male army recruits are HIV infected. Men have brought infection home to their wives, and the disease has penetrated the entire society. As AIDS geographer Peter Gould has written, the magnitude of the AIDS epidemic in Thailand "may well exceed the terror of the killing fields of civil war in neighboring Cambodia. In Thailand a vibrant, yet gentle Buddhist culture is being torn apart and destroyed by the politico-medical equivalent of Pol Pot, except that the destruction is not the result of fanatical, Paris-trained Marxists, but the socio-sexual fabric of the society itself."

A similar story is being repeated virtually everywhere that social, behavioral, and medical conditions provide a heterosexual niche for HIV transmission, although the precise conditions vary from place to place. In Central Africa, where the urbanization of male workers has separated husbands from wives for long periods, and where there is a generally casual attitude toward sex, widespread prostitution, high prevalence of untreated venereal diseases, and low levels of health care generally, AIDS has so saturated some areas that entire nations face the loss of their educated elites. It is also at disastrous levels in some Caribbean nations. India faces a terrible epidemic in coming decades, and parts of China appear poised for a major epidemic as well.

In the mid nineties the rate of new infections began to level off in some heavily saturated nations. Uganda, for example, saw a downward trend in infected young people in certain areas, from 30 percent in the late eighties to around 20 percent in the mid nineties. This followed several years in which up to 150,000 Ugandans died of AIDS annually. But while Ugandan and international prevention programs have been quick to take credit for the decline, citing their intensive AIDS education, it remains unclear how much of the reduction is due to prevention and how much to saturation. A number of prominent African epidemiologists argue that the epidemic there has merely matured, with most of those who engaged in the most risky activity simply dying out. Prevention has certainly provided Ugandans with the knowledge of how HIV is transmitted and the means to prevent it, and many have changed their behavior in dramatic ways. But it may take many years before we learn how much of an impact prevention programs have been able to make.

What is just as striking as where AIDS has spread, however, is where it has not spread. HIV transmission remains extremely low in most countries. In a number of major Middle Eastern cities, for example, HIV seroprevalence at STD clinics remains at 0. It has yet to break out of specific core populations—mostly IDUs—in many other developing nations in eastern Europe, Oceania, South America, and northeast Asia. And as we have seen, in Japan and here in the West it remains largely confined to IDUs, their wives and children, gay men, and blood-product recipients. The factors that characterize those societies where HIV is not spreading exponentially among heterosexuals seem as significant as the factors that characterize its spread: lower levels of sexual partner change, widespread monogamy or at least serial monogamy, better access to health care and less STDs generally, high levels of AIDS prevention funding and information, including access to condoms, fewer or less intense local core groups, little sexual mixing.

None of this is meant to minimize the disaster where it is occurring. The global spread of HIV is one of the great ecological disasters and human tragedies of our time. But the selectivity of AIDS strongly implies that it is not some inevitable force of nature that cannot be stemmed. It seems to result from very specific conditions and human behaviors, conditions and behaviors that many societies seem capable of avoiding.

A Future Heterosexual Epidemic?

Could a self-sustaining heterosexual epidemic arise in developed countries like the United States? The answer is clearly yes, but a number of changes would have to occur before that could happen. For example, if large numbers of heterosexuals increased their sexual contact rate, or if more intense heterosexual core groups developed, or if the amount of sexual mixing between IDUs and the rest of the heterosexual population increased, HIV could spread more widely here. Certainly if several of those things happened simultaneously, a self-sustaining heterosexual epidemic would become much more likely.

Looming over this equation is the fact that HIV appears to be evolving into strains that are more transmissible via vaginal sex. This fact first came to light in the early nineties when researchers studying the epidemic in Thailand noticed something odd. The rate of infection among IV drug users was almost uniform throughout the nation, but the rate of infection from heterosexual sex was from three to ten times higher in northern Thai cities such as Chiang Mai than in the south. Researchers originally surmised that this difference was caused by the sexual contact rate, which they assumed must be higher in the north than the south. But when they looked at rates of other STDs, they found that the north and the south were almost identical, a finding that would be impossible if the northern contact rate was higher. So then they looked at the virus itself, and made a startling discovery. The strain of HIV infecting most drug users and most heterosexuals in the south was subtype B, the same subtype that infects most people in North America, the Caribbean, and Western Europe. But the strain infecting heterosexuals in northern Thailand was subtype E, which had appeared to spawn a relatively new mutation. Could this mutation account for the north's increased rate of heterosexual transmission?

At the Third International Conference on AIDS in Asia and the Pacific in 1995, Harvard retrovirologist Max Essex presented data indicating that this may be what is occurring. Working with teams from Mahidol and Chiang Mai Universities, Essex tested the ease with which various strains of HIV react to Langerhans cells, which are found in the vagina, cervix, breast, mouth, and penile foreskin. He reported that a strain of subtype E that recently emerged in northern Thailand "has a clear propensity for better infection with those cells that line the female genital tract," whereas subtype B has much less propensity for such infection. The implication was that subtype E may be easier to spread via vaginal and oral sex, and easier to spread from a woman to a man during sex, then subtype B. So it seems possible that once subtype E enters developed countries—and there is no doubt amid the conditions of the modern world that it will, if it hasn't already—HIV transmission could increase among sexually active heterosexuals even if other behaviors remain unchanged.

Unfortunately, Essex's findings have been widely misinterpreted to provide fresh ammunition for those clinging to the degaying strategy. According to a popular misinterpretation of the subtype E data, the reason why HIV is not spreading among heterosexuals in the developed world has everything to do with viral biology, nothing to do with sexual ecology. Asia and Africa and Haiti and all the developing societies that have a serious AIDS problem, this thinking goes, were afflicted with the so-called "heterosexual strains" of HIV. These strains have simply not arrived on our shores yet, and the instant they do, the long-awaited explosion of heterosexual AIDS will finally be upon us.

But while subtype E certainly gives pause for the future, it does not explain the past. The strain causing the explosive spread of AIDS in northern Thailand is clearly a recent mutation. However, the vast epidemics of heterosexual AIDS in the rest of the Third World—including the rest of Thailand—were not fueled by northern Thailand's strain of subtype E. On the contrary, we know that many of the most widespread heterosexual epidemics, including those in the Caribbean, Peru, Brazil, and southern Thailand, were caused by the same strain of subtype B that caused the gay AIDS epidemic in the United States. Other heterosexual epidemics in Africa, India, and elsewhere are caused by subtypes A, C, D, and F.

In addition, the idea that a more transmissible strain of HIV will automatically spark a major heterosexual epidemic ignores an obvious fact. That fact is that many long-established venereal diseases in the West—from gonorrhea and syphilis to hepatitis B and CMV—are dozens or even hundreds of times more transmissible than any subtype of HIV, yet we are not sustaining massive, population-wide epidemics of these diseases in the developed world. The theory that new mutations of HIV will someday increase the risk for heterosexuals here is almost certainly correct, and should give pause to anyone who argues that simply because there has been no self-sustaining heterosexual epidemic so far, there can never be one. There can. But to have such an epidemic you need more than an easily transmissible bug. You also need an ecological and behavioral niche. If heterosexuals in developed countries provide such a niche, they will be in serious danger. If they don't, then even a more easily transmitted strain of HIV would have a difficult time building into an epidemic.

Heterosexual AIDS and Gay Men

For American gay men, the fact that AIDS in the world is largely a heterosexual disease has seemed comforting proof that the epidemic in the gay population was a fluke. That belief, in turn, has contributed to our failure to analyze why AIDS struck us so quickly and saturated us so disastrously. But the fact that AIDS is spreading rapidly in some heterosexual populations while barely spreading at all in others hardly sends gay men such a comforting message. True, the global epidemic clearly demonstrates that AIDS is not a "gay disease." Homophobic theories that AIDS proves the inherent "unnaturalness" of homosexuality are belied by global statistics showing that 90 percent of all cases worldwide are spread via heterosexual sex. However, those same statistics illustrate that while AIDS is not a gay disease, it is certainly an ecological disease that will strike with fury at any population whose collective sexual behavior is characterized by high contact rates, active core groups, high levels of sexual mixing, and high carriage of other STDs.

The good news is that the pattern of AIDS in the world illustrates that HIV, like virtually all other microbes, can be contained by human behavior, since it already is being contained by behavior in most places among most populations. The challenging news for gay men is that the behaviors that effectively prevent AIDS across populations seem to have less to do with narrow technological interventions like condoms, although they can be of significant use, and more to do with a sexual ecology characterized by low contact rates, low sexual mixing, and relative absence of core groups.

So for gay men the implications of AIDS in the world are highly challenging rather than comforting. The very traits that many of us have sneered at seem to provide the only sure foundation of a genuine safe sex, while the traits we have often celebrated seem to lead to disaster wherever they occur, without regard to whether the practitioners are straight or gay. The question facing us then is not only whether we can learn these ecological lessons and incorporate them into useful strategies for the gay population but also whether we are psychologically and politically willing to implement such lessons if they tend to fly in the face of cherished ideals about sexual liberation. And even if we can implement them, can we do so quickly enough to prevent the second wave of AIDS from leading inexorably to a third?

CHAPTER   8

Holistic Prevention

At its heart, the condom code is rooted in a simple mechanical analysis of the connection between the biology of HIV transmission and the sexuality of gay men. It tells us that fluid exchange during anal sex spreads HIV between individual gay men, and it stops there. It ignores or glosses over the fact that a whole network of behaviors created, and continue to sustain, epidemic conditions in the gay population. The code's narrow analysis is supposedly rooted in the principles of harm reduction, which advocate that health strategies meet people on their own terms. But in many ways the code is a misuse, or at least misinterpretation, of that concept. Classic harm reduction in the field of drug rehabilitation arose out of many health experts' dissatisfaction with the high-threshold approach of twelve-step programs, which insist that subjects who want help with their substance addictions adopt almost perfect behavior change from the start. Theorists reasoned that while that works fine for most, for some a better strategy would be a low-threshold approach that meets drug users where they are right now, and then helps slowly move them toward harm elimination wherever possible.

This seems eminently sensible, and indeed studies indicate that this approach can work best for some people. In the case of AIDS prevention, however, the harm reduction philosophy has sometimes been twisted into an excuse to avoid ever challenging the larger structure of risk in the gay population. In this view, the goal of AIDS prevention is to advocate the minimum changes to contain the epidemic, and to work to preserve the culture of gay male sexual life as much as possible. The very narrowness of the condom code's focus, which almost always excludes education about the role of multiple partners, core groups, sexual mixing, and any other aspect of unsafe behavior aside from fluid exchange in unprotected anal sex, has been tenaciously defended by some prevention workers who insist that harm reduction demands the most minimal and unobtrusive changes. In that sense, harm reduction, or at least its misuse, has become an excuse for those who want to ignore the impact of the wider web of cause and effect on AIDS transmission.

It is precisely because that philosophy ignores the interconnectedness of environmental causes and effects, however, that it should be viewed suspiciously by ecologists. Indeed, in ecology the general principle of "minimum change" is usually advanced by the foes of environmentalism, who frequently argue that "cultural norms" must not be challenged in the fight against things like environmental degradation and overpopulation. We must not challenge the "culture" of logging, they argue, or the "tradition" of open grazing on public lands, or Americans' "love affair" with the internal combustion engine. In the United Nations some national representatives rail against anyone who challenges cultural traditions such as slaughtering whales, or burning high-sulfur coal in open furnaces, or hunting endangered species such as the rhinoceros to extinction in order to use their body parts as aphrodisiacs—all eminently ancient cultural traditions. In environmental issues, demanding minimum change and placing the primacy of cultural values first often provides an excuse for doing very little—or nothing at all—since cultures and their values and practices are often at the root of ecological crises.

The Technological Fix

Of course, even foes of environmentalism are sometimes forced to acknowledge that certain ecological problems are so acute they simply have to be addressed. But when these eco-skeptics do propose solutions, they generally advocate technological adjustments that fail to address the root causes of problems. Instead of energy conservation, they advocate building more dams and nuclear plants. Instead of better mass transit, they try to make cars a bit more efficient. Instead of generating less waste, they get rid of fussy impediments to waste disposal. These kinds of solutions are often called "technological fixes," and they have very bad reputations among environmentalists, for good reason. It has been found that instead of solving environmental problems, they often make such problems worse.

Consider one example from the annals of air pollution: the effort to reduce the effects of car exhaust on the atmosphere. Twenty years ago one gallon of gasoline produced one pound of smog-causing carbon monoxide. Today, with improved technology, it produces about half a pound, and within a few years it will be down to one tenth. This has significantly reduced smog in major cities, and that, in turn, has greatly reduced public pressure for better mass transit and fewer cars. Partly as a result, there are more cars than ever, and a decreasing sense of urgency to do anything about them. However, one gallon of gas still emits the same amount of carbon dioxide it always has, about five and a half pounds. And it probably always will, since no conceivable technology can prevent petroleum combustion from producing carbon dioxide. CO_2 is a colorless, odorless, invisible gas that doesn't have much of a visible effect on urban air pollution, and as a result people don't notice it. But scientists increasingly believe that it is one of the chief pollutants responsible for the greenhouse effect warming the planet. So the "success" of one technological fix—in this case, more efficient cars that reduce carbon monoxide emissions and visible smog—has reduced the demand that we do something fundamental about limiting cars or replacing the internal combustion engine. And that has worsened the overall ecological crisis that engine efficiency was originally meant to solve. The history of environmentalism is replete with such examples. The more we experiment with technological fixes, the more we discover that the very interconnectedness of things often defeats such narrow approaches.

Some of the most glaring examples of the failure of technological fixes can be found in the realm of sexual behavior. When antibiotics were developed, many believed that science had at last conquered the scourges of syphilis and gonorrhea, and indeed under the onslaught of antibiotics their incidence initially dropped.

But soon it began to rise, and by the eighties both diseases were more common than ever. Sociologists now speculate that antibiotics and the pill contributed to the rise by helping to alleviate the potent force of fear that had once induced people to limit their number of partners. The subsequent increase in partners led to a transmission rate that more than offset the fact that these diseases were now treatable. In that sense, the cure actually contributed to an increase in the disease. Things came full circle in the seventies and eighties when strains of STDs appeared that were antibiotic resistant, and high sexual contact rates produced epidemics of incurable viral diseases such as herpes and AIDS. Hopes that the perennial problem of STDs could be easily fixed with just a shot of penicillin proved utterly naive.

In a similar way, the pill was once expected to limit the number of unwanted pregnancies, but instead the number of unwanted pregnancies has soared, to the extent that it is currently estimated that half of all pregnancies in the United States are unplanned. The reasons are complex, but foremost among them is the fact that the pill, like antibiotics, helped usher in a sexual revolution that lowered the age at which people have sex, increased the incidence of premarital relations, and increased the total number of sexual encounters many people have. Then, since not everybody uses the pill and since not everybody correctly and consistently uses any particular form of contraception, the total number of unwanted pregnancies rose dramatically.

It was partly the enticement of superficial fixes that led Norwegian philosopher Arne Naess to develop the idea of "deep ecology" in the early 1970s. Naess realized that there were two fundamental directions that environmentalism could take as the planet became more crowded and ecological problems grew worse. He called one "shallow ecology," in which environmental problems would be papered over by superficial, nontransformative solutions that focused more on symptoms than root causes. The other was deep ecology, in which underlying causes would be analyzed, addressed, and corrected. Deep ecology does go much further than merely addressing root causes. It argues, controversially, that all life is equally precious and that humans are no more sacred than any beings on earth. But one does not have to buy all aspects of deep ecology to recognize that on a purely practical level it represents perhaps the ultimate expression of ecological consciousness. Deep ecology recognizes that our thoughts, beliefs, and social systems are as much a part of nature's web as any other factor in ecology, and that if we truly want to craft sustainable solutions to the problems that face us, we have to change how we think, challenge our beliefs, and be willing to alter the social systems under which we live. "Deep" solutions to ecological problems are certainly more daunting and less popular than shallow ones, since they require fundamental changes in human organization and philosophy. Yet Naess believed, and many ecologists increasingly agree, that the deep approach is ultimately the only one that can create a sustainable future.

The Condom as Technological Fix

In a sense, condoms are the "technological fix" of AIDS prevention. According to the condom code, gay men have been assured that nothing else needs to change about our sexual culture since latex alone can solve the problem of AIDS transmission. In that sense the safer sex message is a "shallow ecology" message, since it fails to address many of the behavioral elements most responsible for the spread of HIV. And by failing to address them, it actually helps sustain them. Then, since not everybody uses condoms correctly or uses them every time, these lapses occur in the midst of an inherently perilous sexual ecosystem flooded with HIV, and contribute to high rates of transmission. As with antibiotics and the pill, a technological fix designed to solve a problem actually helps perpetuate an entire spectrum of social behaviors that ultimately sustain the problem or even make it worse.

There are several ways the condom code directly promotes behaviors that lead to HIV transmission. Perhaps the most obvious is that the code implicitly and even explicitly encourages gay men to engage in the single riskiest sexual practice of all: anal sex. As we have seen, studies of gay men in the pre-AIDS era indicated that while a majority of gay men practiced receptive anal sex, it was a slim majority. But the central slogan of prevention has been to "use a condom *every* time," implying that anal sex is what all gay men do *every* time. In attempting to make such messages alluring, gay prevention literature has frequently emphasized how "hot" anal sex is. Posters depict beautiful young men holding condoms and exhorting each other to Do It!, reminding themselves that Safe Sex (read: anal sex) Is Hot Sex. No one knows how strongly these messages have influenced young gay men to believe that anal sex is the kind of sex they ought to have, but it would not be surprising if they were very influential.

Thinking Ecologically

To begin the process of envisioning a sustainable gay lifestyle that can encourage gay liberation and avoid epidemic disease over the long haul, we have to learn to think ecologically about sex. Part of that involves challenging not just what we do, but how we think and live sexually. In particular we need to develop a deep ecological approach to sex that takes into account the multiple roots of AIDS. Not just the narrow subject of fluid exchange, but the entire triad of epidemic transmission: prevalence, infectivity, and contact rate. And not just the narrow subject of epidemiology, but the entire spectrum of behaviors and thoughts and feelings and values that made gay culture so susceptible to AIDS. The main ecological goal of this approach would be the same as most ecological goals: to use natural means to restore nature to a healthy equilibrium, and to try to provide room for error so that the same problem will not arise again and again. If it is impossible to contain AIDS solely with technology by getting everyone to use condoms every single time they have sex—and it appears that it is—then we need to create a sexual ecosystem that "forgives" such occasional lapses.

At least two basic steps could help achieve this goal. The first is to attempt to determine what changes in gay sexual ecology would provide this room for error. The second is to determine how to reimagine gay culture in a way that would encourage those changes. In other words, first we have to figure out what to do, and then we need to construct a cultural system that will support us in doing it.

But first things first: To determine what additional changes might provide us with elbow room that would "forgive" occasional lapses in the use of condoms, perhaps the most important issue to address is the fact that new infections are taking place in two basic contexts, and that this requires that we develop strategies to deal with both. Most studies show that HIV transmission in the gay population now occurs both in casual encounters and within long-term relationships when a couple decides to discard condoms, often without realizing that one partner is infected. Since infection happens in both settings, holistic approaches to prevention must consider both.

Prevention in Relationships

As far as relationships are concerned, the level of new infections can be reduced below replacement level in only three basic ways. The first is for couples to abstain from anal sex altogether and the second is for couples who have anal sex to use condoms every single time. Transmission statistics indicate that while such strategies are not absolutely foolproof, they would certainly reduce transmission to extremely low and perhaps even negligible levels. Within mixed or "serodiscordant" couples, totally consistent condom use or no anal sex whatsoever seems easier to achieve when the couple knows that one partner is infected. Many studies indicate that men who know they are HIV positive tend to be safer with their steady partner than either men who are negative or those who do not know their serostatus.

Yet these two strategies have been advocated from the beginning of the epidemic and they are not working terribly well. The main problem is that many couples stop using condoms under the assumption that both are uninfected. This seems eminently human, if for no other reason than that people fall in love and want to trust each other. Unfortunately, this strategy often fails, either because one partner is unknowingly infected from the start or because the partners are not totally monogamous within the relationship and not totally safe outside it.

Prevention education has been unable to halt this behavior, or even to make much of a dent in it. But there is a third strategy that might reduce infection in relationships. Called "negotiated safety," its aim is to offer advice on how partners of the same serostatus can discard condoms within their relationship and still reduce the risk of transmission to negligible levels. The negotiated safety concept is an example of a deep ecology approach to AIDS prevention, although its authors probably did not think of it in those terms. It was pioneered by the Victoria AIDS Council/Gay Men's Health Centre of Australia, which publicized a ten-point list of guidelines that all couples must adhere to if they want to stop using condoms within a relationship. Those ten points, listed in newspaper and magazine ads in the Australian gay press, are as follows:

1. Discuss with your partner how important it is for both of you to fuck without condoms. If it's not that important, keep using condoms.

2. If you'd both really like to fuck each other without condoms, both get tested for HIV antibodies. Be completely honest about your results, or get tested at the same time and collect your results together.

3. Continue to use condoms every time you fuck for three months. It can take this long for the antibodies to show up in a test.

4. After three months, get tested again.

5. If you're HIV negative, discuss and promise each other that you will avoid anal sex outside the relationship, or that if you or your partner fuck anyone else, condoms will be used.

6. Discuss and promise each other that if either of you slips up or has an accident with unsafe sex outside the relationship, you will tell the other immediately and go back to safe sex until you've both been tested again twice three months apart. Or . . .

7. Agree that either partner can insist on using condoms again.

8. Discuss with each other that slip-ups or accidents might happen, and that it won't mean the end of the relationship. Don't punish your partner for being honest. If this feels like too much to expect, then keep using condoms always.

9. If you both have HIV, talk with your doctor about the possible effects of reinfection with another strain of HIV. Discuss the damage to your immune system that might be caused by other STDs that condoms would protect you from and the link between unprotected anal sex and Kaposi's sarcoma cancer.

10. If one of you has HIV and the other does not, continue to use condoms every time you fuck.

Obviously these conditions are not for everybody. It needs to be emphasized that any couple who feels that following every single one would be difficult are wise simply to use condoms every time they have anal sex, or not to have anal sex at all. But it is equally important to point out that many people are already discarding condoms within relationships despite a decade of education urging them not to, and that seems likely to continue. Like it or not, complicated or not, these guidelines represent the minimum requirements for gay men to discard condoms safely in a relationship.

Negotiated safety has not been endorsed by any major American AIDS prevention group. Prevention agencies fear that such an endorsement would give a green light to people in relationships to discard condoms, and that most people who did so would then be unable to follow the guidelines and more new infections would result. This stance bears a striking resemblance to conservative arguments against needle exchange and condom distribution programs—that they will encourage people who would otherwise not engage in drug use or sexual intercourse to do so, with perhaps fatal results. AIDS agencies uniformly reject those arguments in the case of needle exchange and condom availability, maintaining that there is no evidence to support them and much evidence to show that for people already engaging in such behavior, such approaches work. Yet in the case of negotiated safety, these same prevention groups reverse position. What is so striking about this stance is that it seems to be a rare instance in which AIDS prevention groups have abandoned their otherwise firm commitment to their expansive definition of "harm reduction," the idea that if you can't get people to give up a potentially dangerous behavior altogether, at least give them the means and the information to engage in that behavior as safely as possible. This seems particularly misguided because in the ultimate analysis a reduction in the sexual contact rate seems necessary for the long-term containment of AIDS, and a very effective way to reduce the contact rate is to make relationships more attractive. One of the best ways to do that is to show people that there is a way, although an admittedly difficult way, to have intimate and satisfying sex in couples fairly safely.

Prevention in Casual or Anonymous Sex

The strategies of negotiated safety between couples of the same serostatus and absolute condom use or no anal sex whatsoever between mixed couples or couples unable to negotiate safety are both based on the supposition that partners know each other's serostatus. Such strategies obviously cannot work for casual or anonymous encounters, where partners not only do not know each other's serostatus, but frequently do not know each other at all. So entirely different approaches are needed for casual partners.

Up until now the basic advice for casual partners has been that all people should assume their partners are infected and act accordingly, but there are several inherent weaknesses to this approach. One is that people simply do not make that assumption all the time. For most human beings, apparent signs of illness in a partner, such as sores and blisters, symptoms of wasting, jaundice, and so on, are major sexual turnoffs. This is probably a result of evolutionary selection, and seems deeply wired into the human libido. But the same instinct that causes us to be turned off by visible symptoms of illness also seems to lull us into a false sense of security that the absence of such symptoms signifies health. As a result, many people find it easy to dismiss the idea that a handsome, healthy, and vital-looking person is actually harboring a deadly infection.

Combined with this is the fact that the advice to assume all casual sexual partners are potentially infected is based on the concept of self-defense, and is therefore directed almost exclusively at HIV-negative men, who in many places account for only about half the gay population. This self-defense strategy is fine as far as it goes, but it addresses only half of the prevention equation. The other half concerns those who are HIV-positive, and who ought to have an absolute responsibility to protect others. Yet, as we have seen, this call to responsibility is rarely emphasized. People who are HIV-positive are generally advised to practice safer sex for their own protection, mainly to defend themselves against opportunistic infections.

This almost exclusive emphasis on the responsibility of uninfected people to practice sexual self-defense naturally leads to the impression that if they become infected in an unsafe encounter, it's their fault. From that it seems to follow, to some people anyway, that if you are HIV-positive and infect someone else, it's that person's fault, not yours. If someone was stupid enough or lonely enough or drunk enough or inexperienced enough to let safety slide, he or she knew the rules. Many AIDS prevention groups are reluctant to challenge this thinking and emphasize the issue of equal responsibility between negatives and positives for fear of seeming judgmental and stigmatizing people with HIV. The failure to emphasize responsibility has created an ethical hole in the edifice of safer sex large enough to drive a truck through.

The truth is that uninfected people do not always practice self-defense, and infected people do not always take responsibility to avoid infecting others, and that is unlikely to change very much. The experience of gay men in the epidemic and the experience of heterosexual people struggling with birth control strongly indicates that there seems to be a built-in "set point" of unsafe sex for practically everybody. This set point varies in individuals over time, as people cycle in and out of low-risk and higher-risk behavior. But at any given moment a considerable portion of the gay male population is having a considerable amount of unprotected sex, and all the education in the world does not seem to be able to change that.

This, however, is where ecological thinking can make all the difference. Because in fact, HIV transmission between casual partners is not just a function of occasional unsafe sex, but of occasional unsafe sex multiplied by number of partners. And since gay men (and, it bears repeated emphasis, people in general) seem unable to reduce their built-in level of occasional unsafe sex to zero, the other available option is to reduce the other aspects of sexual life that make those occasional lapses so dangerous. Primarily the overall number of partners.

This has been a major missing ingredient in the safer sex equation so far. The condom code seeks to curtail transmission by lowering the level of infectivity per sexual contact, but it ignores the enormous role played by the contact rate itself. More than ignores it, denies it, since a core tenet of the condom code is the idea that so long as everyone uses condoms all the time there is no need to lower the contact rate. People have clung tenaciously to the supposition that the contact rate is irrelevant, but the irrationality of this position can no longer be denied. A set amount of unsafe sex in a population with an average lifetime contact rate of ten partners will have a vastly different result than that same set amount of unsafe sex in a population with an average lifetime contact rate of five hundred partners. Lowering the contact rate alone is no substitute for condom use, but lowering it while maintaining a high level of condom use would likely lead to a significant reduction in transmission. Therefore, one of the most important additions to safer sex regarding casual partners is to reduce them. Preferably to one partner at a time.

Targeting Core Groups

Commercial Sex Establishments. This reduction of partners
alone may seem drastic and sweeping to some, however the evidence argues that gay men must do even more. We have seen that
HIV infection initially began spreading among a core group of gay
men who had very large numbers of partners and engaged in a synergy of risky behaviors. We have also seen strong evidence that
fairly small core groups can, by themselves, sustain STD epidemics
indefinitely in populations in which those diseases would otherwise fade away, and that the harder a disease agent is to transmit,
the more important the role of such core groups becomes. It therefore seems distinctly possible that even if the overwhelming
majority of gay men develop a sexual culture characterized by
condom use, negotiated safety inside relationships, and reduced
partners outside relationships, a fairly small core of individuals
could keep the epidemic going. So to improve chances for success,
gay men would be wise to reduce as much core group behavior as
possible.

Part of that effort must include reaching out to men who engage
in such behavior, helping to educate them and supporting them in
modifying their behavior. This has to be done in ways that not only
prevent an "us versus them" dynamic but also avoid burdening
them with additional stigma or shame. But it must be realized that
people engaging in very high levels of unsafe multipartner sex are
not ideal targets for education or persuasion. Core group behavior
has much in common with compulsive and addictive behavior.
Many of the people involved don't want to stop, and many have
less than total control over what they are doing and would not necessarily be able to stop if they wanted to. For a while in the eighties
it seemed that the kind of extravagantly unsafe behavior characterized by the activity in bathhouses and sex clubs and the "circuit"
would abate by itself due to fear of disease, and for a while it
appears that much of it did. But in the nineties that behavior has
roared back to life. In many New York sex clubs, for example, the
only activities allowed from 1986 to 1988 were kissing and mutual
masturbation. In 1989, some clubs began allowing occasional
unprotected oral sex, and while that initially caused scandal in
some circles it soon became accepted. By the early nineties patrons
were again surprised when some clubs began to allow anal sex with

condoms, but that too quickly became typical, so that by 1993 many clubs were routinely devoted to oral sex without condoms and anal sex with condoms. The only thing that still raised eyebrows was anal sex without condoms, but even this was on the increase. By 1995 one could witness all forms of unprotected sex almost any night of the week in many of the city's most popular sex clubs catering to gay men. The process of escalation was familiar to anyone who experienced the gay seventies, when one behavior quickly pushed the envelope for the next. It seems unlikely that this kind of behavior will curtail itself.

Community Opposition to Regulation. It seems increasingly clear that any form of prevention that expects to contain the AIDS epidemic will have to de-escalate this process as much as possible. This will not be easy—or popular. Core group behavior has traditionally been facilitated by commercial sex establishments, and reducing such behavior necessarily involves regulating such establishments, either by the gay community itself or by health authorities. Yet urban gay culture works against such regulation in many ways. Its ideology and belief systems support the autonomy of such establishments, its economy and media are based in part on perpetuating them, its politics has traditionally defended them. The sense of identity of many gay men, the very thing that sets them apart as gay, is in many cases intricately tied to the behaviors that such establishments facilitate. To many, core group behavior is the ultimate expression of gay sexual liberation, epitomizing the values of freedom, the absolute right to do with one's body what one wishes, and the absolute right to privacy that the gay movement was built upon. As a result, such behavior often receives support even from gay men and lesbians who do not participate in it themselves, but who defend it out of solidarity and a sense that attacks on it are attacks on gay liberation itself.

In addition, entrepreneurs who run sex clubs, bathhouses, backroom bars, and similar venues have the financial and advertising power to encourage the most dangerous kinds of core group behavior and subvert even the most concerted education and prevention efforts. A glance at the "bar rag" newspapers in many gay communities illustrates this point. In any given issue you might find a single lone ad from a prevention agency advocating the use of condoms, surrounded by dozens of alluring and sexy ads from sex clubs and baths and discos with names like Lick it!, Pump, Hard, Blow!, Meat, and Buffed. Some party promoters directly tie their events to conspicuous drug consumption and explicit inducements to unsafe sex. One 1995 ad for a disco party featured a photo depicting two young men engaged in what appeared to be anal sex. The name of the party was High Risk, with the letter *k* in *Risk* printed in a brighter color to advertise that the drug of choice at this party was special K, a popular disco drug often associated with high-risk behavior. The accompanying slogan, a blatant inducement to unsafe sex, read: "Go Ahead. Cross the Line."

To think that mere outreach and education will have much of an impact in such situations is naive. Only direct intervention and regulation by the gay community or, as a last resort, the government, is likely to have any impact at all. In San Francisco, where the gay community is extraordinarily powerful in local politics, a successful attempt at self-monitoring has been mounted. Yet most AIDS agencies vigorously oppose direct intervention, either by the gay community or by health authorities. Educators are reluctant even to criticize such behavior, and where core group behavior is facilitated by sex clubs and bathhouses, prevention workers generally oppose initiatives that would require such places to ban unsafe sex, preferring instead merely to provide patrons with information and condoms and leave the choices up to them. Many of these educators argue that intervention does not work, that it simply drives men away from education and outreach, that it stigmatizes and blames the victim, that it's reminiscent of society's attempts to repress homosexuality itself. Yet this refusal to intervene virtually guarantees that core group behavior will continue to be encouraged by profit-minded entrepreneurs. And since the possibility exists that AIDS can be perpetuated in the gay population through such behavior alone, failure to target that behavior leaves open the possibility that no matter what else we do, the epidemic will rage on and on.

Prove It. Gay AIDS agencies advance a number of arguments against intervention in commercial establishments. One of the most persistent concerns the question of what role, if any, such establishments have played in the epidemic so far. As noted, some epidemiologists theorize that bathhouses and sex clubs played the decisive role in raising the sexual contact rate to the level necessary to spark the epidemic. But most gay AIDS agencies seem convinced that these remain just theories, and that gay men must not take any action against sex establishments based only on theories.

In that light it is worthwhile to note that ecologists have long argued that refusing to act when there is a preponderance of evidence but a lack of absolute proof can be extremely unwise. Absolute proof of any environmental cause and effect is difficult and often even impossible to obtain. Yet while we hesitate and demand proof, the environment may be irretrievably destroyed. A case in point is the current debate about the hole in the ozone layer. The preponderance of evidence indicates that the depletion of atmospheric ozone is largely caused by fluorocarbon emissions, but this falls short of absolute proof. There's a slim chance these theories are wrong. As a result, those who have vested interests in doing nothing about the issue (chemical manufacturers, local governments concerned with economic development, those who believe in the absolute sanctity of private property) constantly argue that we should do nothing until "absolute proof" is in. You might call this the Rush Limbaugh Default Argument about ecology. No proof, no action.

In many developed nations including the United States, however, the pressing nature of environmental damage, combined with the impossibility of absolute proof, led to a revolution in legal thinking over the past forty years. The principle of "innocent until proven guilty," our society's bedrock assumption when applied to individuals in criminal or civil cases, was found to be unacceptably risky when applied to environmental issues. As Garrett Hardin points out in *Living Within Limits*, "Chemists have synthesized more than a million compounds, and a wealth of experience indicates that the effects on human beings of most of the compounds is bad. Society would soon be bankrupted if it had to prove, in courts of law, the harmful effects of every one of these compounds. . . . The most rational policy is to put the burden of proof on the entrepreneur. . . . The cost of proving harmlessness then becomes one of the costs of a profit-oriented business—as it should be." The 1962 Kefauver-Harris amendments to America's food and drug laws ratified this position, and "guilty until proven innocent" became society's baseline principle concerning the introduction of new food products, chemicals, and drugs. The 1970

National Environmental Policy Act extended this principle to environmental changes. Now anyone who wants to fill in a wetland or erect an office building or undertake any project that experience suggests might adversely impact the environment has to file an environmental impact statement proving that what they are doing will not cause irreparable ecological harm.

But when it comes to issues like the impact of commercial sex businesses on the epidemic, most AIDS organizations still operate on the pre-1962 logic, arguing that it is up to society to prove that a venue is dangerous, not for entrepreneurs to prove it is safe. Based on the evidence, I have no doubt that if owners of commercial sex establishments had to file "epidemiological impact statements" proving that they would not harm gay sexual ecology before they could get or renew their licenses, very few would be allowed to operate. Under the same rules of evidence that currently apply to those seeking to build a shopping mall or sell a pesticide, sex club owners would fail to prove that their establishments would do no harm. It seems terribly misguided that the very organizations charged with the responsibility of protecting the gay sexual environment continue to operate on a logic that even the government discarded long ago.

Another argument against intervention in commercial settings is that such intervention would drive core group behavior underground, where it might become even less safe. This has become a virtual article of faith among AIDS prevention agencies, repeatedly trotted out whenever they are pressured to do something about unsafe sex in commercial establishments. "Wholesale closure," says a typical 1995 statement by the board of New York's Gay Men's Health Crisis, "would not cause unsafe sex to disappear but would disperse such activity to parks, alleys, underground clubs and other covert locales where participants would be subject to arrest or violence and where HIV prevention interventions could not easily reach." Yet not only is this "dispersal" theory of unsafe sex completely unsupported by basic economic and behavioral theory, it is also contradicted by recent history.

If anything in economics can be called a law, it is the principle that when the cost of something goes up, demand goes down. This is so powerful a force it barely matters how vital the good or service: Even essential things like food consumption decline when cost goes up, and the effect is considerably stronger on nonessentials. Consider the effect on gun ownership in countries where the "cost" of owning a handgun includes finding a black market supplier, breaking the law to purchase the weapon, and then risking significant penalties by possessing it. The level of handgun ownership in such countries is drastically lower than in the United States, where guns are cheap, plentiful, and legal. Yet the gun lobby argues that banning handguns would have no impact on the handgun murder rate here, since increased cost would provide no deterrence; people would acquire guns anyway. Most of the public dismisses this flawed logic, understanding that by the same logic we might just as well abolish all criminal laws, since they are also based on the principle that raising costs deters unwanted behavior.

Yet this patently absurd argument is often advanced by AIDS prevention groups seeking to defend the gay male commercial sex industry. GMHC's contention that unsafe sex would disperse to parks, alleys, underground clubs, and other covert locales where participants would be subject to arrest or violence presupposes that gay men would be willing to pay enormously higher costs to engage in this kind of behavior. Yet the history of the bathhouse closures in the mid eighties casts strong doubt on this assertion. During and after the closure of sex establishments in New York and San Francisco, detailed cohort studies carefully measured the sexual behavior of gay men and found that there was a huge decline in numbers of partners after closure. One San Francisco study, for example, compared the average number of partners in the last six months before bath closure in 1984 to a six-month period two years later. This "before and after" snapshot documented a 60 percent decrease in the number of men who had ten or more partners in both periods.

The same phenomenon was observed in New York. In a 1995 retrospective study designed to measure as accurately as possible the effect of bathhouse closure on New York City gay men in the mid eighties, researchers at Columbia University reported that "closure and regulation of establishments in New York City did not result in an increase in sexual behaviors in other public places," but rather the opposite. The sexual contact rate not only decreased in commercial settings, it decreased in all other settings as well, including parks and rest rooms. A few years before closure, average New York City gay men had 6 partners per year at home and 35 in "extradomestic settings." A few years after closure, the number of partners at home had registered a slight decline to 4 per year, but there was a huge decline in extradomestic settings, from 35 to 8. Men clearly had not been scared away from sex, but their contact rate had drastically declined. The significance of this decline cannot be overstated. As we saw from Morris and Dean's mathematical model of the New York epidemic, even lowering the average unsafe contact rate by a single person per year can make the difference between a rising epidemic and a declining one. And as we have seen from other studies, preventing a single new infection in a core group might prevent up to ten times as many ultimate new infections over ten years as preventing a single new infection outside a core.

This raises the intriguing question of why gay men in the mid eighties didn't simply relocate to alleys and parks and carry on as before, which is what bathhouse advocates back then loudly argued would happen. One clue may be found in studies that show that most of those who go to baths and sex clubs do so not necessarily because they want to have large numbers of partners (though some do) but because they enjoy the atmosphere of camaraderie. In a bathhouse you can feel safe about being unabashedly gay without worrying about the moral disapproval or the physical dangers of the outside world. For many gay men, particularly closeted ones, the baths have traditionally provided the only sort of gay society they know. These factors are sometimes romanticized by activists, and sometimes looked upon with regret by epidemiologists, since men may not go to the baths specifically to have large numbers of partners, but that's what they often do when they get there. Socializing men into gay life via the baths often ends up socializing them into a life characterized by a high degree of multipartnerism. But in any event, if men are attracted to such places for their safety and comfort and sense of community, they are not likely to engage in the same behaviors in the discomfort of a freezing park or in the danger of a dark alley.

While the record does not imply that closure alone led to a sharp reduction in partners, it decisively disproves the opposite argument: that closure would simply lead to dispersal and would have no impact on the contact rate. Instead it seems likely that if commercial sex establishments are regulated to prevent unsafe sex, a small percentage of determined men will continue to maintain the same contact rate in dangerous, uncomfortable locations (indeed, it shouldn't be forgotten that some people, gay and straight, *prefer* dangerous, uncomfortable locations) but their numbers would be far fewer. And when it comes to core groups and HIV, numbers are the name of the game.

Not all arguments against core group intervention are based on the fear of unintended consequences. Many are frankly ideological. Some prevention workers base their opposition to regulation on civil rights concerns, arguing for an inherent right to unsafe sex in commercial establishments. Some oppose regulation by arguing that personal responsibility in sexual matters conflicts with community intervention in unsafe sex, that by regulating unsafe sex you inherently undermine the principle of personal responsibility. (If this were applied across the board, of course, we should consider abolishing the police, since by this logic law enforcement inherently undermines people's responsibility to obey the laws voluntarily.) Others base their objections on the use, or rather misuse, of the principles of harm reduction, arguing that the regulation of unsafe sex establishments exceeds the minimum necessary response to the epidemic. And some invoke the strong traditions of sexual freedom and libertarianism in gay culture, arguing that nothing should discourage people from exercising that freedom, even overwhelming evidence of communal harm.

Core-Group Behavior and the Gay Sense of Self

This opposition to any intervention that might decrease core group contact rates exposes a central dilemma in gay men's response to the Second Wave of AIDS. For various reasons we are, in effect, defending the behaviors that are killing us. The fact that we did so at the epidemic's outset was fairly understandable. People did not comprehend what was happening, and there was genuine confusion over how to respond. But the fact that we continue to do so far into the epidemic's second decade indicates that this defensive mechanism is immensely powerful and immensely destructive—almost amounting to an unconscious death wish. So part of the future task of prevention must include seeking to understand the internal reasons why so many of us take positions that seem to ensure our collective doom.

For many gay men, adopting an openly gay identity has meant

adopting a whole set of cultural aspirations and assumptions. Many of these are positive and life affirming, and revolve around our attempts to divest ourselves of the legacy of shame that we have been saddled with by an overwhelmingly homophobic culture. Some, however, are more problematic, including the idea that because a gay identity is essentially a sexual identity, anyone embracing that identity is by definition placing sex in the central position in their lives.

Beyond this basic idea are several underlying sexual presumptions in the gay male world that work against an ethic of prevention. These are not necessarily gay assumptions so much as male assumptions, ideas shared to some extent by all men in our culture. One is a belief that sex ought to be without consequence and responsibility. Another is a sense of entitlement about sex. Still another is the notion that males, straight or gay, are at the mercy of biological forces beyond their control, forces that impel us to seek as many partners as possible and that overwhelm whatever feeble cultural roadblocks we place in their way. We are, in this conception, the victims of our hormones.

These beliefs are augmented in some circles by a pervasive suspicion of all forms of restraint, from abstinence to monogamy, a belief that restraint equals repression, and a belief that a major goal of gay liberation is to liberate humanity from such restraint/repression and teach it a lesson about pleasure. Gay men have been singularly unsuccessful spreading this revolutionary concept to others. Author and sex radical John Rechy's assertions in the 1970s that for him "the promiscuous homosexuals are the heroic homosexuals" and that promiscuity was gay men's way of "taking the revolution to the streets" seems pathetic in retrospect. As Ian Young has recently remarked, "The acts in question may indeed have been taken to the streets, but the streets were otherwise deserted; the revolutionaries remained quite invisible to all but themselves and the occasional contingent of undercover police." Certainly the specter of AIDS has done much to discredit the idea that gay men have a lot to teach others about pleasure, since we appear to be dying from the very pleasure we supposedly wanted to educate the world about.

Nonetheless, gay men do continue to teach these lessons to each other. At present, young gay men come out into urban environments in which social status and respect are largely achieved through sexual means. As gay essayist Michael Bronski wrote as recently as 1994, one of the guiding principles of Stonewall is that "gay liberation means sexual freedom. And sexual freedom means more sex, better sex, sex in the bushes, in the toilets, in the baths, sex without love, sex without harassment, sex at home and sex in the streets." Oddly, Bronski was complaining that the AIDS crisis had undermined this basic definition of gay liberation, replacing it with "solipsistic, homophobic theories . . . about why *less* sex was good." But in fact AIDS did not really challenge this male-oriented notion of sexual entitlement. The condom code stoutly defends the primacy of pleasure and the status accorded to sexual adventure seekers. Today's Second Wave of core group behavior in urban gay culture, what some are proudly hailing as the Second Gay Sexual Revolution, is characterized by an immense amount of sexual imagery and multipartner activity. Gay life is flooded with images of the buff and the beautiful, with naked go-go boys in seemingly every disco, with porn videos flickering in neighborhood gay bars, with the return of baths and sex clubs and a rise in contact rates. All of this testifies that the basic values of urban gay life remain much the same as when Michael Callen came to New York in the seventies and found a philosophy proclaiming "that sex was inherently liberating" and that "by a curiously naive calculus, it seemed to follow that more sex was more liberating."

In many ways the prevailing gay urban ethos seems just as overwhelmingly sex-oriented in the 1990s as it was in the clone culture of the 1970s. Although there are now gay churches and community centers and sports clubs, the central gay institutions in large cities remain bars and discos, and much of the urban social scene continues to confer status and self-respect primarily on the basis of looks, muscles, and sexual conquest. This seems so deeply embedded at the heart of the gay male world that virtually all of the behaviors that need to be modified if we are to build a sustainable culture instead continue to be hailed by some leaders as the very essence of gay life. This does not bode well for the future of an ecological approach to AIDS, and certainly not for the likelihood that gay men will successfully intervene in core group behavior. That intervention may be necessary for the physical survival of the gay population, but to many it seems antithetical to their spiritual survival, or to the ideological survival of their core beliefs about gay liberation.

It particularly does not bode well for prevention as new drugs such as protease inhibitors successfully reduce HIV infection to a more manageable condition for many men. In the mid nineties gay sexual life in many urban centers seemed like a vast tidal wave being held in check only by the threat of imminent death. Many believed that the removal of that threat seemed likely to lead to a resurgence of unsafe behavior that could equal the activity that made the seventies a decade of cascading epidemics. Unfortunately, if that threat is only partially removed—if AIDS is made more manageable but HIV continues to saturate the gay ecosystem, poised to mutate into drug-resistant forms—the reestablishment of core group behavior could be unimaginably dangerous. Yet that seems likely if gay men fail to analyze the ecology of core groups and fail to take a strong stand against the reemergence of such behavior.

Blame and Shame. Having argued for intervention, however, let me insert a note of caution. Many gay men are burdened by a sense of shame that permeates their entire lives, especially their sexual lives. We have evolved many strategies for discharging this shame, but one of the most sad and unproductive is the attempt to transfer it to others in the gay community. One frequently hears gay people putting down other gay people for being too out, too in, too flamboyant, too conservative, too effeminate, too butch, too sexual, or not sexual enough. Many of us "blame" the perpetuation of the epidemic on others, and the most obvious targets are those who are engaging in the most obviously self-destructive and promiscuous behaviors.

It is therefore important when approaching these problems to engage in both a careful examination of the public health issues involved and a careful examination of our own motives and tactics. When we do we are likely to find a terrible paradox: that there is indeed a serious problem concerning core group behavior in the gay population, a problem that will not solve itself and that needs intervention of some kind; but also that such intervention has the potential to divert us from the much larger task at hand, which is our own behavior. Ultimately sustainable AIDS prevention is not "us versus them," but simply us. Even if commercial establishments are successfully regulated, the problem will not be solved. We will still have to face our own individual responsibilities, and they will not be any easier than they were before.

Looking at the Long Term

To sum up, it now seems clear that AIDS will not be contained, and future epidemics will not be prevented in the gay population, through the condom code alone. Prevention needs to engage the whole spectrum of activities and behaviors that led to epidemic transmission in the first place. *The use of condoms must continue to be emphasized*, but it must be augmented by other strategies, including negotiated safety for seroconcordant people in relationships, a curtailment of the number of casual partners for those not in relationships, and wherever possible an end to our facilitation and encouragement of unsafe core group behavior. These changes, added to the condom code already in place, could provide the critical margin for error that has so far been lacking in safer sex. This is not to imply that these changes would be foolproof, but they don't have to be. All they have to do is reduce each individual's risk of infection to the point where cumulative risk drops below the epidemic's tipping point. Once that is accomplished, the epidemic will begin to abate, and as it does it will provide increasing room for error.

But before discussing how we might begin implementing such changes, it is important to add a further point: To be effective, these strategies must be considered permanent, not merely temporary deviations from gay sexual life. The reason is that prevention strategies have two basic goals: to bring HIV prevalence down to much lower levels; and to keep it there. That could probably not be accomplished by any strategy envisioned merely as an "emergency" approach, a temporary measure designed to be abandoned at the first signs that the plague was easing or the disease was becoming more manageable.

Restoration Ecology. The task of bringing HIV prevalence down to lower levels is equivalent to what environmentalists call restoration ecology, the goal of which is to return damaged ecosystems to something approximating their "predisturbance state." Restoration ecology is particularly applicable to gay men because levels of HIV prevalence are so high that strategies that might otherwise work in low-prevalence populations—simply reducing the number of partners or using condoms most of the time—cannot work for gay men. High prevalence means high risk, and high risk will continue to face us until we go beyond mere prevention and achieve some measure of restoration to a lower level of prevalence.

But restoration ecology is pointless if it merely leads to a relapse into high-risk behavior the moment it scores some initial success. So prevention's second task is *sustainability*—keeping prevalence low. And that is unlikely to be accomplished if the very strategies employed in restoration inherently undermine sustainability. If restoration requires a broad-based commitment to reduce the entire spectrum of behaviors that led to the problem, sustainability requires doing so in a way designed to prevent a recurrence, a third and fourth and fifth wave.

This is particularly important to grasp because many prevention theorists tend to base their strategies on the immediate problem, treating AIDS like an emergency and ignoring the issue of sustainability. Some argue, for example, that it is fruitless to advocate that gay men reduce their number of partners or attempt to be monogamous because in a population where 25 to 50 percent of all men are HIV infected, a negative man's chances of entering a relationship with a positive man are quite high and monogamy alone would not provide him any reasonable protection. They are absolutely correct. The strategy of monogamy alone has the same kind of drawbacks as the strategy of the condom code alone: unrealistic reliance on just one isolated factor of risk, when in fact the real problem is multifactorial. But those who dismiss monogamy as a strategy fail to consider the long-term consequences of maintaining a culture of promiscuity. Because once HIV prevalence declines, multipartnerism (combined with its seemingly inevitable "set point" of unsafe sex) would again become a very significant issue. Indeed, the lower prevalence drops, the more the contact rate would become *the* issue. If prevention strategies ignored promiscuity, or even encouraged men to be promiscuous, a rising new wave of infections would quickly follow the falling old wave.

This potential of successive "waves" is a key example of why any "nontransformative" strategy that ignores the whole spectrum of sexual behaviors is likely to fail. Assume that we craft a prevention program that goes against the grain of gay culture, so that people adhere to it the way they adhere to crash diets, only reluctantly, pining for the moment when they can chuck the strategy and return to the good old days. So long as AIDS is seen as a looming and immediate threat, people may be motivated to maintain that strategy. (Or they may not be. If the strategy really goes against the grain of cultural values, even fear may not be deterrent enough.) But what happens if the strategy does have some initial success, prevalence declines, and people no longer face an overwhelming risk? Since the strategy goes against the grain of gay sexual culture, and since it is maintained only through crushing fear, many people begin abandoning it as soon as fear abates. They return to the behaviors that led to the crisis in the first place, and plague returns with a vengeance. Within a short time new infections rise until the gay population again faces an overwhelming disaster, at which point people again reluctantly adopt a temporary, against-the-grain strategy to solve the problem. Again that strategy yields results, prevalence declines, fear declines, people return to their old ways, and new infections rise. This "wave" pattern is likely to repeat itself indefinitely so long as gay men condition ourselves to believe that restoration strategies are quick fixes designed to allow us to get back as fast as possible to the gay sexual culture of the seventies.

Suspended Extinction. In a purely ecological sense, this wave pattern describes a situation that might be called suspended extinction. Gay men are experiencing a form of extinction as devastating as that inflicted upon any dying species. Of course, we are a social species, not a biotic one, but the process of our numerical decline parallels or even exceeds that of other extinctions and the overall analogy is apt. If things continued this way for any other biotic population, that population would be erased or completely transformed fairly quickly. Species that fail in such a spectacular way either die out or evolve some adaptation that allows them to claw their way back to survival. The factor that prevents gay men from following this course is the unique way gay society replenishes itself. Gay men don't produce children who become the next generation of gay men, and whose existence is therefore dependent on the reproductive success of the older generation. Each new homosexual generation is replenished by heterosexuals, whose production of gay sons is entirely unrelated to the dynamics of the epidemic. AIDS can therefore keep mowing down gay men, and rather than dying out, phalanx after phalanx will emerge from the trenches, ready to be mowed down anew. This might seem hopeful to some, since it implies that there will always be gay people and that we will therefore survive. But it also means that the natural mechanisms of evolution, including the mechanisms that help ter-minate epidemics, don't really apply to gay men. Extinction is not an option, and neither is unconscious evolution: There won't be a small number of people who survived either through genetic immu-nity or behavioral and cultural adaptation, and who then produced healthy and immune future generations. Instead, the epidemic could literally go on forever, each generation taking its place in the line of fire, rising up, going down. This is why conscious evolution is so necessary for gay men to contain AIDS. Things won't get better by themselves.

For those who doubt that increased sexual restraint could pro-duce a long-term sustainable gay lifestyle, supporting evidence is all around us. There is no sexually transmitted heterosexual HIV epi-demic anywhere in the developed world except among crack cocaine users, yet heterosexuals engage in virtually all of the behav-iors that led to AIDS in the gay population. The difference is that among heterosexuals these behaviors are relatively moderate and fairly diffuse. Many gay men are understandably loath to take a lesson in prevention from heterosexuals, but that lesson stands nonetheless. There is no need to equate sex with an endless epi-demic or have sexual lives wrapped forever in latex. The answer is not condoms alone (although condoms will always play a role in prevention). The answer is moderation. Balance.

Where's the Plan?

Is there a fully articulated plan for achieving this revolution? No. The task of creating a new gay culture will be vast and daunting, and it will proceed in an evolutionary fashion. It's impossible to have the whole thing figured out in advance. Just as gay liberation itself is a work in progress, drawing from the best and the brightest among our resourceful community, so too will be our adaptation to the biological disaster of AIDS.

Some might argue that if there is no grand master plan, we should shelve discussion of the whole problem until there is and stick with the condom code. But the example of recent adapta-tions—such as the revolution in attitudes toward smoking—argues strongly against this. In 1963, when the U.S. surgeon general issued his landmark report linking cigarette smoking with cancer, he had no plan for getting all Americans to quit. No one did. No one does. But Americans would not and could not have even confronted the problem of smoking, much less created strategies to move toward a smoke-free society, unless we first realized there was a problem. The surgeon general's report was a prerequisite, a call to action. Only after we understood the connection between smoking and disease could we begin devising ways to induce people to quit. More than three decades later that evolution is still under way, and still incomplete. But it would never have begun if the surgeon general had decided not to release his report until he could simultaneously release a program that would get all Americans to quit.

In much the same way, understanding the link between gay sexual ecology and epidemic AIDS is merely a prerequisite. First comes understanding and a recognition of the full dimensions of the problem. Only then can people devise new approaches, and slowly, through an evolutionary process of trial and error, can we grope our way to a new equilibrium with nature.

CHAPTER 9

Imagining a
Sustainable Culture

The Population Analogy

Ecologist Paul Ehrlich uses the term *conscious evolution* to describe how humans must adapt in the increasingly technological future if our species is to survive. Ehrlich argues that humanity can no longer expect to muddle through the environmental crises that face us and expect things to turn out fine. Instead, people must learn to analyze our interactions with the environment, design sustainable solutions to our problems, and then implement those solutions on a broad scale, across cultures, nations, even the planet itself. The environmental movement is devoted to—and is itself a form of—conscious evolution. So is the gay movement, which arose when people realized that society was arbitrarily stigmatizing an entire category of people based on ancient misconceptions and biases about sex and gender. And so, too, must be the movement to create a sustainable gay sexual ecology.

The connections between environmentalism and AIDS prevention are more than merely rhetorical. A whole way of thinking about environmental issues can be applied to AIDS, starting with the idea that lasting remedies require not technological fixes but changes in basic aspects of the way we live. From that ecological realization springs perhaps the central challenge of environmentalism, which is the question of how we change the way we live. How do individual people and entire cultures go about altering their behavior once they discover how that behavior is harming them or their habitats? Especially when that behavior contains elements they value, things that have cultural or historical meaning, things sometimes steeped in desire or pleasure? No one has easy answers to these questions, but they have been the subject of decades of thinking by environmentalists, and certain basic principles have emerged that can be applied by those looking for signposts to a sustainable gay future.

The ecological issue most analogous to AIDS prevention is one that many ecologists consider to be the single gravest challenge haunting humankind: the population explosion. When Malthus first proposed in 1798 that the earth's resources are finite and cannot support an endlessly increasing population, no one realized that for several centuries the "set point" of population sustainability would dramatically rise as industrialization and then the green revolution increased the earth's carrying capacity for the human race. As a result, many were lulled into thinking that the world can accommodate an infinitely growing population. But it is increasingly clear that if global growth does not eventually halt, catastrophes will ensue that will make AIDS and other epidemics pale in comparison. The question is not whether the earth's population will eventually stop growing—it certainly will. The question is whether it will stop growing in time to preserve its ecosystems, or whether it will overshoot that point (if it hasn't already) and stop growing at a level of sustained ecological ruin. The famous $I = PAT$ equation has codified the problem in an easily understandable way. Impact on the environment (I) is a function of Population (P) *times* Affluence (A) *times* Technology (T). According to this equation, all three factors—population, wealth, and technology—have impacts on the environment, so that if one factor is reduced but another increased, the result can be a wash. For example, a country with a large population that's extremely poor and has little technology might have a similar ecological effect to that of a country with a much smaller population that has greater wealth and a higher level of technology. Since few people want to preserve the environment by abolishing technology and reducing affluence, the solution to many of the greatest challenges facing us, from the greenhouse effect to the depletion of the ozone layer, from massive desertification to the destruction of the rain forests, from species extinction to the kind of relentless poverty that impels immigration and wars, must include reducing the earth's rapidly growing population. As a result, many brilliant minds have pondered what, in essence, is a question very similar to the question facing this generation of gay men: How do you motivate people to modify their sexual and reproductive behavior in order to prevent both personal and ecological catastrophe?

There are, of course, significant differences between population control and AIDS prevention (aside from the obvious one that population planning is concerned with too much birth, AIDS prevention with too much untimely death). Birth control offers people far more options than AIDS prevention, and many of its techniques—including implants and the pill—allow for full sexual intimacy and do not need to be considered each time a couple has sex. Even more important, birth control has a crucial escape hatch. While abortion is not always available or affordable, and while it is morally unacceptable to many women and psychologically untenable for others, it does exist as an option for millions. Indeed, it is one of the chief means of birth control in many parts of the world. There is simply no equivalent if you fail at safer sex. In comparing the two, it seems safe to say that as difficult as birth control is, it is significantly easier to achieve than successful AIDS prevention, at least within populations that have a high prevalence of HIV.

Nonetheless, the similarities between population control and AIDS prevention are in many ways more striking than the differences. Both deal with the unwanted side effects of human sexual desire and behavior (getting pregnant, getting AIDS), effects that have both a personal and ecological impact. The solutions to both require that people modify their personal and sexual behavior in ways that many individuals would prefer not to, partly in order to alleviate ecological problems that many people don't feel personally responsible for. The proposed solutions to both often conflict with deeply held cultural values, as well as with many individuals' immediate and powerful psychological and biological desires. Both are influenced by the fact that individuals often receive the full immediate reward of their actions while dividing the cost among a much larger group.

The approaches to the two issues, though, have been strikingly different. Whereas AIDS prevention has focused primarily on individual behavior and on the question of why individuals, or at most couples, engage in safe or unsafe sex, population theorists tend to examine sexual behavior at the cultural level. In this they have an obvious advantage: While population dynamics differ from culture to culture, their general principles apply to all, and population planners can easily see that some cultures produce uniformly high rates of population growth while others produce zero growth or even shrinking populations. Translated into our epidemic terms, some populations are consistently "above threshold" and others are consistently below. So rather than ponder why an individual couple chooses to have four children and another couple decides to have only a single child, population planners can ask why some entire cultures produce couple after couple who all seem to have an average of four kids, while other cultures produce couples who average only one. And what they find is that cultural factors are extremely powerful determinants of people's sexual and reproductive choices. Individuals don't make decisions about sex in a vacuum, but rather act in their own interests as cultures define and shape those interests.

Perhaps the most consistent finding in the field of population control is that "rewards influence behavior." Even in the highly charged and often seemingly irrational area of sex, people act in ways that reward them most and punish them least. Applied to the population issue, cultures that "reward" small families tend to produce small families, and those that "reward" large ones produce large ones. Societies that have attempted to alter their cultural incentive systems in a way that combines family planning education with distinct rewards and penalties favoring small families have managed to lower their population growth quite dramatically, even in the face of ancient and powerful cultural values that favor large families. Those that have merely relied on education and persuasion but left the old reward system unchallenged, however, have not succeeded in reducing population growth very much, if at all. The conclusion of these experiments has been evident for some decades now: When it comes to changing reproductive behavior, merely educating people and then leaving things up to individual choice is not enough.

Education

Education remains perhaps the most crucial component of changing sexual behavior. In the case of population control, for example, people need a clear understanding of the importance of reducing family size and a clear understanding of how to practice birth control. They need both the *why* and the *how*. How is fairly easily communicated, and involves a growing range of behavioral and technical options from the rhythm method and condoms to the pill, diaphragms, IUDs, implants, and vasectomies. But the why is often less clear, and the more sophisticated and educated the population, the more sophisticated and educated must be the why part of education. You cannot simply tell people what they ought to do and explain how to do it. You must also explain why in ways they find compelling and believable.

Thus far AIDS prevention has concentrated on a fairly narrow reading of education's first task. It has provided people with technical information on how to reduce transmission through the use of condoms, which is vital and must continue to be emphasized. But it has ignored the broader educational goals of convincing gay men they need to change gay sexual culture in more fundamental ways, and of convincing them that such changes are *possible*. The first step in that process would be self-education.

In the next chapter I will argue that self-education of gay men needs to be directed toward a broad shift in gay culture, one in which sex and sexuality remain a major part, but only one part, of a more balanced gay life. I will argue that to create a sustainable gay culture requires a paradigm shift in many of the most basic aspects of the way gay men relate to each other and the world. But first I want to focus on just one narrow aspect of self-education, namely self-education about sexual ecology itself. I focus on that first not because I believe that if gay men have a better understanding of the ways that AIDS happened to us and the reasons it is continuing, we will automatically be able to and willing to build a safer culture. We will probably not. Rather, I focus on it first because I believe that without a better understanding of sexual ecology and epidemiology, we will not see the reasons why we need to change more basic aspects of our culture. The same is true throughout the environmental movement. Before populations became motivated to stop the destruction of the ozone layer, people had to educate themselves about the relationship between fluorocarbons and ozone. It may seem ridiculous to expect the public to learn about or care about such technical things, but such understanding is an essential prerequisite to action. In the same way, as long as gay men do not understand basic connections between AIDS and concepts such as epidemic threshold, core groups, sexual concurrency, and so on, most of us will be perfectly justified in resisting attempts to change those behaviors. You have to understand how something is hurting you before you're motivated to do anything about it. So the first task of self-education is self-education about sexual ecology itself.

Self-education is hardly new to gay men in the AIDS epidemic. In the early and mid eighties many became experts in volunteerism, quickly learning how to take care of the ill and dying, how to organize and raise money and build effective community-based organizations, how to provide basic prevention information, how to comfort and bear witness. In the late eighties many others successfully tackled the intricate medical aspects of AIDS, the financial workings of drug companies and research institutions, the complex politics of AIDS funding and ways to counter right-wing responses to the epidemic, and the techniques of direct action. Until now, however, self-education in the field of sexual ecology has been the exception rather than the rule. Gay men who are experts at the wily ways of the virus, adept at the politics of AIDS, compassionate caregivers to the afflicted, remain surprisingly ignorant of the ways that the epidemic itself proceeds among us. That needs to change quickly. Environmental progress is based on ecological self-awareness, and so sexual ecology must become as familiar as any other aspect of the epidemic.

As part of this process, gay men must become researchers ourselves, as we have with other aspects of AIDS. We also need to encourage professional researchers to speak plainly. Unfortunately, we have often done the opposite, and as a result many epidemiologists have been reluctant to share their insights with gay men. Social scientists and medical researchers have long understood that they need the respect, trust, and cooperation of the communities they study in order to carry out their work. Researchers who become lightning rods for controversy often lose the respect and trust of many of those they study, and when that happens it can become impossible for them to continue their work. Unfortunately, in the case of AIDS and gay men it has often been extremely difficult for researchers to speak honestly about epidemiological matters without giving offense to some, since many of the most important causes of the epidemic are directly related to highly sensitive factors within the gay world. Researchers who speak plainly are likely to find themselves embroiled in controversy and accused of unscientific bias. During the heyday of AIDS activism many activists sought to silence epidemiological studies they felt implicitly "blamed" gay men, studies that might have an adverse impact on funding, or those that merely seemed insensitive to gay men's feelings. One of the most public examples occurred in New York City in 1988, when Health Commissioner Stephen Joseph, acting on the best available epidemiological information, reduced the city's estimate of people infected with HIV from 400,000 to 200,000. Activists suspected that the reduction was motivated by the Koch administration's desire to reduce expenditures on AIDS, and Joseph was vilified, picketed, called a murderer, and publicly compared to Nazi torturer Josef Mengele. Yet Joseph's revised figures are now accepted as having been, if anything, too high, not too low. Current estimates are that 100,000 New Yorkers are HIV infected. The furor lasted months, and was a vivid public example of the perils that any epidemiologist faced for speaking about AIDS in ways that ran counter to the perceived interests of the gay and AIDS activist establishment. Across the nation some respected researchers simply withdrew from AIDS work altogether, while others shifted their attention to the epidemic in Africa or Thailand or other areas where basic research was less controversial. Still others continued studying the gay epidemic, but in whispers, presenting their findings to each other in by-invitation-only symposia and private meetings but keeping the data out of print and nervously avoiding any publicity, especially publicity that might attract the attention of AIDS activists. This situation is by no means over—as of this writing, stories still abound of academicians, mathematical modelers, field researchers being shouted down and insulted, or having their professionalism questioned, when presenting basic epidemiological information about gay men and AIDS.

It may seem an overstatement to call this approach to research on the part of gay men suicidal, but imagine a scenario in which a patient suffering from a potentially terminal illness shouted down his doctor and stormed from the clinic each time the physician attempted to explain the role that his two packs a day and his excess two hundred pounds played in the disease, convinced the doctor was pushing some "closet moralism" instead of offering sound medical advice. The idea that the AIDS community would prefer enforced ignorance rather than bitter truths amounts to a form of self-harm. If education and self-empowerment are crucial to the containment of AIDS, then epidemiologists will by the nature of their business be among the chief educators. The process of learning must include learning from them, however unpleasant their diagnosis.

Self-education, however, is just a first step. Another necessary step involves helping to educate those who are less interested and less likely to make an effort to educate themselves. The message of holistic prevention must permeate the whole of gay society if it is to have any chance of changing the course of AIDS, and most gay men, like most people generally, are unlikely to take the time to embark on a major course of detailed self-education. This is why groups that battle scourges such as lung cancer and heart disease engage in a continuous process of public education, emphasizing and reemphasizing the link between smoking and cancer, or demonstrating for the umpteenth time the coronary benefits of a low-fat diet or daily exercise. No population is likely to accept the need to make major behavioral changes unless that need is presented with compelling evidence and then repeated constantly. Gay men have done that about condoms. We must do it about the rest of the AIDS equation as well.

Transgression and the Will to Change

When trying to communicate the need to change gay sexual culture, educators almost immediately come up against two enormous roadblocks. One is a widespread belief in the gay world that gay male culture should not be changed, and the other is the pervasive belief that gay male culture *cannot* change.

To some gay men, the idea that gay culture needs to change is seen as heretical, especially when those changes seem to mimic aspects of the heterosexual world. The outlaw aspect of gay sexual culture, its transgressiveness, is seen by many men as one of its greatest attributes. To this way of thinking, the answer to Harry Hay's famous question, What are gay people for? is that we are here to challenge the sexual hypocrisy, smugness, and repression of the heterosexual world. The fact that gay men's culture is so overtly sexual is seen as its purpose. The rest of the world would do itself a favor if it copied us.

Any move to modify that transgressive stance is seen by some as treason.

This opinion is obviously a very difficult obstruction to the creation of a gay culture in which sex would become more integrated and balanced, especially since it is held by many of the most articulate, talented, and vocal members of the gay community. But it is here that ecological education could make an impact. While I have no doubt that some determined gay men will remain proponents of sexual libertinism no matter what, I also believe that many who adhere to that cause do so because they have never understood the facts of sexual ecology. And those facts are that many of the very behaviors gay men celebrated as transgressive and revolutionary—the behaviors bound up in the "brotherhood of promiscuity"—proved to be the very behaviors that spread HIV among us and that continue to do so. This may seem obvious to some readers, who see a clear cause-and-effect relationship. But it is not obvious to many gay men. Indeed, many of us have worked long and hard to obscure the connection.

Of course, making the connection more explicit will not impress everybody. Katherine Haynes-Sanstad of the University of California's Center for AIDS Prevention Studies has compared the strength of some gay men's visceral attitudes about their status as sexual outlaws to an attitude common among minority youth. "Consider the African-American adolescent who lives in the projects and is seen walking down the corridor with his books," she writes. "Home boys see him and say: 'What? You tryin' the be white?' Implicit in this is the assumption that to be white is to study and to play by the rules, and to be black is to hang, skip school and be tough. The gangsta identity is precisely the internalization, amplification and reflection of a caricature that was fostered on negative, racist stereotypes."

She goes on to suggest that some of the gay resistance to change may come from this same process, an internalization of society's stereotypes. If so, a way to combat that attitude is to combat the stereotype in the larger culture. If people are not treated like outlaws, they may not internalize that stereotype. But here things get very circular, because society is unlikely to eliminate a stereotype that is being celebrated and defended by some of the most articulate members of the minority it is attributed to. Obviously, then, the fact that many gay men do not want to change many of the basic factors that led to AIDS will remain a major impediment to constructing a sustainable gay culture.

State vs. Trait: The Ability to Change

Another major roadblock is a pervasive belief in the gay world that gay male culture *cannot* change. One frequently hears the view that the way gay men constructed their sexuality in the seventies and early eighties constitutes a sort of "default sexuality" for homosexual men. Things had to happen the way they did, it is said, because human males are inherently promiscuous, and a sexual society consisting only of men must, by an implacable law of nature, lead to the kind of promiscuity we experienced in the seventies.

If this is true, gay men can do little for themselves but hope for an early and complete cure for AIDS, and hope further that if the gay population produces epidemic after epidemic of other diseases, science will always be one step ahead—a rather forlorn hope if recent medical history is any example. However, if this concept is not true, it is vital to say so, because the very belief that it is may make change impossible. The reason lies in something psychologists call state vs. trait. It has long been noted that when people believe they must act a certain way because of some inborn "trait," they tend to believe that change is impossible and as a result don't even make an effort to change. But if people are convinced that their actions or feelings arise from a transitory "state" that they happen to be in at the moment, they tend to believe that change is possible. This psychology applies to communities as well as individuals, so it is crucial that gay men, both as individuals and as a community, closely scrutinize any theory that argues that we must act a certain way because of an inborn trait.

According to the "trait" argument, the behaviors that swept the gay world after Stonewall were inevitable not so much because of features intrinsic to homosexuals but because of traits intrinsic to men. Promiscuity, it is argued, is simply what must happen when males are free to pursue their erotic natures in a sexual culture devoid of women. This is an extension of a centuries-old belief that males were the only ones who had any sexual drive at all and that women were merely the objects of male desire. In this century the pendulum swung quite far in the other direction as feminist thinkers argued that most of the differences between the sexes are cultural rather than biological. So when gay activists, who often tend to be feminists, make the trait argument about male promiscuity, they seem to contradict themselves, arguing that patriarchal men control the world and control women, but that when it comes to the most powerful aspects of desire, women have managed to arrange things to their own liking and thwart heterosexual men's deepest promiscuous impulses. Why patriarchs throughout history haven't simply turned women into sex slaves to satisfy their apparently insatiable and universal male desire to have unlimited promiscuous adventures is usually left unexplained.

Feminist contradictions aside, those who argue that men innately are more interested in sexual variety than women do seem to have an increasing body of literature and theory on their side. Evolutionary psychologists now argue that the environment of our hunter-gatherer ancestors strongly predisposed males to be more promiscuous than females for basic evolutionary reasons. According to this theory, children require a huge maternal investment, so a hunter-gatherer mom's best strategy for passing her genes to future generations was to select carefully a reliable mate who would help her raise her young. But while it was in a woman's biological interests to be very picky about her mate, hunter-gatherer dads had dual strategies for maximizing their chances of passing their genes on to the next generation. One was to select a female carefully and help her raise a family, since children raised by two parents had a better chance of survival than those raised by one. But the other part of the strategy was to mate with as many additional females as possible, since a quick fling required no long-term investment on the part of the father and the more offspring you have, the more likely that a few will survive. As a result, modern humans are descended from women who were extremely selective about their mates and from men who were good at selecting reliable mates and then cheating on them as often as possible. This, it is argued, has left men with very different sexual natures than women.

If this is so, and it seems likely that it is, then it stands to reason that an exclusively male sexual society will tend to be more promiscuous than either a society of heterosexuals or a society of lesbians. Which is precisely what we see today. From this it is further argued that liberated gay men must always end up behaving pretty much like gay American men behaved in the seventies, and that there's nothing much anyone can do about it except get out of the way. But that second part of the equation actually amounts to an unwarranted leap, because the question is not whether gay men will always be somewhat more promiscuous than other populations. Let us assume, for the sake of argument, that we will be. The question is, must gay men always be so much *more* promiscuous that our behavior will inevitably spiral out of control, leading to epidemic disasters? In other words, must liberated gay men always tend toward biological self-destruction unless continually rescued by modern science? And here the answer seems to be no.

Throughout history the voluntary control of sexuality has been a major preoccupation of all religions, all cultures, all peoples. Every society on record has attempted to channel sexual drive in ways that promote stability, usually by enacting explicit rules about whom you can and cannot have sex with, and then backing up those rules with powerful rewards and penalties, social customs, religious beliefs, laws, and taboos. Men have usually been allowed more sexual leeway than women, but sexual restrictions have always applied to men as well as women, often in ways that tremendously constrained male freedom. One obvious example is the almost universal ban against committing adultery with another man's wife. This protects each man's investment in his own life partner and helps assure that the children he raises are his own, but only at the expense of ruling off limits the vast majority of eligible and desirable sexual partners, a pretty overwhelming constraint. Since men have dominated women in most societies, this raises the question of why men would make rules that so restrict their ability to have sex with as many partners as possible. Without digressing into all the theories as to why (see the evolutionary psychologists for that), it is fair to say that they have. And they still do. All of this seems to undercut the idea that men are biologically incapable of sexual restraint. They seem quite capable of it. In fact, self-imposed male sexual restraint has been the norm in virtually every society.

Some then argue that while this may be true, it's also true that the whole business of restraint gets a huge boost from women, who exert a monogamist and stabilizing influence on men, and from inheritance and property considerations, all of which provide incentives to moderate male sexual behavior. Since gay men don't generally have the incentive of trying to maintain a stable family environment for the sake of wives, children, and property, those kinds of influences are unavailable to us, and as a result, gay men cannot create a sexually moderate society.

This may be true, but it's not a *biological* argument. In fact, it tends to disprove the biological argument. What it argues instead is that men can indeed control their sexual behavior provided they live in a culture that provides them sufficient incentives to do so. There have to be things in men's lives that are worth more than absolute sexual freedom, things they might have to sacrifice if they practiced absolute sexual freedom. That, of course, is not necessarily good news for gay men, since there is nothing in gay culture at the moment that conflicts with absolute sexual freedom the way spouses and children and property do for straight men. Even long-term gay relationships don't necessarily conflict with the freedom to play around, since so many relationships are "open." But it certainly undermines the idea that gay men, as men, are biologically incapable of restraint.

Still another theory places more emphasis on the absence of women. It argues that without women's moderating influence a synergy occurs as sexually adventurous men pursue equally sexually adventurous men, producing a sort of feedback loop that turns an otherwise controllable energy into a tornado. According to this argument, each individual gay man might be capable of restraint if he were operating in a culture of restraint. But a community of all men operates like a chain reaction out of control, creating a critical mass and eventual meltdown: AIDS as China Syndrome.

If that were biologically inevitable, however, we would expect it to be universally true. After all, if homosexual men who are free to pursue their sexual natures *must* end up creating a promiscuous culture, then every society in which homosexual men have been free to pursue their sexual natures must have produced such a culture. Yet the historic record does not support this contention. In ancient Greek civilization, for example, men were free to love youths and, if examples such as Alexander the Great and his lifelong lover Hephastion are any indication, other men, yet they evolved a complex form of courtship and loyalty that seems the antithesis of promiscuity. Far from encouraging men to be, in Michael Callen's phrase, "sex pigs," the Greeks emphasized romantic qualities of selfless devotion and sacrifice in homosexual and pederastic love. As David Greenberg writes of the Greeks in *The Construction of Homosexuality*, "Homosexual love inspired by male beauty had the potential to develop into the most exalted love for ideal beauty and truth. By comparison, the object of heterosexual love lacked the special qualities that could inspire a spiritual or philosophical quest."

The Greeks may have accepted homosexuality, but they hardly condoned promiscuity. Immoderation and lack of restraint were among their chief horrors, not because of moralism but because, like good ecologists, they believed in moderation in all things. Greek thinkers had a theory that sexuality was so important that nature had endowed it with an extremely intense pleasure, and that because of this intensity people were naturally induced to go beyond their needs. Michel Foucault writes that Greeks were deeply aware that this passion could "overturn the hierarchy, placing these appetites and their satisfaction uppermost, and giving them absolute power over the soul. Also because of it, people were led to go beyond the satisfaction of needs and continue looking for pleasure" after they had been otherwise satisfied.

"One understands why, in these conditions, sexual activity required a moral discrimination," Foucault continues. "If it was necessary, as Plato said, to bridle it with the three strongest restraints: fear, law, and true reason; if it was necessary, as Aristotle thought, for desire to obey reason the way a child obeyed his tutor . . . the reason was not that sexual activity was a vice, nor that it might deviate from a canonical model; it was because sexual activity was associated with a force, an *energia*, that was itself liable to be excessive."

In discussing Foucault's analysis of Greek homosexuality, David M. Halperin writes that the Greek elite developed an ethic governing the usage of pleasures that "takes the form of a kind of calculated economy of sexual spending: limit yourself to what you really need; wait until the most opportune moment to consume; and take into account your social, political and economic status. Sexual morality is thus subsumed by the more general practice of self-regulation with regard to enjoyment that constituted for free upper-class Greek males an art of living, a technique for maintaining personal equilibrium, 'an aesthetics of being.' " Greek men went so far as to (in theory anyway) largely restrict their homosexual activity to a single mode of copulation: "intercrural," or intercourse between the thighs. No glory holes or fisting orgies for them, no psychological musings on the "meaning of semen exchange" in homosexual relations. With no apparent evidence of homosexually transmitted epidemics looming before them, the Greeks nonetheless seem to have practiced a form of "safer sex" almost identical to the one that modern gay men need to adopt: moderation within the relationship, and few or no outside partners. To the Greeks, the purpose of this restraint was not moralistic piety but freedom, while the danger of succumbing to pleasure was not dishonor but slavery, slavery to the passions of the body. "The most kingly man," wrote Plato, "was king of himself."

The idea that self-restraint and male homosexuality are quite compatible is seen in the historical records of several cultures that tolerated and celebrated homosexual love. The late Roman author Pseudo-Lucian, writing centuries after Plato, wrote that "wisdom coupled with knowledge has after frequent experiments chosen what is best, and has formed the opinion that gay love is the most stable of loves." Samurai warriors in feudal Japan had male youths as lovers and Greenberg writes that Japanese literary sources "depict the relationships as highly romantic, sustained by undying loyalty." Indeed, there is no record of any culture that accepted both homosexuality and unlimited homosexual promiscuity. Far from being the universal default mode of male homosexuality, the lifestyle of American gay men in the seventies and eighties appears unique in history. Which, of course, is what gay academics frequently argue when they advance the theory of social constructionism. So to the question, Must liberated homosexual males always produce a culture of promiscuity? the answer appears to be no. If we have never been this way before, it makes little sense to argue that there is some immutable law that says we must remain this way forever.

Admittedly, the record of cultures that accepted homosexuality is not very extensive, but for our purposes it doesn't have to be. For scientific theories to be considered tenable, they must survive refutation. In other words, if we hypothesize something—the classic example is to hypothesize that all swans are white—and then someone finds even one exception—a single black swan—our theory is disproved. If we are to accept the theory that men who are liberated to engage in homosexual activity must always become extremely promiscuous, the moment we find a single society in which men weren't, the theory is out the window. And that is the case.

This is not, by the way, to suggest that modern gay men ought to look to ancient Greece or samurai Japan as models of any kind. Such vanished cultures operated under belief systems so utterly different from ours that such a proposition is absurd. There's a passage in *Borrowed Time* where Paul Monette, traveling with his lover in Greece, rhapsodizes about what ancient Greek homoeroticism means for him as a modern gay man, and then wryly remarks, "Hopeless romance, I know: they kept slaves, their women were powerless, they sacrificed in blood." The point of citing Greece is not to suggest how we might be, but to apply the black swan rule to an unsupported and potentially dangerous theory of how we must be.

What the historical record shows is that people are not insects blindly following some genetic script. This point is raised because the existence of free will in gay male sexual behavior is hotly disputed, surprisingly not only by homophobes but by many gay men. Both camps contain people who argue that gay men are programmed to act as if they were sleepwalkers in a sexual dream. It's easy to understand why homophobes advance this argument. To them homosexuality is either a mental illness, which connotes loss of control, or a sinful and immoral choice, which connotes willful transgression and excess. Either way they naturally think of gay men as innately and uncontrollably promiscuous. But why would so many gay men subscribe to this idea, especially in a community where social constructionism is the intellectual fashion? After all, consider the implications of an argument stating that whenever you have gay liberation and free homosexual men to be themselves, a very large proportion of them will act like lemmings racing to the sea, engaging in a form of sexual self-indulgence almost unparalleled in human experience, a form that tends inherently to spiral out of control and produce epidemics that require the continuous intervention of medical science? This is hardly a pro-gay argument. Indeed, one can scarcely imagine a more anti-gay argument.

It is especially ironic that so many gay men believe this since the experience of gay men in this century is one of such amazing sexual evolution. Gay men have gone from living within a totally heterosexual and heterosexist culture, in which most people believed that only "fairies" or "queers" could desire members of the same sex, to the revolution of the sixties and seventies, when gay men carved out and defended great urban enclaves in which an unprecedented level of egalitarian promiscuity became acceptable. Male homosexuality has changed much more than heterosexuality in this century.

Of course, the obvious riposte is that gay men were simply evolving naturally toward their default state, and in the specific context of late-twentieth-century America that may be true. The way we were in the sixties and seventies and eighties is possibly the way we had to be, given the tenor of the times. But that very unfolding vividly illustrates that different states of homosexuality are possible, that cultures evolve, that gay men's sexual behavior, like humanity's in general, is subject to change.

We don't even need to examine earlier decades of this century to see gay sexual behavior turn on its heel: We have seen it quite recently. The fact that today the majority of gay men who have anal sex use condoms most of the time is eloquent proof of gay men's ability to adapt. Such a shift in mores would not have been predicted by any theory arguing that gay sexuality is fixed. But it not only happened, it happened consciously and deliberately, the result of an obvious ecological threat and a clear message, not of some unfathomable shift in the larger culture. True, this revolution in gay men's use of condoms does not seem to have been enough by itself to contain the epidemic, but that does not diminish the significance of the fact that it occurred. Combined with other evidence, the record seems abundantly clear: Gay male sexual behavior has changed many times. No one can say that implacable biology ordains failure, that gay social organization is fixed, promiscuous, and doomed. So long as we believe that ourselves, however, we take what might be our only hope of survival and rule it out of bounds. And as a result of that, our belief that we cannot change becomes a prophesy destined to fulfill itself, a case of an imagined "trait" creating its own implacable state.

Strangers in a Strange Land

Youth. The "trait" belief is not the only obstacle to gay men imagining that we can change our culture. Another is the idea that because we are a minority, we are not really in control of our own destiny. That we bob around on a sea of cultural enemies, objects acted upon by the malign majority, incapable of influencing much about our lives because we are so scattered, disunited, and diffused within the larger majority.

It is true that gay people, more than most minorities, are directly shaped by the majority, since we grow up within heterosexual families, imbibing homophobic values from childhood. The influence of those values often becomes pronounced during adolescence, which for many gay men and lesbians is a time made immensely complex and traumatic both by homophobia itself and by our inability to progress through phases of personal development that heterosexuals take for granted. Young gay adolescents rarely get to be open about their most basic desires and crushes on others. They don't get to go on dates or go steady, to dream of adult relationships and marriage. They rarely get to confide these problems to supportive parents or siblings, or to anybody. Instead, many experience deep shame and revulsion concerning their sexuality, and end up cultivating a secretiveness that often reinforces self-perceptions as undesirable and disgusting. In adulthood many lesbians and gay men attempt to throw off the shackles of shame and reimagine ourselves in a positive light, and many succeed, some more so than others. But having failed to undergo an open course of development as adolescents and having missed the opportunity to integrate sex with social approval and intimacy, many gay men face great difficulties in attempting to forge those connections in adulthood.

Unfortunately, the very process of ridding ourselves of shame and developing a more positive self-image is made infinitely more complicated by AIDS itself. The epidemic is now so associated with male homosexuality that when a group of junior high school students was asked to write down the first thing that came to mind when they heard the word *gay*, the vast majority immediately wrote *AIDS*. Now, in addition to the stereotypical images of gays as immoral and mentally ill, young gay kids are saddled with a new stereotype, one of infection, wasting, and death. As time passes and AIDS fails to permeate the rest of society while continuing to devastate gay men, such associations may grow even stronger. And so we face another terrible synergy: AIDS deprives many gay young men of hope, and hopeless young men help perpetuate AIDS.

The traditionally low level of monogamy among gay men and the unfortunate association between sex and self-destruction may well have many of their roots in adolescent experiences. If so, however, this suggests that one promising strategy for creating a sustainable gay ecology is to work to improve the lives of gay youth. The question is, How can we go about doing this? Some argue that by fighting for adult rights, we inevitably fight for youth as well, but this seems increasingly self-serving and myopic. The serious problems facing gay kids—particularly safety in schools; coming out and dealing with hostile reactions it can engender; shame, homelessness, and suicide; AIDS education and social skills to put that education to use; confronting the fear of AIDS; and negative self-images generally—will not be solved by trickle-down liberation. If gay adults, and for that matter straight adults, want to improve the self-images of gay kids, we have to address those problems directly.

Thankfully, more and more people are working to do just that. Around two hundred groups now address gay youth issues, from P-FLAG to the Gay Lesbian Straight Teachers Network, from New York's Hetrick-Martin Institute to dozens of local drop-in centers. Gay men and lesbians are running for school boards, fighting for the inclusion of positive gay images in curricula, demanding honest AIDS education. Those who do this work say it's compelling, rewarding, and can make a big difference. The problem is that so few are doing it. There may be two hundred groups dedicated to these issues, but we need two thousand. Even more, activists need to make youth issues central to the groups we already have, not afterthoughts.

Every population recognizes its obligation to its youth. Some gay men and lesbians may perhaps feel less of an obligation, partly because we don't actually parent the next generation of gay kids and partly because we've been accused of "recruiting" for so long that many of us shy away from the whole painful subject. But in the age of AIDS these excuses cannot stand. The world of gay adults is having a massive impact on gay youth, and that means we have an obligation not only to fight against homophobia in the adult world and hope that will trickle down to gay kids, but also to fight just as hard against the major problems that confront gay youth, especially safety in schools, homelessness, suicide, AIDS prevention, and lack of a belief in the future.

Victims. Another product of homophobia is the sense that gays have been victimized by AIDS. Theories of victimization come naturally to movements that were founded to fight oppression and unfairness. It seemed eminently reasonable to apply that same analysis and rhetoric to the AIDS epidemic itself, and we have done so with gusto since the mid-eighties. Although some of the theories of how AIDS was foisted upon gay men seem plainly paranoid—HIV as deliberate germ warfare; AIDS as planned genocide—others have been far easier to accept because they were partially true. Many of us have argued that neglect of the epidemic was caused by the radical right, by the uncaring media, by the general climate of hostility that society directs against homosexuals. As part of this rhetoric of blame, we accused uncaring public officials of being "AIDS murderers." In AIDS discourse homophobia itself was commonly cited as the "cause" of the epidemic. This was a hallmark of the intense activism of the late eighties, when it was often confidently asserted that elimination of homophobia would, in and of itself, quickly solve the problem.

This rage against society's infuriatingly lackluster response to AIDS was often quite effective, since it pricked the conscience of the nation and ultimately increased the attention and funding directed at the epidemic. But for those of us who believed our own rhetoric perhaps too well, in many ways it also became a comforting deflection of responsibility. Now the epidemic became the "fault" of straight people who didn't do enough to inform gay men of the danger, finance services for the afflicted, and produce a cure. It came to be considered "pro-gay" to blame AIDS on homophobes, and "homophobic" to mention our own epidemiological role in the whole mess. That would be "blaming the victim."

This is not to diminish the roles that homophobia played or continues to play in exacerbating the problem. For one thing, homophobia has contributed to the fact that AIDS prevention remains critically underfunded and the vast preponderance of funding is not directed where the need really lies. For another, by constantly attacking the very legitimacy of gay identity, homophobes place gay men in a defensive posture from which it becomes exceedingly difficult to engage in an honest discussion of the very problems that are destroying so many of us. Every embattled minority tends to fear that disclosing its internal problems might provide ammunition to the enemy, and there seems to be an almost universal tendency to avoid airing dirty laundry in public. Unfortunately, sometimes when sensitive problems remain unaddressed they have the potential to cause far more harm than open discussions ever would, and in such situations far more can be lost than gained by hushing things up.

Reluctance to discuss the problems of gay sexual ecology is not, however, confined only to gay men or lesbians. Very often progressives and the heterosexual friends of gay people are just as anxious to avoid providing ammunition to homophobes, and thus frequently feel skittish about giving offense to gay people by analyzing how aspects of gay sexual culture contribute to AIDS. As a result, very little honest discussion exists between gay men and our straight allies about the perpetuation of AIDS in the gay population. Not long ago I discussed the state of the AIDS epidemic at a P-FLAG meeting, and while the members were attentive and polite, several people came up to me afterward and said that while they were certainly concerned about the facts I had presented, they were equally concerned that such facts not get in the hands of the anti-gay right. I certainly understood their worry. Folks in groups like P-FLAG can easily be so overwhelmed with the task of countering ugly myths and stereotypes about gays that it seems self-defeating to admit that there are serious problems in the community they are defending, much less that some of those problems relate to the very sexual behaviors that moralists love to criticize. It's almost as though one has a choice: either to fight against homophobia or fight for genuine AIDS prevention—one can't do both.

That, it seems to me, is inaccurate, since one of the most effective ways to fight homophobia is to engage in genuine AIDS prevention. It's also a shame. The gay male population could profit from the commonsense perspective of supportive friends who are not caught in the midst of the epidemic. Common sense can be hard to come by in a holocaust.

No one can deny that homophobia and gay men's minority status place significant obstacles in the way of conscious evolution, and these problems should not be minimized. But the history of the modern gay movement seems to demolish the widely held theory that gay men are incapable of moderating their sexual culture. It may be true that men tend to be sexually more adventurous than women, and it is certainly true that gays are outnumbered in this society. But gay culture has been remarkably pliant, the history of past gay cultures shows amazingly little automatic attachment to promiscuity, and gay men have been notably successful in developing a very distinctive culture with its own institutions and norms.

Perhaps the biggest obstacle to change is gay men's belief in our own social victimization and inability to change. Such ideas can be more damaging than anything real. Indeed, by believing in them we can make them real, allowing us to forgo a search for real answers. True, most of these beliefs contain grains of truth, but their omnipotent power does not survive close scrutiny. So a principle task of sexual ecology is to challenge sloppy arguments that purport to explain why gay men cannot create a healthy and sustainable culture, and to foster instead a vision of the future in which we are empowered to save ourselves.

Building Incentives into Gay Culture

n order to develop a sustainable sexual culture, gay men need
detailed education on how to change our behavior and need to
be convinced of the possibility of change. But those are only prerequisites. Ultimately, the situation is unlikely to improve unless
the broader gay culture supports the necessary changes. To return
to the birth control analogy, population experts have long noted
that culture exerts a powerful influence on human sexual behavior,
and that a significant part of culture's power takes the form of what
is called the "selection principle," which states that rewards influence behavior. Sometimes this principle operates fairly transpar-
ently, as in the profit motive. Other times its operation is less
obvious, as when people do things that seem to cause them harm
but which, on closer examination, seem rewarding to those
involved. Addiction is perhaps the starkest example of this. When
addicted people light up cigarettes, or inject heroin, they satisfy a
powerful immediate craving. While the results of that satisfaction
may be terribly detrimental in the long run, the long-term detri-
ment just does not outweigh the short-term reward. In a similar
way, for many people who consistently overeat, the immediate
positive rewards of eating outbalance the negative consequences of
being overweight. Or looked at another way, the negative consequences of suffering through the deprivation of a diet outbalance
the positive rewards of being thinner. Even the most literal forms

of punishment, those meted out to criminals, do not always out-weigh crime's perceived benefits. Criminals may appear to behave irrationally, but as Garrett Hardin points out, for certain individuals the positive rewards for criminal activity outweigh the negative reinforcements of apprehension and conviction, which in any case are only probable, not certain. "If society aspires to change criminal behavior—not merely to punish it when the offender is caught," writes Hardin, "it must identify the total reward system" that influences individuals' choices.

The same can be said when society aspires to change reproductive and environmental behavior. Population planners have found that it is not enough simply to educate people on how to change, or to convince them that they can change, even though both of those things are crucial prerequisites. The "total reward system" of the culture must be structured so that the rewards of the desired behavior considerably outweigh the penalties.

This is not to say, by the way, that altering a population's total reward system is, by itself, sufficient to alter people's behavior. The factors that go into personal decision making are complex, and cultural incentives form only a part of the total equation by which people order their lives and make day-to-day decisions. Indeed, some individuals are quite impervious to cultural incentives, or even take pleasure in flouting them. Because of the complexity of human decision making, altering a culture's reward system will not by itself produce automatic change, nor can it ever hope to produce change in everyone. But the experience of population control indicates that it is a prerequisite to producing change, and that so long as the cultural system continues to reward the wrong kind of behavior, change is virtually impossible. Attempts to influence population growth that have ignored this principle have uniformly failed. And it seems likely that attempts to contain AIDS transmission that ignore this principle will fail as well.

The Tragedy of the Commons

In an influential essay in the journal *Science* in 1968, Garrett Hardin sketched out a dilemma concerning overpopulation and environmental destruction that illustrates the error of supposing that some "invisible hand" will always direct people to do what is best for the common good. He calls this dilemma the tragedy of the commons.

Hardin asks us to imagine a town commons like the ones in old New England villages. All the villagers have a legal right to graze their cattle on the commons, and this arrangement benefits everyone equally. But there's a built-in problem: Each time a new cow is added to the commons, it places stress on the environment, and only a finite number of cows can graze without destroying the ecology of the commons for everyone. The "tragedy" lies in the fact that it is in each individual farmer's interest to add another cow, since each farmer receives the full benefit of that cow, while the loss in grazing capacity is shared equally by everyone. In Hardin's equation, the "positive utility" of adding another cow equals roughly 1 for each farmer, but the "negative utility" is spread equally among everyone, and is therefore far less than 1 for any individual farmer. So the only sensible course for each farmer is to add another cow. Everyone does, and the commons is destroyed.

The relevance of this principle to AIDS and gay men was first pointed out by Martina Morris and Laura Dean in their famous paper on the effects of behavior change on the spread of HIV. They found, you recall, that if the average gay man in New York reduced his sexual contact rate to one "unsafe contact" per year, the level of HIV in that population would probably drop to less than 5 percent in thirty-five years. But if the average rose to two unsafe contacts per year, HIV prevalence would rise to 60 percent. "The implications of temporary returns to unsafe practices are not simply an increase in individual risk," they wrote, "but also the persistence of HIV transmission at epidemic levels in the [gay] population. This result is a classic example of . . . the 'Tragedy of the Commons,' where the disjunction between individual and population level effects leads to the potential for worst-case outcomes. Here the increment in individual risk from a slight increase in contact rate is negligible, assuming the individual acts alone. If all individuals make this choice, however, the aggregate impact is nonnegligible, and the result is a phase shift in the population dynamics of the disease, dramatically increasing everyone's risk."

The problem is rooted in the difference between individual and aggregate risk. What each man gains by having occasional risky sex is, from his perspective, potentially much greater than what he loses, especially if his activity is not really very risky. "I can have plenty of sexual partners and do so perfectly safely," someone will typically say. "I always have safe sex, or at least almost always. Why should I change?" From his perspective, of course, he shouldn't. That's the "tragedy" part of the tragedy of the commons. Each person sees no need to change a system where his individual choices are indeed logical and beneficial for him. But all those "logical" choices add up and tip the entire system into disaster. By helping to facilitate a system that produces disaster, each person contributes to the disaster, even if he remains uninfected himself.

Many people cannot fathom what we mean by "commons" when we speak of gay men and AIDS. Most people think of sex as a private affair, and in the gay movement the concept of sexual privacy is elevated to almost a sacred principle, since much of the gay movement is based on the idea that sex is and ought to be nobody's business but your own. But biology is under no obligation to respect ideology, and the gay commons is as biologically real as the commons in an old colonial village. The play *Six Degrees of Separation* proposed that no two people on earth are separated by the acquaintance of more than six others. In a biological sense, no two sexually active gay men within a given sexual ecosystem are separated by anywhere near that much. Every gay man who has "private" sex joins together in a visceral, biological stream that flows through our blood and our bodily fluids both in time, connecting us to the private sexual acts of gay men years ago, and in space, linking us to the sexual acts of those all around us. By becoming sexually active, each of us influences the fate of our brothers, and is influenced by them as well. The question is not whether there is a gay commons; the question is whether that commons will remain polluted with HIV in such a way that it will continue to pose extreme danger even for those who make only modest contact with it, including gay youth who are just becoming sexually active and cannot be expected to be as sophisticated in the practice of safer sex as their more experienced elders.

However, the tragedy of the commons is neither inevitable nor immutable. All societies can, if they choose, negate the tragedy by altering the reward system. In the literal case of the town commons, the village can pass a law limiting how many cattle each villager can graze, or charge an escalating grazing fee that makes overgrazing unprofitable, or hire a manager with power to oversee the commons. The same principle has been effective in the case of population control. All the education in the world cannot slow or reverse population expansion when the reward structure or status structure of society favors large families. But conversely, even long-standing cultural beliefs and deeply held religious convictions operating in favor of large families or against birth control don't seem to have much impact if the reward structure of a society changes to favor small families.

An interesting case in point is modern Italy. By most measures Italy would seem a poor candidate for population control. For centuries Italians touted the large family as the social ideal, seeing it as a measure both of male and female status. In addition, Catholicism forbids modern methods of birth control, and 98 percent of Italians are Catholic. Yet Italy today has reduced its "average completed family size" to a point where the Italian population will actually begin shrinking in a few years, once baby boomers have passed reproductive age. Planners believe that this happened because over the past few decades the reward and status system of Italian society was transformed. Perhaps most important, the level of Italian women's education and liberation rose sharply, giving them sources of status other than children. Meanwhile, Italians' incomes and standard of living rose dramatically, but the cost of raising a child rose even faster. Suddenly Italians of both sexes were tempted with all sorts of financial and cultural rewards, including an unprecedented high standard of living and meaningful sources of prestige and status, provided they had very small families. Conversely, they were punished with a lower standard of living and consequent lower status if they chose to have large ones. Faced with this tectonic shift in the reward and status structure of society, family size dropped so dramatically that long-standing cultural values and religious prohibitions on birth control appear almost inconsequential. A similar process has occurred in many developed countries, from Japan to Sweden.

Fortunately, for most developed countries, low population growth occurred more or less spontaneously, but there was nothing inevitable about this lucky state of affairs. Indeed it has not happened that way in many Third World countries such as India and China, where prosperity and women's emancipation have not occurred soon enough to provide a demographic brake. As a result, populations in these countries are now so large that a high standard of living for everyone would cause environmental disaster.

Chinese demographers have estimated that to attain a modern Western standard of living without destroying the environment, China ought to have no more than about 650 million people. It currently has over a billion, so it needs negative population growth for decades to attain a sustainable prosperity. Since China has a strong and repressive central government, it has been able to implement perhaps the harshest population control program in the world, and its rate of growth has fallen dramatically. But interestingly, China's strict and repressive governmental policy, like Italy's benign and "natural" one, is still based primarily on rewards and penalties. The Chinese have developed a complex system of financial, cultural, and political incentives to encourage small families, including a major stress on women's equality (no small task given women's traditionally low status in Chinese society), tied to an intensely punitive system of financial, cultural, and sometimes legal punishments for those who have more than a single child. The difference is that China's penalties are far more cruel and coercive, and its rewards more meager, than Italy's, where the process occurred naturally without imminent threat of catastrophe.

It may seem unfortunate, even tragic, but looking around the world at the record of successful and unsuccessful population control, those are essentially the choices we see. Much of the developed world has achieved very low population growth, and some developing countries have made impressive gains as well, through a combination of education, women's liberation, and strong rewards and penalties that attempt literally to change the society's status system so that it favors small families. But there is no example anywhere of a society where education and birth control availability alone have made much progress in reducing population growth. India, for example, whose population problem is more severe than China's, has relied primarily on education, birth control availability, and persuasion to induce behavior change. It has failed catastrophically, say the experts, for a simple reason: The reward system of Indian society still favors large families in many ways. The health-care system is very poor and infant mortality is very high, so people feel the need to have lots of kids in order to be sure that any survive into adulthood. There is little or no social safety net, so parents' old-age insurance consists primarily of the security provided by their offspring. Women remain severely oppressed and see their status primarily in terms of children. And while the rewards for having a large family are great, the penalties are minuscule, since amid India's great poverty and limited educational opportunities it costs relatively little to raise a child. Indeed, the penalties mostly accrue to people who have small families. Given that, there could hardly be any other outcome than a steep continued rise in population, and blaming individual Indians utterly misses the point. The only blame that can be assigned is to the society as a whole for maintaining a system that is so obviously headed for disaster. As Hardin points out, the tragedy in these instances "is brought on not by individual sin ('greed'), but by the system itself; or by clinging to a system that won't work once the carrying capacity has been reached."

The record of population control seems clear: If a society wants to change ingrained behavior to avert ecological disaster, it has to do more than educate; it has to create a system of direct rewards to encourage that behavior. It is important to note how sharply this ecological principle clashes with the modified "harm reduction" philosophy that motivates much of AIDS prevention in the gay world. According to that philosophy, prevention should encourage only the minimum necessary changes in gay men's behavior that would give them the means to protect themselves from HIV, and it should specifically avoid advocating changes in larger aspects of gay culture. Yet as the experience of successful population control attests, it is precisely the larger aspects of culture that most influence whether people will change their behavior. By ignoring this principle and attempting to interject the techniques of safe sex into a culture of inherent unsafety, we make the same error that India makes in its approach to population control. We ignore the maxim that rewards influence behavior, and then act surprised when people continue to behave in a way that serves what they perceive as their immediate best interests.

The Logic of Unsafe Sex

The idea that some gay men perceive risky sex to be in their immediate best interests and need some cultural incentive to practice safer sex may strike some as absurd. What greater incentive could there be than the negative incentive of avoiding infection with one of nature's deadliest viruses? And if health and life are not incentive enough, what could possibly provide greater motivation?

That argument might make sense if unsafe sex automatically or even usually led to HIV infection, and if HIV quickly and invariably led to illness and death. In that case such penalties would surely provide enormous incentive. But the cause-and-effect relationship between unsafe sex and negative consequences is nowhere near that direct. An attempt to identify the "total reward system" that influences gay male behavior reveals that as things currently stand, the penalties meted out to those who have occasional unsafe sex are relatively uncertain and abstract, while the rewards are often powerful, enticing, and immediate. It might sound odd, but in many ways gay men who have occasional unsafe sex are acting quite logically.

Weak Penalties. First of all, unsafe sex is not followed by the swift and sure penalty of infection. Given the statistical infectivity of HIV, one can expect to have unsafe anal intercourse dozens of times before becoming infected, even with an HIV-infected partner, and one can expect to have unprotected oral sex perhaps hundreds of times with an infected partner and still avoid infection. Biostaticians grimly point out that the cumulative result of all these individual risks is continued high prevalence in gay communities, and that's true. But for each individual, the immediate risk of one unsafe encounter—the one they are about to have right now—often seems quite low and escapable, and statistically speaking they're right. As long as the odds are with you—and at odds of 1 in 50 to 1 in several hundred they are indeed with you—many people will decide to take a chance.

A second weakness is that even when infection does occur, illness is postponed for many years, perhaps even decades. HIV's long incubation period has been one of its most bedeviling characteristics, and this is just one more example. A twenty-year-old gay man having unsafe sex today can quite logically assume that if he does get infected, he probably won't get sick until he reaches his thirties or, with today's improved drug therapies, even later. To many twenty-year-olds, the age of thirty-five seems like a lifetime away. In addition, any becoming infected today can certainly hope that before infection proceeds to the point where they would get sick, AIDS will have become a "manageable" syndrome and may even be cured. Indeed, as of this writing many argue that HIV infection is already a manageable syndrome, at least for those who can afford and can tolerate the expensive combination therapies. In addition, even before the advent of protease inhibitors there was an ongoing effort in AIDS discourse to refute the idea that AIDS is an automatic death sentence. On the one hand, AIDS activists pointed to plenty of "long-term nonprogressors" infected for ten years or more who showed no signs of immune depletion whatsoever, and "long-term survivors" infected for more than a decade who lead fairly healthy lives despite occasional illness. On the other hand, even when infection progressed along the usual lines, many argued that there was no reason to rule out a high quality of life. People are said to be "living with AIDS," not dying from it. Gay magazines and newspapers are filled with articles that celebrate the ability of healthy-looking HIV-infected men to lead rewarding lives, and stories abound of men who experienced meaningful personal growth only after they found out they were infected, at which point shame and sexual compulsion and substance abuse were swept away, replaced by a new spirit of hope and purpose and determination to get the most out of life. Many of the publications that engage in this kind of well-intentioned boosterism often carefully avoid images of wasting or illness or gruesome deathbed scenes, considering such journalism "intrusive." A stranger to gay culture, unaware of the reality of AIDS, might believe from much of the gay press that HIV infection was a sort of elixir that produced high self-esteem, solved long-standing psychological and substance abuse problems, and enhanced physical appearance. This, of course, is hardly the reality for most HIV-infected people, who scoff at any supposed "benefits," wish that they had never become infected, and pray desperately for a cure. But such messages, which are primarily aimed at the already infected, inevitably reach the uninfected as well, often inadvertently creating the subconscious impression that infection—the "penalty" of unsafe sex—is really not so bad after all.

An additional, if frequently unspoken, factor limiting the "penalty" of infection is the fact that once infected, many people believe they no longer need to practice safer sex for their own protection. Of course, prudence dictates that infected individuals should avoid contracting other STDs or opportunistic infections, and it has been theorized (although not yet convincingly proved) that reinfection with different strains of HIV can hasten illness and death. But for many, once they become infected the primary reason for struggling with safer sex is now eliminated. This was eloquently expressed by Scott O'Hara, the HIV-positive editor of a defunct gay sexual publication called *Steam* magazine, in an editorial in the autumn 1995 issue entitled "Exit the Rubberman":

> One of the most liberating comments I've heard in recent years came from a friend who's also been positive since the early years of the epidemic. "I'm so sick and tired of these Negatives whining about how difficult it is to stay safe. Why don't they just get over it and get Positive?" This was the first time I'd heard it in those words, but I realized that I agreed, wholeheartedly. Men who orient their entire life around a desperate struggle to stay negative—and then have the gall to complain about it!—are akin, in my mind, to those unhappily married men who spend their whole lives struggling to avoid acknowledging their attraction to men. It's an effort to deliberately eliminate pleasure from life . . . which is not, in my far-from-humble opinion, the object of the game. One of my primary goals is the Maximization of Pleasure, and just as I believe that Gay Men Have More Fun, so too do I believe that Positives have learned to have much more fun than Negatives. I'm delighted to be Positive. . . . The Negative world is defined by fear, ours by pleasure. . . .

This is followed by what O'Hara calls his Declaration of Independence: "I'm tired of using condoms," he writes, "and I won't."

Some might be shocked at his audacity, but O'Hara is at least being honest. And the view he expresses is not necessarily confined to a subset of HIV-infected men, but is shared by many gay men who are not infected, and who envy the ability of their positive but still healthy friends to engage unabashedly in the very behaviors that once defined, and in theory still define, what gay male liberation is supposedly all about. In the weird logic of modern "sex-positivity," only those who are HIV infected can, without fear or inhibition, fully experience the ultimate meaning of gay liberation as it has been defined by much of gay male culture since the sixties. Negative men, struggling to stay negative, are like closeted men: plainly less free, less liberated, and, according to the "total reward system" of gay life, less gay.

Mainstream society contributes to this problem as well. From childhood on, gay men and lesbians are bombarded with the message that they are sick and disgusting. Polls consistently show that about 75 percent of Americans believe that homosexuality is, in the words of one poll, "always wrong." But once you're infected with HIV, matters frequently change. Governments that deny basic civil rights to homosexuals often provide housing, income support, and health care to those with AIDS. Companies that are allowed to fire employees simply for being homosexual are often forbidden by law to discriminate against those disabled by HIV. Clergy who revile homosexuality from the pulpit often turn around and take up collections and provide care for AIDS sufferers. Families who throw out their gay sons often take them back when they're dying. The same mainstream culture that decries homosexuality as "always wrong" produces volumes of red ribbons and home-delivered meals and fund-raising benefits for ailing homosexuals. It's almost as if society is saying to HIV-positive gay men: Now that you're infected, you're forgiven.

This is not to say that people with AIDS are adequately taken care of, or that there is little stigma against those with the disease. But many people and many mainstream institutions exhibit deep compassion for homosexuals dying of AIDS while continuing to respond with unabashed contempt to those struggling to stay healthy, and, God forbid, healthily sexual. If you're merely gay, the subliminal message goes, you're "always wrong." If you get sick, however, people will love you again. You will be cared for, and find meaning and community. You will be mourned. It is not illogical for some gay men to conclude, at least subconsciously, that they're better off, if not dead, at least dying.

Strong Rewards. As a result of all of these factors, the "penalty" meted out to any given incidence of unsafe sex is fairly weak. Arrayed against it are the powerful immediate rewards for having risky sex. First and foremost, unprotected sex is good old-fashioned sex, without inhibitions and restraints, which to many people is the whole point of sex. In addition, sexual intimacy is a way of connecting with other gay men, a way of creating community, a source of psychological meaning. In a gay world in which sex itself provides the sense of meaning and community that marriage and children provide for others, a world in which many influential forces continue to extol sexual freedom and pleasure as its highest values, the surprising thing is not how much unsafe sex is occurring but how little. Within the structure of gay society, those who have occasional unsafe sex are acting in full accord with the total reward system they find themselves in.

Logic would therefore suggest that if gay men want to create a sustainable culture, this reward system has to be turned upside down. Taking a lesson from environmentalism and population control, immediate and tangible social rewards need to be implemented to encourage safety and restraint. And these rewards will have to be built right into the structure of gay society if they are to effectively counterbalance the weak penalties and strong rewards that currently help to foster a culture of risk among many gay men.

I hasten to add that this is not to suggest that such a reward system would automatically lead to widespread behavior change by itself, or that it would, by itself, solve the many long-standing problems that contribute to our unstable sexual ecology. Behaviorist theories that presume that people act entirely on the basis of outside rewards and penalties were never very convincing in their heyday in the middle of the century and seem far less so today. It seems clear that human behavior is influenced by a wide constellation of factors, and immediate rewards and penalties can often be overshadowed by many other things. What it does suggest is that while a system that encourages safety will not guarantee a culture of safety, it is probably a prerequisite for creating such a culture. All of our other efforts may come to little if we perpetuate a social system that undercuts those efforts.

Providing Incentives

If the central task of the new gay male culture is the integration of sexuality into a whole life, a life that respects sex but does not make it the central point of existence, gay culture needs to embrace the whole human being, his spiritual and personal self, his humanity, his vocations, his dreams, and not just his muscles or his libido or his penis. It has to draw explicit connections between sex and intimacy, and needs to reward self-restraint and end the pervasive belief that those who are living at the most extreme fringes of gay sexual life are somehow the most liberated and the most gay.

The construction of a gay culture that validates sexual moderation and constraint will be a daunting task. The tendency so far has been for the most visible and seemingly representative members of the tribe to veer rather wildly between extremes: intense core group activity in the seventies and early eighties, intense fear and a shutting down of sexuality in the mid to late eighties, and today a powerful revival of the external aspects of core group behavior. Many observers feel that only the specter of illness and death has prevented the full resurgence of gay sexual extremism in intensely active core groups, and that as AIDS becomes a more manageable disease the old disastrous lifestyle will fully reassert itself, with devastatingly predictable results. It therefore seems incumbent on gay men that if we want to avoid the continuation of the AIDS epidemic or the fostering of new epidemics, we will have to provide ourselves with incentives to live a life that is both openly and proudly gay on the one hand, and that reduces as much as possible the dangerous imbalances of the past.

The emphasis on condoms during anal sex will remain a major component of safer sex for as far into the future as we can imagine. But beyond that, a new gay culture of safety will also have to aim for the integration of sex into a wider fabric of private intimacy and public community. There will be many ideas about ways to accomplish this, and the ideas presented here are just a few out of many possibilities. Many readers may agree that such a shift in gay culture is necessary, but disagree strongly with my tentative suggestions for accomplishing it. Fine. What is offered here are simply ideas meant to help initiate a broader debate.

Respect Relationships and Fidelity. One of the most basic ways to make gay culture more sustainable is to create an honored place for relationships and fidelity. By this I mean that we need to encourage a new gay ideal that validates and supports relationships rather than one that validates and honors sexual adventurism, sexual consumerism, and risk taking. Some might complain that this implies aping a heterosexual model, the very model that many gay men argue they came out of the closet to escape. But that seems to prejudice the enterprise deliberately from the start. In fact, one could just as accurately say that the values I'm talking about are found in the lesbian world more than among heterosexuals. Indeed, if gay men want a model at all, the lesbian model seems much more appropriate to our condition than a heterosexual model, since lesbians are in much the same political and social boat as gay men. They cannot marry, and are therefore free to enter and leave relationships usually without an entangling web of legal or cultural impediments. As members of the same sex they do not enter relationships with predetermined power imbalances based simply on the sex of one partner. Yet lesbian society tends to honor fidelity in relationships as the ideal. Far more than gay men, lesbians tend to be monogamous, if not for life then at least for the duration of the relationship. It is worthwhile to note that lesbians have constructed such an ethic without feeling that they are mimicking straight people. Rather, their respect for the integrity of their relationships seems to arise from a basic respect for themselves and each other.

Of course, lesbians are dealing with a very different set of biological urges and cultural assumptions than gay men. A gay male culture that placed sex in more perspective still would not, and could not, look just like lesbian culture. But lesbians have shown gay men the possibility of creating such a culture without necessarily aping or mimicking heterosexuals, or developing automatic power imbalances within relationships based on sex. They also demonstrate that there is an alternative to promiscuity on the one hand, and an ideal of absolute lifetime monogamy on the other. That alternative is a culture in which serially monogamous partners expect and reward fidelity while they remain partners, but are ultimately free to dissolve the partnership, and tend to do so several times over the course of a lifetime. This kind of balance between fidelity and freedom would probably be important for gay men who seek to build a culture that is safe but not smothering, that still leaves open the possibility of sexual freedom while respecting relationships and encouraging fidelity.

Alternative Spaces. Building a more embracing gay culture would also seem to require that we develop alternatives to bars and discos as the prime meeting ground for gay male life. When I came out in the seventies, virtually the only places you could go to socialize as an openly gay man were bars, nightclubs, and bathhouses, places that inevitably connected gay life with cruising, with consumption of alcohol or drugs, and with racking up large numbers of casual partners. From a purely practical point of view, there were few alternatives. If you were gay and wanted to interact with others socially, those were the main, indeed almost the only, places to go.

So if gay men are ever going to place sex within the context of a larger cultural life, we need to create a larger array of spaces where people can be gay, be social, and do so in environments that are not focused exclusively around sex, cruising, and drug and alcohol consumption. Perhaps the most promising example of this kind of institution is the gay community center. From a humble beginning in the seventies, usually in rundown or abandoned buildings, a network of lesbian and gay community centers has now blossomed across the nation, and many of these institutions are now united in a national network dedicated to creating even more such spaces for social interaction. They provide meeting rooms for all sorts of groups, switchboard services, community bulletin boards, they host dances and parties as well as lectures and meetings, and generally provide a focus for gay life that respects sexuality but is not primarily sexual. In addition, there has been a huge increase in the past decade of gay sports teams, political groups, social service groups, volunteer organizations, and all sorts of recreational groups that also provide ways for gay people to be openly and socially themselves outside of an exclusively sexual context. All of these kinds of alternatives need to be encouraged and expanded, and a host of similar alternatives need to be explored.

Spirituality. In addition, there are growing networks of gay religious organizations that provide places for gay people to express their spirituality. These groups—ranging from gay synagogues and churches to New Age groups and meditation centers—reach out to the spiritual aspirations of gay men and lesbians that were often ignored or repressed in the heyday of the gay sexual revolution. In many instances, the sexual outpourings of those days were the only form of spiritual connection and intimacy men had. Today, a whole literature has appeared seeking to connect gay men to their spiritual and religious cores, and this needs to be encouraged and nurtured.

Integration. A major part of an integrated life for many people involves interaction with different generations, which provides a sense of connection to both the past and the future. Yet in many urban gay male settings, life is segregated by age to an almost astonishing degree. Not only are there virtually no children, but in many cases there are few friendships that span more than a decade or so. One gay venue may be filled with twenty-year-olds while another down the block may contain mostly people in their fifties and older. While this reflects modern American culture to some extent, the phenomenon is mitigated in the larger culture by fact that heterosexual adults often have plenty of contact with their children's generation, and kids interact with their parents and their parents' generation. In the case of the gay world, where most gay adults don't have children and most gay kids don't have gay parents, the age segregation seems more absolute, and more alienating. As gay men grow older they have little to connect them to the vibrancy and hope of a younger generation. And as gay youth enter the community, they have little to connect them to the wisdom and the assistance of an older generation.

So perhaps another way to foster a more sustainable gay culture would be to create institutions that promote intergenerational interaction. And in fact this is already happening. Older gay men are helping to sponsor gay youth, helping to shepherd young gay men through the often difficult process of coming out and finding a place in the world. Younger gay men are volunteering in gay agencies, often helping the elderly. Across the spectrum of gay life, in each institution and each gay family, people can encourage this process, making a point of trying to foster intergenerational contact and communication.

Valuing Both Youth and Age. I have already mentioned the need to promote greater self-esteem among gay youth generally. Still another way of promoting a more embracing gay culture is to make old age more attractive. The heavy emphasis on sex and looks and body culture in gay male life has produced a sometimes obsessive focus on maintaining youthfulness, leading in some cases to an almost desperate attempt by gay men to stave off the aging process. In a seemingly direct internalization of one of the worst anti-gay stereotypes, many younger men despair that since, to them, being gay is mostly about having lots of sex, which is facilitated by being young and looking good, life must lose much of its meaning after youth and looks have faded. One result is the cult of the gym. A much less healthy response is the sense of fear that some gay men report they feel when they contemplate growing older, sometimes resulting in at least a subconscious feeling that you might as well live fast and die young.

What is so ironic about this is that it does not conform with what many older gay men report about their lives. Counter to the stereotype of the lonely older gay men, many researchers argue that older gay men tend to be happier and better adjusted even than their heterosexual peers, largely because they have spent their lives learning how to be self-sufficient. As a result, gay men are already used to many of the things that straight people also find so frightening about growing older. But the inspiring resilience of older gay people is rarely communicated to gay youth. In fact, the vibrancy of gay seniors is one of the gay community's best-kept secrets—kept secret even from itself. In a culture that glorifies the humpy, hunky twenty-two-year-old as its ideal, how could the gray-haired elderly man seem anything but slightly pathetic? For those who see gay life reflected almost solely through the prism of physical beauty, it's not surprising that gay old age seems like an inherently empty place.

Talking It Through. Since long before Stonewall, gay men have engaged in a process of self-invention. The very fact that the larger society rejects homosexuality has meant that there has been no template, no norm or accepted life path for gay people. And this has meant that we have to invent our own way instead. Today this process remains difficult, since we must grapple with issues that face us both as gay men and as people surviving in the midst of an epidemic. Gay men are writing and thinking and proposing ideas as we have always have, often with vision and intelligence. Gay groups and AIDS prevention groups are beginning to experiment with different kinds of messages. All of this needs to be encouraged and strengthened.

Some Thoughts on Social Rewards

All of these changes could have an impact on helping to develop a more balanced gay life by encouraging and rewarding those who integrate sex more holistically into their lives. But they might not be enough by themselves. One could easily imagine a gay culture that had constructed thousands of community centers, had all sorts of programs and activities for people based on nonsexual pursuits, honored relationships, encouraged generational interaction, and yet still produced an amount of behavior that generated major epidemics and spread such epidemics across the gay population. And so we might have to go even further. If so, what might that entail?

All societies, from small tribal groups to modern industrial civilizations, have moderated sexual behavior through a system that provides direct benefits for those who exercise sexual restraint. The anthropological record shows that every single culture on earth encouraged people to settle down in structured sexual relationships, usually with a single partner. Societies seem to have universally recognized that while many individuals may desire sexual variety, unstructured sexual license leads to considerable social destabilization and is particularly disruptive to the process of raising children. You can't, it seems, be absolutely free to mate with anyone you wish while at the same time maintaining a stable family, which generally requires a strong central relationship with a long-term mate. Aside from providing a stable environment for children, the purpose of encouraging strong families has generally been to clarify inheritance and property rights and to avoid the social disruptions and distractions that seem to accompany promiscuity. There is little evidence that societies have consciously encouraged strong families in order to prevent the transmission of STDs, but the culture of restraint inherent in family life clearly served that purpose.

The core institution that encourages sexual restraint and monogamy is marriage. In most societies an essential part of the marriage contract, perhaps the most essential part, is the expectation that married partners will remain sexually faithful to each other. Partners exert strong pressure on each other to stay faithful, under the implicit threat that if one partner commits adultery and gets caught, the other has the right to terminate the union. The reward for exercising sexual restraint and remaining faithful is that marriage and family are maintained. The expected punishment of not remaining faithful (and getting caught) is marital discord and the possible breakup of the family. Some have argued that this arrangement has been imposed upon women by patriarchal men, and some say it has been imposed upon men by naturally more monogamous women, and a case can be made for both arguments. Until recently marriage was an inherently patriarchal institution in Western society (and still is in most societies), with men owning all the property, including, in a very real sense, the wife. And yet it is also evident that men are, as is sometimes said, "tamed" by their wives, who exert a sexually moderating influence. In fact both sexes seem to support marriage and monogamy for their own purposes, and both tend to be unforgiving of mates who stray.

Even so, marriage is hardly a foolproof enforcer of monogamy. There have always been cultures in which males, especially upper-class males, were allowed to play around so long as they remained fairly discreet. In addition, many people commit adultery in the belief that they can evade the expected penalty simply by not get-ting caught—although implicit in such a strategy is the recognition that if the adulterer does get caught there may be a serious price to pay. And some married relationships are deliberately and frankly "open." It is also true that even in cultures where marriage serves to enforce monogamy, the entire system can easily break down when one partner is unhappy in the relationship and wants to escape. In such cases, maintaining the family no longer functions as a reward, and its dissolution no longer serves as a penalty. The rewards and penalties can actually get reversed: Some people commit adultery precisely because they want to be "rewarded" with divorce. In general, however, the benefits of family life and the threatened punishment of familial breakup have, at least in many modern cultures, provided a major incentive for people to try to remain faithful, and in many cases are quite literally the bonds that hold many marriages together.

The restraining influence of marriage on couples is, however, hardly natural or automatic. It is a deliberate artifact of culture, and is socially constructed in myriad ways. The larger society propa-gates the rule that married partners are supposed to remain faithful, a rule that is accepted by most people and then operates from within the marriage as an internal check. If boys and girls were told that when they grew up and got married both they and their spouse would still be free to have sex with anyone they wanted whenever they wanted, marriage might not serve a moder-ating function at all.

In addition, some societies impose a system of even more direct external rewards and penalties to keep couples as monogamous as possible. One way they do this is by playing two seemingly "essen-tial" male desires off each other: the desire for sexual freedom versus the desire for social status. Many societies have used these twin desires to encourage sexual stability by saying to men that you can't have it both ways. If you choose sexual freedom over family and stability, that's fine, but you will not be afforded the same social status and respect as someone who chooses marriage and family. Conversely, if you choose family and stability you can expect the social status that comes with it, but obviously at the expense of the absolute sexual freedom enjoyed by a Casanova. In a system like that men are free to forgo status if they choose, and some Casanovas certainly do, flouting convention and boastfully racking up all the conquests they can—which among certain circles has a status of its own, the status of stud. But interestingly, when faced with that choice, the vast majority of people seem to have chosen conventional status and family over freedom.

Of course there's always been the famous double standard, the fact that men have not been expected to be as faithful as women. But even though many societies allow men more leeway, men have traditionally been expected to fulfill at least two conditions: remain discreet about their extramarital affairs and remain married. As a result, in many countries including this one until very recently, no man who had been divorced, or who had a public reputation for philandering, or who had been named in someone else's divorce proceedings, could aspire to the highest political office or many major positions of public or corporate trust. As recently as the mid sixties, for example, Nelson Rockefeller was considered disqualified for the presidency simply because he had once been divorced, even though he had long since remarried. An ambitious lawyer or corporate executive might soon discover that he would never make partner in the firm, or vice president of the company, until he was suitably married. As recently as the mid eighties Gary Hart was considered disqualified for the presidency after being caught in an adulterous affair, and in the nineties Bill Clinton continuously suffered in the polls for his alleged adulteries, even though it clearly seemed that he and his wife had some kind of arrangement. Such sanctions permeated society and popped up even in the most unlikely places. U.S. marines may have had a reputation for boasting about their sexual exploits, but any marine who contracted an STD was automatically disqualified for the officers' corps. Society did not exactly forbid male philandering, but any philandering that destabilized the core institution of marriage exacted a price to be paid in a currency almost every male could understand. That currency was, and to a significant extent still is, status.

Given the balance between these incentives, it stands to reason that if society relaxes the reward system favoring marriage, then divorce and premarital sex might increase. And the trends of the past few decades seem to confirm that prediction. As society has progressively lowered the stigma against divorce (a process that reached a sort of official culmination in the election of Ronald Reagan as America's first divorced president), rates of divorce have dramatically risen. Of course there may be other confounding reasons for this change. Indeed, society may have lowered the stigma against divorce in part because of other factors that have made marriages more difficult to sustain. In any case, a century ago most people remained married for life, no matter how unhappily. Today half of all marriages end in divorce.

Tying Incentives to Rewards. Marriage illustrates another fact about social reward systems. For social incentives to work there must be a direct connection between the reward (status) and the behavior society is attempting to encourage (marriage), so that those who play by the rules directly enjoy the fruits of their behavior. This crucial point is often lost on AIDS prevention workers who talk about trying to reduce unsafe sex simply by raising the self-esteem and happiness of gay men. If there were less homophobia, this argument goes, gay men would be less likely to take occasional risks, or have so many casual partners. This may be true in some cases, but the cultural record strongly suggests that unless the reward is directly tied to the benefit, what you'll generally get by making people happier are happier people who still have little incentive to change their behavior.

Any gay man doubting the power of social rewards and punishments should consider the recent development of gay men's "gym culture." There has probably always been a small clique of bodybuilders in the gay population, but right up through the seventies most gay men did not spend a lot of time pumping their muscles. Even the idealized bodies in sixties and seventies gay erotica were not necessarily "buffed." Then in the eighties, as disease swept the gay population, perceptions began to change. Perhaps in an effort to avoid the wasted look of many AIDS sufferers, more and more men joined gyms, went on strict diets, began trying to build the ideal body, and gym culture took off. It might be defined as a lifestyle that emphasizes strict, sometimes even fanatical addiction to exercise, weight control, and bodybuilding, combined with close attention to diet, nutrition, and other healthy regimens. Gay culture has developed a powerful, even merciless system of rewards and penalties based on body image. Those that stay in shape are socially valued, desirable, able to attract a lover, able to feel a sense of pride and self-esteem. Those who are flabby and out of shape are stigmatized, made to feel undesirable, have difficulty attracting a lover, and feel a powerful lack of validation, even a sense of invisibility. These standards are built right into gay culture, and operate in thousands of ways.

The strictures of gay men's gym culture often sound a lot like the advice that doctors urge most Americans to follow. But since most women do not impose particularly stringent rewards and penalties on their husbands and boyfriends based on looks (though men frequently impose them on women) the benefits of participating in gym culture for most straight men are more vague and theoretical: You'll live longer and be healthier. Sort of like the benefits of safer sex for gay men, and not, apparently, much more compelling when arrayed against the inducements to eat a greasy burger or drive instead of walk. As a result, American men today are more out of shape than at any time in modern history. In urban gay culture, however, the benefits of participating in gym culture and the penalties imposed on those who do not are immediate and tangible. A glance at the hard-bodied, flat-tummied musclemen in most gay neighborhoods illustrates how powerfully such social inducements can work among gay men, and how quickly they can produce shifts in behavior that under most circumstances people would consider extremely difficult if not impossible to maintain.

Developing a Reward System

What kinds of rewards might encourage gay men to adopt a culture of sexual restraint and responsibility, one in which they will be likely to reduce their contact rate and be as safe as possible within relationships? No one knows for sure, but since gay men are not a different species, it seems likely that these rewards are the same that influence most people: a culture that grants status to those who exercise restraint and responsibility, and by implication withholds status from those who don't. Since this is established for most people through the institution of marriage and the responsibility of raising children, one way to accomplish it in the gay world might be to establish the right of gay people to same-sex marriage and the right to raise children, and then encourage gay men to do both.

Many societies recognize that marriage is central to social and sexual stability—as the growing panic about the breakdown of families in our society attests. And it is overwhelmingly clear from the anthropological record that human sexual relationships that are not recognized and validated by society are nowhere near as durable as those that are. Try to imagine the heterosexual world with no marriage and no children. Many people feel that such a society would be far less stable and that large numbers of people would naturally engage in higher levels of promiscuity, and they're probably right.

In addition to marriage, many people say that raising children is perhaps the single most maturing experience in their adult lives. The selflessness involved in raising children, the need to make sacrifices and place others' interests ahead of your own, the sheer work involved, are powerful factors fueling personal growth and maturity. For many people, being a parent is their most important life's work, giving them a palpable link to the future and a strong sense of worth and self-esteem. Adults facing death often cite as their greatest regrets that they may not see the graduation of a daughter, or the marriage of a son, or the birth of a grandchild. And the project of raising children often ties couples together, providing a common purpose for couples who might otherwise drift apart. This may be why in most societies, including ours, the divorce rate for childless couples is significantly higher than for those with children.

In childbearing the interests of children must obviously come first, and it would be unconscionable to advocate a social order that benefited parents while harming their kids. Yet study after study consistently shows that children raised by lesbian moms and gay dads—and there are now thousands of such kids, many already grown to adulthood—are just as healthy and well adjusted as other children. Indeed, the only consistent difference is that kids raised by gay parents tend to be more tolerant of human diversity than other children, perhaps because they grow up recognizing the injustice that mindless bigotry has heaped upon their parents.

The idea that marriage would play a stabilizing role in gay male society has long been acknowledged within gay culture itself. Ironically, it is one of the chief reasons why many gay liberationists have vehemently opposed legalized same-sex marriage. Ever since Stonewall a furious debate has raged within the gay world over this issue, and one of the main objections of gay and lesbian radicals has been that such legalization would inherently undermine a major goal of gay liberation, which is to validate all kinds of relationships and all forms of sexual expression and experimentation, not to mimic an outmoded and oppressive heterosexual norm. Legalization of same-sex marriage, they argue, would create a two-tiered gay society in which married couples would be viewed within gay society as legitimate, while those who were unmarried would be considered social outcasts. This seems wildly exaggerated, since unmarried heterosexuals are not exactly seen as "outcasts." But the core of the objection—that marriage would provide status to those who married and thus implicitly penalize those who did not—seems essentially correct. Indeed, that's a key point. In a culture where unrestrained multipartnerism has produced ecological catastrophe, precisely what is needed is a self-sustaining culture in which people feel socially supported *within their identities as gay men* to settle down with individual partners for significant periods of time.

The anti-marriage sentiment in the gay and lesbian political world has abated in recent years, and the legalization of same-sex marriage is now an accepted focus of gay liberation. Yet it is rarely posed as a major issue of AIDS prevention. Prevention activists generally don't include marriage as a goal because they generally don't include monogamy as a goal. Belief in the condom code seems to render the subject moot. Meanwhile, most advocates of same-sex marriage generally fail to make the case for AIDS prevention because such advocates are generally careful not to make the case for marriage, but simply for the *right* to marriage. This rights-based approach is similar to the one taken by activists during the debate on gays in the military, when no one argued that gay men and lesbians should join up and serve their country, but simply that those who wished to do so should be allowed. In seeking to build the broadest possible coalition, advocates for marriage rights advance the same kind of argument. This is undoubtedly good practical politics, since many if not most of the major gay and lesbian organizations who have signed on to the fight for same-sex marriage would instantly sign off at any suggestion that they were actually encouraging gay men and lesbians to marry. But while practical, it leaves unarticulated the argument that winning the legalization of same-sex marriage and the right of homosexuals to adopt and raise children would create a solid foundation upon which a sustainable gay culture could arise. Fighting for those rights may turn out to be among the most important things gay men can do to assure our own survival.

Of course, it would be simpleminded to expect that legalized marriage and the ability to raise children would, by themselves, somehow magically solve the problem of AIDS transmission. They would not. But it seems equally absurd to expect gay men to develop a more stable and responsible culture without any social inducements at all. Gay male society is often "blamed" for being promiscuous as if it were possible for a male society whose members have no sanctioned relationships and no responsibility to anyone but themselves to be otherwise. If anything, gay male culture, being a culture without women, almost certainly needs *greater* social and cultural incentives for sexual restraint, not fewer. So it seems likely that fully legalized same-sex marriage, and the full right to raise children, are not cure-alls but prerequisites in any serious attempt to create a sustainable culture among gay men.

Think Publicly, Act Personally

Although the ideas presented above may ultimately aid in the creation of an overall culture of responsibility, they are offered only as suggestions. I expect readers will disagree with many of them, some perhaps violently. I hope that many of those readers might be prompted to offer their own ideas. But while specific approaches are wide open to debate, gay men's experience of both the First and the Second Waves of AIDS ought to convince us that the need to look at the problem ecologically is not so wide open. The fact that the challenge we face is an ecological challenge, with all that that implies, is not so much suggested by theory as, it seems to me, dictated by biology.

In any event, the enactment of things like same-sex marriage and the right to raise kids is not within the power of gay men and lesbians alone. These rights may be a long time coming, and we can hardly afford to wait until we have achieved victory before beginning the work of trying to create a more balanced gay life. As already noted, there are plenty of things we can do in the meantime. And most of them begin at home, with ourselves and our closest circle of friends.

Until now many gay men have grown used to the idea that AIDS prevention is something devised and promoted by folks at prevention organizations and then propounded to the gay population as a sort of techno/behavioral party line. People in the prevention movement speak of "crafting programs," "designing interventions," "developing strategies" that will impact this or that subpopulation, often in a hierarchical way. To be successful, however, sexual ecology needs to go further. Each person who supports its goals needs to demonstrate, by his own actions, that prevention can work in his own life. And each person needs to try to develop ways to build a structure of safety into his own personal version of a gay life. A fundamental precept of environmentalism is René Dubos's maxim that people should "think globally, act locally." A corollary precept of holistic prevention is that gay men need to "think publicly, act personally." To recognize that the transformation of gay culture begins at home.

There's a story about an ecologist visiting a college dorm and being peppered by the students with elaborate theoretical questions about what they could do to save the rain forests, halt global warming, and so on. Looking around at the mess of a typical dorm, he replied wryly that the first thing they could do was to clean up their rooms. What he meant was that environmentalism on the macro scale mirrors environmentalism on the personal scale; respect for balance in the world cannot be separated from respect for balance within our own lives. As it is with ecology generally, so it is with sexual ecology. Gay men who come to appreciate the necessity of building a sustainable gay culture must be willing first and foremost to apply such principles to themselves. The first step in ecological consciousness is to make a commitment to adopt holistic prevention yourself, knowing that the world will be delivered from AIDS one person at a time.

We need to embody such values not in order to mimic straight people or placate moral conservatives, but to save our own gay culture and our own collective lives. Some gay men may react with outrage to that. They may argue that the current approach to AIDS prevention already lays too heavy a moral claim upon gay men, and that this moral claim contributes to unsafe sex by shaming people into silence about the unsafe sex they have, or want to have. Indeed, one of the primary tenets of some new prevention thinking is that the condom code has failed because it has been too moralistic, and that "moralism" must never be employed in the service of AIDS prevention. Yet most people, gay or straight, inherently understand that to risk infecting another person or themselves with a deadly virus is morally wrong. They don't need AIDS prevention brochures to tell them that. And such moral feelings are not necessarily counterproductive. Cultures have always deemed certain behaviors right or wrong, and have always sought to encourage their collective survival by granting status to those who promote survival and withdrawing it from those who don't. In a sense, one of the very things that might make people who have had unsafe sex feel bad about it is the fear that they might lose status in the eyes of their peers, and that might be a mechanism that helps many people avoid unsafe behavior in the first place.

There is, however, a problem with overemphasizing morality as a way to bolster gay sexual ecology. Shame is one of the great enforcers of moral codes, but it seems highly unlikely that shame by itself would be a successful tool to change gay sexual behavior. Shame, after all, is the force that larger society has traditionally used to try to prevent gay people from being gay in the first place. One of the primary evils of homophobia is the way it has instilled a sense of shame in gay men and lesbians around the most basic sense of self and identity. The legacy of shame permeates our attitudes toward ourselves and toward each other, and so poisons individuals and the entire gay culture that in a sense the struggle for self-acceptance and gay liberation is a struggle against shame. It is therefore extremely unlikely that gay men could construct a sustainable sexual ecology primarily based on a foundation of shame, and even if we could, most of us probably wouldn't want to. Our challenge lies far more in encouraging the kind of culture we want rather than in discouraging the kind we don't want. But that does not imply that we should throw out the baby of morality with the bathwater of shame. The entire gay movement rests on at least one moral imperative, namely that society ought to treat sexual and other minorities with dignity and fairness. In some senses, the more radically we demand gay liberation, the more extravagant our moral claims on society and each other. It would be self-defeating in the extreme if the one instance in which we refused to make a moral claim was the instance where our physical survival was at stake.

Still, there is a crucial difference between being moral and being "moralistic." AIDS prevention has to avoid becoming censorious about sex itself, especially in a community whose sexual behavior has been and still is the focus of so much shame. And many people might not see how to disentangle the morality of AIDS prevention from the older morality that has oppressed gay people for centuries. Perhaps one way is to return to ecology and base our morality in that. There is a basic ecological principle that the morality of an action is based on the state of the system at the time the action occurs. I have already mentioned the classic example, which is that ecologists consider it perfectly moral to build a small bonfire on an empty prairie, since that does not damage the environment, while it is plainly immoral to burn millions of tons of urban refuse in unfiltered incinerators, since that would lead to ecological disaster. That same principal can be applied, nonjudgmentally, to sexual and reproductive behavior. The point is that the activity itself, in this case combustion, is not by itself moral or immoral. No one says fire is morally wrong, and those who burn things are not inherently immoral. What is immoral is polluting an ecosystem in a harmful and unsustainable way, especially in a way that is almost certain to destroy human life. In the same way, individual sexual behaviors that traditional moralists might consider "always wrong" can still be considered perfectly moral so long as they don't produce widespread harm. But those behaviors must be considered immoral when they do. Harm is the key—ecological harm. This principle will come to be employed more and more as the earth gets increasingly crowded and its ecosystems increasingly strained. It does not seem regressive to put it to use in the service of gay survival as well.

With this principle in mind, one can even imagine that behaviors that today cause harm and are therefore "immoral" will be perfectly moral at some time in the future. After all, given the overall progress of science and technology a day may someday dawn when microbial illness will be an artifact of the past, and when that day arrives the behaviors that cause disaster today will no longer be harmful. In that sense, the "moralistic" idea that nature will always punish sexual promiscuity, that biology will always demand a culture of sexual restraint, does not seem likely to stand the test of time. When the last microbe is tamed, when the problem of mutation is solved, people will be free to decide how to behave based on ethical and social considerations, not epidemiological ones.

All this is almost irrelevant right now. Indeed, at the moment the microbes seem to be winning. But those who feel oppressed by the moral dimension of sexual ecology might be comforted to know that such morality is not an absolute, and is based on effect rather than some concept of original sin. To change the state of the system is to alter the moral dimension of the activity. Someday homosexual men will be able to behave as gay men did in the seventies, and do so without promulgating epidemics. When that day dawns it will be up to that generation to decide how to behave, and they may just decide that such behaviors, being without biological harm, are justifiable, moral, and rewarding. Someone may then pick up the yellowed pages of this book and wonder what all the fuss was about.

The Stakes

The late nineties has become an era of new hope about medical treatments for HIV infection. Perhaps more than at any time since the epidemic began, this moment demands that we train ourselves to think about sex in ecological terms, and to do so now, before another window of opportunity passes us by.

At the International AIDS Conference in Vancouver in July of 1996, studies showed that combinations of drugs could successfully suppress HIV replication in most patients, reducing viral load in many to undetectable levels. Some researchers began to speculate that if these treatments worked for long enough, they might actually rid the body of HIV. For the first time since the epidemic began, experts began openly musing on the possibility of an actual cure for AIDS, at least for some people under some conditions. As of this writing much is still unknown about this prospect. It could be that HIV will remain hidden in so-called sanctuary sites in the body, away from the reach of drugs, ready to burst back into full bloom as soon as therapy ends. It could be that the drugs will become ineffective over time because of the body's decreased ability to absorb or tolerate them. It could be—in fact it's considered almost inevitable—that HIV will mutate into drug-resistant strains that evade combination therapies, at least in some people. Still, despite these possibilities, things look better than they ever have for people with AIDS, or at least for those who can tolerate and afford these compounds.

But while the development of new drugs that slow or halt the progression of disease is a triumph for medicine, it may be a mixed blessing for medical ecology. There are certain scenarios in which society's complex reaction to these therapies could actually make the epidemic more intractable than it already is. And these scenarios are not being spun by crackpots. They're being proposed by medical historians, who point to the fact that we have declared victory over STDs in the past, only to be brought up short when our own reaction to our supposed victory contributed to a worsening of the situation.

Antibiotics: The Short-Lived Miracle

Perhaps the most salient case in point is the relationship between antibiotics and venereal disease. In the mid-forties when penicillin began to be widely used as a treatment for syphilis and gonorrhea, some experts confidently predicted that these two diseases would soon be eradicated. After all, penicillin cured both diseases quickly and with 100 percent effectiveness. It seemed natural to assume that once large cohorts of infected people were cured and the prevalence of the diseases declined, and once newly infected people were routinely treated and cured before they could infect others, the problem of VD would be permanently solved. And from the late forties until the mid sixties, as rates of infection dropped dramatically across the nation, that rosy prediction seemed to come true. But as people got used to the idea that they no longer needed to worry about life-threatening infection from casual sexual encounters, attitudes about such encounters began to change. And not just among individuals. Government itself slashed its prevention budget, and routine education about VD disappeared from the national landscape. After the birth control pill was introduced, attitudes began to change even more dramatically. By the mid sixties most people believed that the two most compelling biological impediments to casual sex—the fear of unwanted pregnancy and incurable disease—were solved, and partly as a result, a sexual revolution swept the Western world. As it did, cases of syphilis and gonorrhea began to rise. What happened was an entirely predictable result of the fact that rates of STD infection are a function of three factors: infectivity per sex act, prevalence of the disease in the population, and the rate of partner change. In this instance, antibiotics initially reduced prevalence by curing most of those who were infected, and that drove down the infection rate. But as the sexual revolution picked up steam, the increase in the rate of partner change began to outbalance the drop in prevalence. At some point, that increase in partner change pushed the incidence of new infections past the epidemic threshold at which the average infected person infects slightly more than one other person, and epidemic amplification began. Between 1965 and 1975 the incidence of gonorrhea tripled and the incidence of syphilis quadrupled, so that by the early eighties 2.5 million Americans were contracting gonorrhea every year and syphilis ranked as the third most common infectious disease in the nation. Many sexually active people did not seem to mind, however, since both diseases were still easily curable. Then things took a more ominous turn when the casual use of antibiotics produced drug-resistant strains of gonorrhea that rendered antibiotics useless. And things really got bleak when incurable viral diseases such as herpes and AIDS began to take advantage of microbial highways we had created. By the mid eighties the myth that sex had been liberated from biological consequences came crashing down in a blizzard of statistics about incurable and fatal STDs, in much the same way that myths about the atmosphere's ability to absorb pollution were swamped by news about global warming and the hole in the ozone layer.

This is not to disparage the miraculous benefits of antibiotics, which saved and continue to save millions of lives. In fact, it's important to point out that drugs did not cause the resurgence of disease, but rather society's reaction to them. The tragic magnitude of that mistake can be gleaned from statistics showing that before the introduction of antibiotics, only a few thousand Americans died each year of syphilis, whereas hundreds of thousands have died of AIDS, and around the world tens of millions are expected to die of AIDS in the next few decades.

Is it possible that good news about AIDS treatments could produce the same social reaction as the good news about penicillin fifty years ago? And could that reaction lead to a more intractable epidemic, fueled by strains of HIV that have evolved resistance to even our most effective drugs? The answer to both is surely yes. If anything, such results seem more likely today than back then, for several reasons.

The Biological Risk of Mutation

HIV is by far the most mutable retrovirus ever encountered by medicine. Within an infected person's body it spawns up to 10 billion virus particles per day, and an entirely new generation every two days. Because retroviruses do things backward, their replication tends to be sloppy, and up to 10 percent of the new virus created by HIV is mutant. That means that a person can produce up to 1 billion viral mutations per day. While this may seem wildly inefficient, it is actually one of HIV's cleverest characteristics. It means that the virus is constantly producing strains that have the ability to adapt to all sorts of environmental challenges.

Some of those challenges consist of the drugs that we throw at it. HIV has so far found a way to stumble around every compound mobilized against it, and many drug combinations as well. By the mid nineties, for example, up to 10 percent of all newly infected gay men in the United States were infected with a virus that was preresistant to AZT, the most commonly used AIDS antiviral drug, even though they had never taken it. And HIV does not just mutate to evade drugs. It also appears to mutate to take advantage of different transmission routes, as the emergence of subtype E in northern Thailand, which shows greater ability to infect Langerhans cells, seems to imply.

The success of combination therapy lies in the fact that several drugs used together require more simultaneous mutations than HIV can handle. And once the drugs suppress viral replication from billions per day to mere thousands, HIV's opportunities to stumble upon a mutation that evades all the drugs are greatly reduced. So if everyone who was infected was able to take these therapies consistently, and absorb them and tolerate them well, they might mark the beginning of the end of the epidemic. Unfortunately, there's a major evolutionary catch. If patients stop taking these medications, even for relatively brief periods, the remaining virus in their bodies can reproduce quickly and swarm back through the bloodstream. Worse, there is the distinct possibility—many virologists consider it a certainty—that when people use these drugs in an on-again, off-again fashion, it will prompt HIV to mutate into strains that resist all the drugs in the combination cocktails. Once that happens such patients will no longer be able to benefit from the drugs, and if they infect others, those people will presumably never be able to benefit from these drugs at all.

How likely is this to happen? Quite likely, for at least two major reasons. First, most AIDS therapies are so expensive they are primarily available to wealthy people in developed nations with access to health insurance, a fact that effectively rules them off-limits to almost 90 percent of all infected people around the world. Mutation aside, this could worsen the global epidemic simply because developed nations provide most of the money for global prevention programs and the search for better and cheaper drugs, and they could lose their sense of urgency once their own citizens have access to fairly effective treatments. If so, those with HIV in the rest of the world may be left out in the cold, unable to afford the new compounds and without much hope that cheaper ones will become available. But economic inequities also make viral mutation more likely. Many poor people, desperate for treatment, may cobble together the money to get drugs for a while, but will be unable to afford them for long periods. The result will be a pattern of use most conducive to the mutation of multiple-drug-resistant strains.

But even for those who can afford these drugs, there are factors that make such mutations seem likely. The drug combinations are difficult to tolerate for many people. Some individuals have periods of intense nausea, pain, physical discomfort. The drugs can produce kidney stones and other painful and serious side effects. Pharmacists normally consider a 70 to 80 percent rate of drug compliance to be acceptable for people on long-term medications, but the severity of the side effects probably means that these drugs will be taken with less consistency by many people. Yet in order to minimize the risk of mutation they have to be taken with almost 100 percent consistency on a rigid daily schedule with no real breaks. Even a few days off provides the virus with a window to quickly multiply and mutate.

Put all of this together and you have a situation that is far less hopeful than the one that faced the medical world when penicillin and other antibiotics were first deployed against VD. The new AIDS drugs do not necessarily cure all those who take them. They're expensive and not well tolerated, yet they need to be taken according to a strict daily regimen. And if patients falter, the virus comes roaring back, possibly in resistant forms.

Of course, we can always keep developing better and different drugs. But at the moment humanity is barely able to keep pace with the evolution of antibiotic-resistant strains of simple bacterial diseases, which mutate much more slowly than viruses and immensely more slowly than HIV. The idea that we can keep one step ahead of HIV by constantly coming up with newer and newer compounds seems naive, at least in the short term.

What all this implies is that while these new drugs are indeed miraculous, they are unlikely to be successful in containing the epidemic unless they are used ecologically. By that I mean unless they are used in context with behaviors that minimize the risk of mutation, and minimize the chance that when drug-resistant mutations occur, or when mutations occur that are transmitted more easily through different primary routes, they will be rapidly transmitted along new viral highways. If we do not approach things this way, if we make the same mistake we made with penicillin and syphilis, presuming that we have been rescued from the web of ecology by the miracles of a technological fix, we will very likely make the situation worse.

Can History Repeat Itself?

So what might this portend for gay men? Are gay men and AIDS prevention organizations prepared to adapt the ecological lessons of the past to the new situation? Or are we drifting into a further sense of complacency about AIDS that might even exacerbate the problem?

As AIDS evolves into a more manageable disease, many gay men are debating whether or not this will portend a return to the sexual culture of the seventies, and whether or not it should. Some argue that it probably won't, that the experience of AIDS and the maturing of gay institutions in the wake of AIDS make such a return highly unlikely. They point to an increased percentage of gay men in stable relationships, a new attitude toward sex and relationships among the young, a rise in non-sex-based institutions like gay sports teams, churches, professional groups, racial and ethnic organizations, choirs, political groups. Perhaps, they argue, now that gay men are no longer so reliant on sexual networking for their sense of self or their feeling of community, things will be different.

Others point to opposite omens. The outward manifestations of the urban gay world are still as overtly sexual as ever despite fifteen years of AIDS. If anything, even more so. With a few major exceptions, an uninformed reader of the gay press might assume that the gay world consists almost entirely of extremely handsome naked men aged twenty to thirty. This profusion of beefy temptation is used not only to sell all manner of products, as it is throughout our culture, but to sell sex itself in the form of commercialized sex, porn, and prostitution. Drug use in urban gay settings remains high, and popular drugs have undergone a nasty evolution from the relatively benign ecstasy to the much more hellish crystal meth. There has been an increased fixation on body culture throughout the nineties, and the cult of the gym has soared to new heights. Old-fashioned bathhouses and sex clubs—some devoted to safe sex, many not—have staged a return. The sense of entitlement around sex has certainly not abated. If anything, gay culture's very male view of sexual entitlement has been intellectualized by gay academics in ways that would be considered scandalous if they were coming from straight men talking about women. There is little in gay culture to support a spirit of sacrifice or self-denial, little to encourage a sense of wider responsibility, few things, aside from caring for the AIDS-afflicted, that impel gay men to take responsibility for others. And then there is the well-documented Second Wave of new infections, which was fully under way before the new drug therapies sparked new hope. According to this argument, if large numbers of gay men had already begun slipping back into the old patterns even when AIDS was still considered absolutely incurable, just imagine what will happen when it is seen as more manageable.

It is impossible to predict how gay male culture will react, but it did not take long after the good news about combination drugs for men to begin reporting, at least anecdotally, an increase in unsafe sex based on reaction to the new therapies. Many of these reports seemed to fall into the divisions noted earlier in the epidemic by researchers Levine and Siegel—either excuses or justifications. Some men began reporting that while they wanted to continue having safe sex, it was becoming more difficult now that the element of fear was abating. Others seemed to be using the news about therapies to construct their own sometimes elaborate justifications for unsafe sex. There were reports of HIV-infected men who had decided that since their viral load had been reduced to undetectable levels in their blood, they must be noninfectious, and could therefore return to unsafe sex. There were reports of uninfected men who believed that since so many infected men had reduced their viral loads, the chances of running into someone who's highly infectious were now extremely low, and so they, too, could have unsafe sex. One enthusiast told me that having unprotected anal sex with strangers in epicenters like New York and San Francisco was now "low risk." That did not mean, he hastened to add, that it was zero risk. I should think of it, he said, the way AIDS groups tell us to think of oral sex—there's still some risk, but it's low.

One gay New Yorker announced to friends perhaps the ultimate in an anti-ecological approach to combining survival with unsafe sex. He pointed out that there were newly marketed home tests for HIV that yield a totally anonymous result whenever you want. He also pointed out that many prominent AIDS researchers have speculated that the best chance of eliminating HIV infection from the body is to begin treating it immediately after initial infection has occurred. So, he proposed, from now on we can have all the unsafe sex we want, take the home test every few weeks, and the instant we get infected, begin taking the combination therapy and wipe out the infection. This may seem painfully naive and dangerous, but it's not that far from the common practice among bathhouse denizens in the seventies to swallow a few penicillin tablets before a night at the baths, just for insurance. All in all, the anecdotal signs from gay men are not initially encouraging. Based on the limited evidence, there seems every reason to expect that the natural tendency of gay sexual life is to slide back into a posture of unsafe sex with multiple partners, unless that trend is strongly counteracted by some other force.

Gay Groups and Ecology

A primary force would have to be gay AIDS prevention organizations. Their initial reaction to the development of more effective AIDS drugs was to caution gay men that nothing had really changed and that prevention had to continue as before. But that message was clearly not working even when the level of fear was very high. It seems much less likely to work as fear abates. It seems likely that what they need to do is incorporate ecology into their message, to help explain why certain behaviors may be safe, or at least safer, when practiced with knowledge, balance, negotiation, self-awareness. And why those same behaviors can become extremely unsafe if practiced the way we practiced them in the seventies.

Have gay groups demonstrated this kind of ecological awareness so far? Unfortunately, not really. Perhaps the best example of how far they remain from an ecological approach is their new policy on unprotected oral sex. As mentioned, a movement began among American gay AIDS groups in the wake of the Second Wave to promote unprotected oral sex as a form of prevention. It was argued that if men became more confident that they could suck with safety, they would be less inclined to fuck unsafely. As a result, no less an organization than the Gay and Lesbian Medical Association has declared unprotected oral sex to be "low risk." The activity is now aggressively marketed that way, and a significant goal of AIDS prevention is to reduce gay men's anxiety about the practice as much as possible.

On the face of it, this seems reasonable as far as it goes. Even though unprotected oral sex may carry a higher risk than many gay men and prevention workers would prefer to admit, it is still unquestionably far less risky than unprotected anal sex. If it could be shown that there is a direct cause-and-effect relationship between promoting oral sex and reducing unprotected anal sex, a strong case could be made that oral sex should be promoted as a form of AIDS prevention. But to be responsible, the promotion of unprotected oral sex would have to be ecological. By that I mean that it would need to emphasize that unprotected oral sex is relatively safer under many circumstances, but highly dangerous under others. Unfortunately, no such message is being conveyed. Oral sex is advertised as "low risk," period. AIDS groups send no message about ways in which the number of partners might impact risk, no message about the inherent dangers of fostering core groups, no message about other diseases that are highly transmissible via oral sex, no message about other strains of HIV that might be more transmissible via oral sex, no message about communal responsibility to make sure we do not create conditions for epidemic relapse. They send no message about the sexual ecology of oral sex at all. Their message is simple: Unprotected oral sex is safe sex.

This message has led to a predictable result. Many gay men have decided that since oral sex is apparently "safe," it doesn't matter under what conditions you have it, or with how many partners, or who those partners are. So why not have it with 300 people a year? Why not commercialize it? Why not create venues for new core groups centered on unprotected oral sex, venues in which promoters stand to gain financially by fostering this activity? The result is an ecological disaster waiting to happen, one that gay and AIDS prevention groups are both facilitating and defending.

Consider, for example, the case of San Francisco's Blow Buddies, a new-style sex club for gay men devoted, as its name implies, almost exclusively to oral sex. It and many others like it across the nation came into being in large part because of the argument that oral sex is safe, and have been defended as models of safe sex by gay AIDS prevention workers. AIDS educator Eric Rofes, a prominent figure in the "new prevention" movement and former head of San Francisco's Shanti Project, described a visit to Blow Buddies in *Reviving the Tribe*, his book about gay men and AIDS prevention:

[M]y eyes took a moment to adjust. I was in a large space filled with small wooden cubicles, like cupboards, in which men were apparently expected to kneel and give head. Glory holes were drilled into these closets, and other men came by, hoisted out their dicks, and inserted them into the holes in the cubicles. In another part of the room, men stepped up on a raised platform and other men stood below, eager to suck them off in a standing position.

While there may have been thirty men in the room, none were talking. The only sounds were the throb of the music and the sounds of cocksucking—slurps, gagging, coughing, moans of relief. . . . I moved toward the next room and discovered more cupboards, aligned along an elaborate maze filled with several dozen men moving, glancing, stopping, moving, kneeling, sucking, moving, unzipping. . . . As my eyes adjusted, I recognized more and more people—colleagues from political work, neighbors from my apartment building, friends from the gym. Everyone seemed plugged into the same intense energy and focused on the same thing—oral sex.

I remained at Blow Buddies until three in the morning. During that time, I gave head to three different men. Seven men sucked my dick. I did not witness a single condom in use during oral sex. I did not encounter a single man who refused to participate in unprotected oral sex, and four of the men who sucked me asked me to reach orgasm in their mouths. Of the men I sucked, one came in my mouth.

What Rofes describes is, in the opinion of many prominent AIDS educators and prevention workers, a model scene, an example of what sex-positive gay life ought to be like in the age of AIDS. Blow Buddies, they point out, is gay owned and operated. It has an excellent record of cooperation with San Francisco's Coalition for Healthy Sex, a community-based group dedicated to the self-monitoring of the city's sex clubs. Blow Buddies earns high marks from the coalition for not allowing unprotected anal sex on its premises, for providing plenty of AIDS materials and condoms and brochures, and for providing guidelines that encourage patrons to use condoms during oral sex—although as Rofes points out, no one does. But what does that matter? In light of the message that oral sex is safer sex, Blow Buddies is indeed an exemplary institution. While Rofes, who is a thoughtful and honest voice in the new prevention movement, writes that after his visit he was confused about why so many people ignore the club's advice to use condoms and avoid ejaculate, he nonetheless writes that he "left Blow Buddies that evening sexually satisfied, and happy with the ability of gay men to create environments which encourage men to enjoy a lot of sex."

Unfortunately, the picture described by Rofes is of a microbial disaster area waiting to explode. Set aside for a moment the fact that oral sex is emphatically not safe for a host of diseases that became epidemic in the gay world just before AIDS—from herpes to antibiotic-resistant gonorrhea—diseases with the potential to kill and the potential to mutate into worse strains under precisely these kinds of conditions. Put aside the fact that oral sex is not even safe for HIV, merely safer than anal sex, a fact that doesn't necessarily mean much considering that anal sex efficiently infected almost half of the entire gay male population in just a few years. Put aside the fact that under the conditions of Blow Buddies a regular customer who is highly infectious, someone with a viral load of several millions as opposed to several thousand—is in a perfect position to infect a wide swath of gay men.

Put all of that aside and consider a simple fact of AIDS ecology. That fact is that oral sex is relatively safer than anal sex based on studies of subtype B, the type most prevalent in the United States *so far*. As noted in Chapter 7, molecular biologists have demonstrated that subtype B is easily transmitted during anal sex, but has a hard time infecting Langerhans cells, which abound in the vagina, penile foreskin, and mouth. However, we have evidence that a strain of subtype E that originated in Thailand may have a much greater affinity toward infecting the Langerhans cells. Such a viral mutation was probably inevitable under the selective pressure of the modern world.

Why should the appearance of a subtype in Thailand whose primary infection route is Langerhans cells matter to gay men in a sex club in San Francisco? Because just as drug-resistant gonorrhea originated in far-flung locales in the seventies and then raced across the planet, new strains of HIV are mutating everywhere and then spreading everywhere. Data presented at the International AIDS Conference in Vancouver in 1996 indicates that as people travel around the world HIV is mixing together rapidly. This point was driven home when, as the Vancouver conference was about to get under way, health officials announced that the rarest and most mysterious type of HIV, type O, had finally entered the United States. There was a minor panic when it was revealed that type O is so unusual that it doesn't even show up in standard antibody tests, a fact that seemed to threaten the integrity of the nation's blood supply and forced blood banks to assure the public they would begin screening for it.

Based on experience, we must assume that the aggressive subtype E will soon enter this country, if it hasn't already. (Indeed, it almost certainly has.) Once here, it shouldn't take long to enter the gay male population. Once it does, it shouldn't take long for someone carrying that strain to walk into a place like Blow Buddies. If he hasn't already.

This scenario, like many ecological scenarios, cannot be reduced to a simple mechanical question of whether oral sex is safe. It can't be reduced to a question of individual risk. The danger is ecological more than mechanical, communal more than personal. It is true, as the Gay and Lesbian Medical Association insists, that each individual instance of oral sex is still safer than each individual instance of anal sex. But the Gay and Lesbian Ecological Association, if one existed, would be duty bound to point out that reconstructing networks and core groups that facilitate the rapid spread of orally transmitted infections to thousands of interconnected gay men is not safe. There has to be a way to communicate both of these ideas, and groups like GMHC and the Gay and Lesbian Medical Association should be at the forefront of communicating them, instead of touting only the happy half of the equation.

The limits of AIDS groups' collective thinking on this subject was illustrated at a public forum at the 1996 Vancouver AIDS conference. Sponsored by GMHC, the forum was clearly designed to support the new official line that oral sex is a form of safe sex, and to proselytize it to AIDS prevention workers around the world. The speakers on the dais, gay male AIDS researchers, educators, and administrators from the United States, enumerated all the reasons why oral sex ought to be considered safe, and why prevention workers are duty bound to promote it. Blow Buddies, in fact, was touted as a model institution. The clear sense of the panel was that "they" were trying to take oral sex away from "us"—they being either traitorous, sex-negative gay men (one panelist criticized my article on oral sex in *Out*) or homophobic government leaders. Things continued in this vein until a gentleman from the audience raised the scenario concerning subtype B. Might it be, he asked, that the panel's confident recommendations about oral safety were only narrowly applicable to the American subtype B? What about the rest of the world? And what about the near future, as aggressive subtype E looks for new niches, and finds them? The panel appeared flustered, as though this possibility had not occurred to them.

"Certainly," one panelist replied, "it would be important, as the E strain moves around, to be able to find out if there might be differences" that make it easier to transmit orally. But after all, he protested, nobody has yet proven that some strains are more easily transmitted orally. "We have to keep an open mind" to that possibility, he said, but "in the meantime, we can't put our lives on hold."

Another panelist remarked that this scenario might make a good topic for further research. "But I also would say," he added, "that if indeed it's the case that the strain that's predominant in the United States and Western Europe is a strain that's more difficult to transmit orally, thank God there is something good that happened for us."

The response sounded eerily similar to those at the very beginning of the AIDS epidemic. There was the same insistence that no matter how likely a scenario may be, it has to be decisively proven before we take action. There was the same reluctance to issue seemingly commonsense advice. The same defensive feeling that a recommendation of sexual restraint somehow amounted to asking gay men to "put our lives on hold." The same lack of ecological context, of understanding that if we re-create the ecosystems of disaster, disaster will likely ensue.

The fact that gay AIDS organizations have so far ignored ecology in their approach to oral sex may not yet be very important, as of this writing anyway. I mention it because it is a current example of the kind of ecological thinking, or lack thereof, that gay AIDS groups are displaying as we enter a new era of combination drugs and a rapidly shifting situation around prevention. If their approach to oral sex is any indication of their approach to prevention in the new era, we're in trouble. There seems to be every reason to think that the messages going out to gay men will be mechanical messages about individual risk, not ecological messages that emphasize context and the interconnectedness of everything with everything else. There is every reason to fear that gay culture will be encouraged to return to the unsafe practices of the seventies on the narrowest possible evidence. Every reason to think we will not look both ways before we cross the river of unsafe sex. And given the biological hazards of viral mutation, every reason to think that this will lead to disaster.

Could Treatment Become Prevention?

The thing that is so unfortunate about a drift back to this behavior is the fact that these new drugs actually offer the very real chance of containing the epidemic, if they're used judiciously in context with behavioral efforts. The reason is simple. HIV transmission in the gay population is probably never very far above epidemic threshold. As a result, anything that would significantly and permanently lower transmission could be decisive in containing the epidemic. If a very large percentage of infected gay men began to take the drug combinations, lowering their viral load and making it less likely that they could infect others, this would lower the infectivity of HIV per episode, which is one of the three key elements that determine the population's overall transmission rate. So provided that there was no increase in either of the other two factors—prevalence (which we have no control over) and the contact rate (which we do)—this by itself could lower transmission below the tipping point. Treatment itself could become a key form of prevention.

Of course, this is what would have happened with penicillin and syphilis, if people had not reacted by increasing the contact rate. So the lesson of the past is to somehow obtain the benefits of technological treatments—in this case combination therapies—without responding by raising the contact rate. This does not seem an impossible goal. Indeed, all that this optimistic scenario requires is that we maintain the contact rate where it is right now. We know that this is possible, because we're doing it. But the only way we can keep doing it is if we start to think like ecologists, to educate ourselves about the consequences of relapse, and emphasize our responsibility to community. If we do not, then our tendency will probably be to reenact the tragedy of the commons. Many of us will be tempted to interpret the news about new therapies by calculating our own best interests as individuals. Under a reduced threat of AIDS, it will certainly seem in the immediate best interests of many of us to take more risks. And as we do, our rosy scenario may turn to ashes. The decline in infectivity could easily be outbalanced by a rise in the unsafe contact rate. Indeed, the very factor that caused reduced infectivity, the drugs themselves, could prompt a rise in the unsafe contact rate. We will have lost our last best chance of containing the epidemic. And we will be opening the door to new epidemics.

The Three Pillars of Defense

While gay men have not been able so far to stave off biological disaster, we have staved off political disaster. At the outset of the epidemic, all sorts of doomsayers predicted all sorts of terrible things in store for us. Concentration camps. AIDS tattoos. Re-criminalization of gay sex. It was widely believed that gay liberation itself would falter and that people would return to the closet in droves. Even the coolest heads predicted that AIDS laws would be draconian. There would be mandatory testing, quarantine, legal discrimination against the infected. And in fact all of these measures were proposed by right-wingers and sometimes by public health authorities in the early years of AIDS, and attempts were made to enact many of them into law in various places. But such attempts were almost uniformly unsuccessful. Gay men, with the strong support of lesbians, of civil liberties organizations, and of liberal and progressive political groups and leaders, managed to stave off almost all of the worst scenarios, often after waging bitter political battles.

Our success was based on a few main arguments that proved to be solid pillars of self-defense against blame and repression. One was our appeal to the public's sympathy. We argued that the vast majority of HIV-infected gay men were stricken before anyone knew about the epidemic, and that once we learned about the danger of infection we successfully reduced new infections to negligible levels. Therefore, draconian measures were not only punitive but unnecessary. We had solved the problem ourselves. Of course this appeal was problematic for many gay men, since it seemed to carry with it the implied admission that there had been something unhealthy about our sexual behavior in the past, something that we had found it necessary to reform. In effect, we seemed to be arguing that we deserved support because we had now become desexualized "good gays" who had stopped having that nasty anal sex. Nonetheless, this argument was aggressively promoted by gay and AIDS activists, in part because it seemed effective, in part because it seemed undeniably true. Most gay men had indeed been infected before they knew what was happening, and the statistics seemed to show that by the mid to late eighties new infections had dropped to negligible levels because gay men were practicing safer sex, or no sex at all. In a homophobic society in which many people wanted gay men to stop having sex, it was a very effective message, and it worked.

Another strategy was to prick the public's sense of guilt by arguing that society ignored and covered up the epidemic just when it was spreading most rapidly, and then refused to invest adequately in a cure or vaccine or in prevention. According to this argument, the epidemic was essentially society's fault. At best, we argued, the major institutions of society had participated in a deadly form of homophobic and racist neglect. At worst they had acquiesced in a form of passive genocide. In this interpretation, AIDS was "caused" by homophobia, and things would only get worse so long as people continued to propose restrictive, homophobic measures to contain the epidemic, measures that were doomed to failure. Again, there was enough truth to this argument to make it convincing to many people. The record of society's dismal response to AIDS, reported in best-selling books like *And the Band Played On*, reiterated with anger by activists and public health officials and journalists, was too blatant and well documented to deny. And so that argument, too, was effective.

Finally, we appealed to people's sense of fear by arguing that it was only a fluke of fate that AIDS hit gay men first. Sooner or later, we warned, it would strike heterosexuals in the same devastating way. As we have already noted, the degaying of AIDS and the promotion of the idea that everyone was equally at risk was a strategy eagerly embraced by the most disparate elements of society, from the far right to the far left and including the gay and AIDS movements themselves. Look at Africa, we said, or Thailand. For that matter, look at the frightening statistics about "heterosexual AIDS" in this country. And after you've taken a good look, don't be so quick to propose punitive and probably ineffective strategies. You just might find yourself or your loved ones caught in your own ill-conceived proposals. This, too, was a highly effective argument.

By and large these appeals prevailed with enough of the public and the political establishment to prevent the worst predictions of backlash from materializing. There are no concentration camps for HIV-infected men. No mandatory tattoos. No quarantine. Bathhouses and sex clubs were closed as a public health response to AIDS in some places, but that was never followed by the closing of bars and other gay businesses. Jackbooted police do not routinely pound down the bedroom doors of gay men, as once predicted. As of this writing, no state that had previously decriminalized sodomy has recriminalized it—although the Supreme Court's notorious Hardwick decision affirmed the right of states to do so. There is extensive, if often vague, AIDS education throughout society. While many contend that it remains underfunded, most experts now argue that its major problem is that its funding is misdirected toward convincing us that everyone is equally at risk, rather than being concentrated on those most at risk. Condoms are widely available, although the battle to make them freely available to teenagers still rages. Bigotry and discrimination against people with AIDS still exists, but those who are discriminated against often have recourse to the law, and often win. The media pay as much sporadic and cyclical attention to AIDS as they do to most comparable issues. The demise of the kind of AIDS activism made famous by

ACT UP has been attributed to many factors, among them burnout and the death of key activists. But another major reason is that most of the things activists lobbied for—expanded access to drugs, more and better drugs, a say in the drug development process—they achieved. It has almost become difficult, in the late nineties, to remember how dire the situation was back in the early and mid eighties, when there was no money, no publicity, no public sense of urgency, no drugs, only threats of the loss of civil liberties and the eclipse of community.

If all of this is testament to the success of AIDS advocates in forcefully advancing our cause, it is also testament to the strength of our arguments. Most of our advocacy would probably have come to naught if our appeals has not resonated with the public. But many liberals and moderates and even some conservatives were moved by the innocence of those who had been infected before they knew an epidemic was afoot, felt guilty for society's ineffective and homophobic response, and were terrified that if a cure wasn't quickly found they or their loved ones would be next. In the end, it was not just that AIDS advocates were better debaters than people like William F. Buckley, Jr., who once proposed that people with HIV be branded with mandatory tattoos. We had better debating points.

The Erosion of Our Arguments

Today, however, most of those debating points are unraveling. There is the distinct possibility that if AIDS transmission continues at high rates, or if the epidemic shifts into some even more fearsome form, people with AIDS in particular, and gay men in general, will lose much of the tenuous progress we have gained, and that many of the more extreme reactions that we feared may loom again as real possibilities.

Consider the argument that almost all infected gay men were exposed to the virus before anybody knew about the epidemic. As it currently stands, a very large proportion of today's HIV-positive gay men became infected *after* the epidemic became widely recognized. Among those in their twenties and younger, the overwhelming majority were infected after safer sex became the watchword of gay life. That percentage grows with each passing day. At current rates of new infection, the overwhelming majority of all HIV-positive gay men will fall into that category within a decade.

In April of 1994 an article appeared in the *New York Times Magazine* by Stephen Beachy, a young HIV-positive gay man, that seemed a harbinger of things to come. GREETINGS FROM THE SECOND WAVE, read the headline, YOUNG MEN WITH "NO EXCUSE" INFECTED IN AN AGE OF SAFE SEX, FREE CONDOMS, AND FEAR. The article was well written, artful, full of rage, and horrifying:

> We're called the "second wave," young gay men still seroconverting at an impressive rate. Seroconversion: sort of sounds like a weird religious ritual, doesn't it? Are you going to the seroconversion tomorrow night in the basement of the abandoned church? Be sure to wear black. What we lose in peace of mind, we gain in credibility at ACT UP meetings. At this point, let's face it, we're the least innocent of "victims"— we have no excuse, the barrage of safe sex information, the free condoms, blah blah blah. . . . Maybe the image of death, a dark, sexy man in black, is something we find exciting. That's death as metaphor, of course, not sickness and putrefaction.

For several weeks after it appeared, AIDS activists around the country spoke of the article in hushed whispers. The fact that the *Times* editors had singled out the young man's phrase "no excuse" and put it in the headline made people shiver. The worry is that if new transmissions continue at current levels, this kind of reaction is just a prologue. Of course, the counterargument is that most diseases have a behavioral component, that smokers and the overweight and those who fail to exercise also have "no excuse," and society does not turn its back on them. We can, and will, advance that argument, and it may help stem the tide of backlash. But it remains to be seen whether the liberal and moderate allies of gay people will feel compelled to fight the AIDS battles of the future, or fight them very hard, when the vast majority of sufferers are perceived, even by themselves, to have "no excuse."

Then there is our argument that society did virtually nothing to help in those tragic early years. The terrible stories of governmental neglect, pharmaceutical industry negligence, and media disinterest in the early and mid eighties were both tragic and true, and ought to instill forever a sense of outrage and regret. But how long will an appeal to the past rescue us from the future? Society's response to AIDS today is a far cry from the days when epidemiologists were setting up shop in hallways with borrowed equipment, a far cry from the days when the president and top government officials refused even to mention the word *AIDS* in public, a far cry from the days when the press refused to cover the subject because homosexuality was considered inappropriate for family newspapers. Indeed, it is now sometimes argued that society spends more on AIDS on a per capita basis than on the other major killers of Americans, and this accusation has become a political issue in its own right. Rather than disagreeing, AIDS advocates often justify this apparent discrepancy by arguing that unlike most major killers, AIDS strikes people when they are comparatively young, robbing them of productive and fulfilling years, and that therefore it deserves more funding. It's a good argument, but to many cancer and heart disease sufferers it's not that good. Given that, it's probably safe to say that strategies based on appeals to the public's guilty conscience are not likely to be as successful as in the past.

As for perhaps our most effective argument, that AIDS exceptionalism is justified because the epidemic is poised to spread among the heterosexual population, the evidence so far indicates that this is not happening. We have already mentioned scenarios in which this could occur. Much more transmissible subtypes of HIV-1 will surely enter the developed world, and if heterosexuals increase their level of unsafe behaviors as these new strains enter the population, a heterosexual epidemic could easily ensue. But at the moment, despite the dire predictions of fifteen years, the disease is stuck where it began, among gay men, injection drug users, crack cocaine users, and their female sexual partners and children, with only the occasional incursion into other groups. As a result, the old appeal to fear no longer instills much terror, and would no longer seem a potent argument in the face of repressive proposals.

All this seems to add up to a frightening conclusion: that gay men face the risk of significant backlash in the future. As the changing face of the epidemic becomes more widely understood, it seems likely that moderates and liberals will not only have less ammunition to counter conservative attacks, but many may feel less motivated to counter them. This is already occurring in some ways. Editorial boards of certain newspapers have moved to distance themselves from gay-run AIDS groups they once unquestioningly supported. Liberal politicians have begun asking tough questions in private while becoming noncommittal in public. Friends of gay people have begun to wonder aloud at the high rates of unsafe sex and transmission. The truth of an epidemic cannot be hidden for very long, and once it has sunk in, the consequences may be more politically damaging than anything that has happened so far.

The first to suffer could be the HIV infected themselves. The amounts spent on the care of those afflicted may decrease as conservatives becomes more successful in pressing home their argument that gay men have "no excuse." A decrease in public sympathy will likely translate into a decrease in public funding and assistance. A comparable situation is the way society cares for substance abusers. There the need is also obviously great, and public expenditures in helping such people quit drugs and build productive lives would probably pay off handsomely in reduced crime, medical expenses, and other related costs. But most of the public tends to consider drug addiction a personal failure, and as a result compassion for drug users is low. This translates into very low public expenditures on the problem.

Of course, people with AIDS tend to have more articulate advocates than drug users do. But the power of AIDS advocacy has rested largely on its moral suasion, precisely the thing being eroded by the way the epidemic is evolving. Many people reasonably expected that AIDS advocates would show heightened alarm over unsafe sex and a heightened determination to do whatever is necessary to reduce it. After all, these are the same advocates who have screamed for years that AIDS is a supreme emergency and that desperate times require desperate measures. Yet in the face of the Second Wave many activists appear ambivalent, asking little of gay men, seeming to accept the situation, making the case for sexual freedom and the right to choose to take risks, privileging civil liberties concerns over prevention. For example, in the mid nineties when a new debate over bathhouses and sex clubs erupted in some cities, New York City officials proposed a law that would remove doors on private cubicles in sex clubs so that health inspectors could monitor for unsafe behavior. The board of directors of Gay Men's Health Crisis passed a policy resolution opposing this legislation. That resolution read, in part, as follows:

Some have suggested that [New York City] enact legislation requiring the removal of doors on all cubicles in commercial sex establishments. Such an approach might suggest to the uninformed that the City had taken aggressive action to fight AIDS. Prevention, however, isn't a question of doors. At the point when a door closes and persons choose to engage in intimate behavior in private, GMHC believes that the City's jurisdiction ends, and personal responsibility must govern.

This was seconded and signed by a coalition of almost every major gay-run AIDS organization in New York.

Such sentiments shocked many moderates and liberals who had long led fights for AIDS funding and battled right-wing attempts to blame AIDS on gay men. Many privately saw the coalition's stance as a defense of unsafe multipartner sex and HIV transmission, but coalition members scornfully dismissed these concerns as veiled homophobia and as indications that heterosexual liberals have never really understood or sympathized with gay men. As these discordant perceptions continue to crystallize in the future, the moral suasion of AIDS groups may be deeply eroded among the very people they most rely upon for support. Instead of being seen as stalwart fighters against the epidemic, they will increasingly be seen as wishy-washy apologists for unacceptable, even inexplicable, behaviors that transmit HIV. And once their moral authority is gone, they may stand helpless against the conservative onslaught.

Along with decreased aid, society may adopt a more punitive approach to the epidemic and its sufferers. The great debates in the eighties about forced testing, contact tracing, quarantine, and the like were generally successfully rolled back by a coalition of AIDS activists, libertarians, liberals, and moderates who convinced legislatures and judges that such traditional public health approaches would be ineffective in containing HIV. But these victories were often won by razor-thin margins, and the pressure for such nostrums has remained just under the surface. Any erosion of the coalition may provide opportunities for the reintroduction of such measures.

Broader Implications

Beyond its impact on AIDS, continued HIV transmission is liable to have a powerfully adverse impact on the social acceptance of homosexuality itself, or at least male homosexuality. At the beginning of the epidemic many thought that AIDS would signal the end of the fledgling public acceptance of gay rights, but instead the gay cause made enormous strides under the shadow of the epidemic, both in the realm of politics and culture at large. While AIDS was devastating for gay men individually, it was oddly beneficial for the movement, forcing gay men out of the closet and into the streets, and forcing society to confront its homophobia. The cost was tragically and unacceptably high, but many now argue that public acceptance of homosexuality would be far less advanced if AIDS had not radicalized a generation of gay men and lesbians and provoked a wider wave of sympathy and under-standing. What remains to be seen, though, is how sympathetic the great moderate to conservative center of society will be to a social movement many of whose most articulate members seem compla-cent about risking death on a massive scale, and whose very source of difference—sexuality—is seen as the behavior leading to the problem.

The battle may become especially intense over the issue of gay and lesbian youth. One of the central goals of the gay movement has been to create a social atmosphere in which young homo-sexuals can grow up without shame, free to express themselves and their sexuality as openly as heterosexual young people do. As we have seen, this goal has become even more pressing in the age of AIDS, since internalized shame and confusion about sexuality contribute to the risk facing young gay men. Conversely, one of the central goals of those opposed to homosexuality has been to prevent this normalization of gayness in the eyes of youth. The anti-gay argument was summarized by E. L. Pattullo in a widely noted essay in *Commentary* in 1993. Pattullo argued that although violent anti-gay prejudice is deplorable, social disapproval of homosexuality is necessary to discourage young people who "are born with the potential to live either straight or gay lives" from becoming gay. He called such people "waverers" and argued that society has an obligation to try to prevent waverers from becoming full-fledged homosexuals. To that end he wrote that all sorts of anti-gay discrimination should be allowed. Gay couples should not be permitted to adopt. In custody cases involving natural parents discrimination "in favor of a straight parent over a gay one" should be encouraged. Public institutions such as the Boy Scouts should actively exclude gay members. Schools should prohibit gay student groups and dismiss gay teachers who "flaunt their sexual orientation." He did not support mandatory discrimination against gays in the private sector, but argued that such discrimination should be allowed and left to the discretion of "individuals and institutions." In essence he called for a return to a pre-Stonewall social order, all in an attempt to prevent young waverers from succumbing "to the temptations of homosexuality in a social climate that was entirely evenhanded in its treatment of the two orientations."

Pattullo cited no specific studies supporting his contention that a more accepting society would produce more open homosexuals, but there is an enormous body of evidence that supports such a claim: the modern gay world itself. A half century ago when gay people bore the full force of stigma, the choice that faced most was not between a life that affirmed their sexual desires and one that did not. It was a much more frightening choice between the security and respectability of the mainstream world or a mysterious, mostly invisible queer world rumored to be full of mental illness and tragedy, in which one might attain sexual fulfillment but only at the expense of sacrificing almost everything else meaningful in life. It's hardly surprising that few people with homosexual inclinations chose that route, that most chose the closet, marrying, living conventional lives, and conducting a lifelong effort to repress sexual urges that could never be openly affirmed.

One of the central strategies of the gay movement has been to remove that stigma so that people can express their sexuality freely. In that sense, the very thing that Pattullo fears is what gay liberationists hope for: that removing the stigma from homosexuality will prompt closeted homosexuals to come out, free at last to lead openly gay lives. Until now Pattullo and company have had great difficulty explaining precisely why this is so bad that it is worth denying basic civil rights to an entire class of citizens in order to make examples of them to children. Encouraging everyone to procreate is an absurd argument in an overcrowded world, and arguing that gay rights is part of a general moral decline that erodes the family makes little sense in the face of a gay movement whose members are demanding the right to marry, to serve in the military, and generally to lead the kinds of mainstream lives that moralists wish everybody would lead. So while Pattullo's flimsy arguments may resonate with religious extremists and moral conservatives (no small faction), they have some difficulty convincing anybody else why gay rights are a threat.

But in a world in which gay liberation has unleashed what seems to be an endless epidemic that swallows up its own, such anti-liberation arguments would make sense to otherwise compassionate people. Who wants to encourage their kids to engage in a life that exposes them to a 50 percent chance of HIV infection? Who even wants to be neutral about such a possibility? If the rationale behind social toleration of homosexuality is that it allows gay kids an equal shot at the pursuit of happiness, that rationale is hopelessly undermined by an endless epidemic that negates happiness.

In a 1995 interview in the *Harvard Gay and Lesbian Review*, gay leader and author Urvashi Vaid expressed one of the primary goals of the gay movement when she said, "We have an agenda to create a society in which homosexuality is regarded as healthy, natural and normal. To me that is the most important agenda item." From as early as the turn of the century gay advocates have agreed that a foundation of both social acceptance of gay people and personal acceptance of ourselves lies in disproving the old canard that there is something inherently sick or diseased about homosexuality. But an endless AIDS epidemic would essentially hand anti-gay forces their greatest gift: seeming proof that liberated homosexuality inevitably leads to disease and self-destruction.

Given this inherent danger, one has to wonder why so many gay and AIDS organizations and gay theorists in the new prevention movement argue that the containment of AIDS may be impossible, that continued epidemic transmission may simply be unavoidable, and that the best thing gay society can do for itself is get used to the epidemic. While this is presented as a form of pragmatism, it skirts dangerously close to an acceptance of the homophobic idea that to be gay is to be sick. One can only shudder at the aid and comfort this idea gives to those who have made that argument all along.

Gay Backlash

If the continuation and "normalization" of AIDS in gay populations is likely to prompt a heterosexual backlash, it is also likely to prompt one within the gay community itself. Indeed, it already has.

The fault lines are everywhere, only starting with those between positives and negatives. Young gay men "blame" the older generation for bequeathing them a world of disease, and older gay men complain that the young do not appreciate the world of openness they now enjoy. Prevention activists who want to take stronger action against core group behavior battle those who argue that this is a mere transference of panic onto others, or who advocate passionately for individual rights. Those who emphasize sexual responsibility are arrayed against those who believe that talk of responsibility is stigmatizing and implicitly blames positive men. These arguments and others like them are the inevitable consequence of the pressures of a seemingly endless epidemic, and they can only get worse with time. Indeed, the gay world may experience a general cleavage between those who adopt a lifestyle of sexual restraint and those who drift further into an acceptance of a homosexuality that is inevitably diseased and death-ridden. How this will affect AIDS organizations and the direction of prevention, and which part of the community will be seen by gay society and gay youth as representing the "average" gay male, remains to be seen. But if such an "us versus them" cleavage takes place, the advocates of sexual freedom will probably be the more vocal and prominent faction. For one thing, those who choose to withdraw from the sexual fast lane and settle down tend, as a rule, to be less outspoken than self-proclaimed sex radicals. For another, the values espoused by those who choose a life of sexual moderation and monogamy expose them to charges of internalized homophobia and "sex negativity." As a result, those who argue against seventies values can easily be pegged as being anti-gay, and since this is a label no gay person relishes, such people would be more likely to keep their opinions to themselves. So a possible result of such an internal backlash is the withdrawal of the most ecologically responsible elements of the gay world from the main stage of gay life.

Another area that holds the potential for acute backlash in the gay population is the always fragile relationship between gay men and lesbians. "As I listened to my brothers speak of unprotected sex and the rise of drug use," Virginia Appuzzo told the 1994 Dallas HIV Prevention Summit, "I asked myself what my response would be if they were straight men speaking of unprotected sex with women. I know I would be enraged. . . . I must say to you—we cannot afford to ignore the issue of taking responsibility."

Appuzzo's has not been the only prominent lesbian voice raising hard questions about the direction the epidemic is taking. Lesbians have played an enormous role in AIDS service and activism since the dawn of the epidemic. A strong sense of solidarity and care led many lesbians to defer their own considerable health issues in the face of what was clearly an extreme social and medical emergency, and during the first decade of AIDS lesbians and gay men drew closer than the two groups had ever been.

A distinct danger remains that many lesbians will withdraw from such close support if new infections and continued saturation remain a part of the male landscape. Rumblings have already begun in the lesbian world that this is simply unacceptable. Former NGLTF executive director Torie Osborne summed up the thinking of many in her *Advocate* column in late 1994:

> Over the past fifteen years, our fierce reaction to the sexphobia of the vanquishing right, along with a dissolution of the dialogue between gay politics and feminism, have enshrined sexual self-expression as our underlying community ethos. The radicals won the "sex wars," but we lost the truly radical vision of full human liberation in the process. The idea of sex as salvation and as self, which dominates gay male—and now young lesbian—culture, holds no promise for real change; it is consumeristic and ultimately hollow.

Perhaps the deepest and most damaging backlash, though, is the one that occurs within the hearts and minds of individual gay men who increasingly associate their own deepest desires, and the fate of their community, with illness and death. As AIDS ceases to be a crisis and becomes a permanent part of the gay landscape, it will likely exacerbate the sense of shame that is at the very root of the psychological problems that gay liberation seeks to alleviate. The first goal of gay liberation, after all, is the liberation of the self. This process began only when early activists were able to throw off at least some of the debilitating legacy of shame that oppressed them and make the revolutionary claim that Gay Is Good. But the liberation of gay people from shame is an ongoing and lifetime task, and nobody who grows up in the homophobic climate of the modern Western world ever fully achieves this self-liberation. Indeed, it sometimes seems that the most self-aware among us are those who are most aware of how their own shame and self-loathing remain with them, and who are conscious of their daily battle to reimagine themselves as fully healthy, fully sexual, and fully whole. AIDS complicates this to a tremendous degree. For many gay men the epidemic only confirms subconscious and deeply held views of sexuality as diseased, of themselves as guilty. Its perpetuation cannot help but confirm further subconscious stereotypes of ourselves as compulsive, doomed people who do not take life and living seriously.

The Greening of Gay America

As the previous chapters attempt to show, constructing a sustainable sexual ecology for gay men will not be easy. The formidable obstacles begin with the difficult task of convincing ourselves we need to fundamentally alter the very parts of a lifestyle that seem synonymous with freedom and liberation, and which many of us feel compelled to defend. The idea of altering that lifestyle in the cause of sexual restraint will strike many as reactionary, anti-sex, homophobic, a repudiation of the freedom that Stonewall was all about.

Yet the creation of a sustainable gay culture is almost by definition the opposite of reactionary. A reactionary agenda would call for gay men to return to lives of shame and fear in our place of psychic exile, the closet. Indeed, that is essentially the conservative agenda for gay people. Send them back into the closet. Make them stop having sex. Bring back the silence and invisibility of the past. Sexual ecology calls instead for us to move forward into a world that has never existed before, one in which we apply two of our most precious and hard-fought inheritances, sexual self-awareness and ecological knowledge, to the purpose of living openly and with dignity and health in a supportive world—as gay men, as sexual beings, as human beings. This is not a reactionary vision but a revolutionary one, not "sex negativity" but the only sustainable kind of sex positivity, the kind that would demonstrate to ourselves and others our ability to be both sexual and healthy. Sexual ecology calls us to come fully out of the half-shadows of plague and partial liberation, to apply the ageless lessons of social cohesion to our own queer condition, to respect the intense *energia* of sexual desire and our imperfections as human beings, and to work with those forces to craft a sexuality that is both fulfilling and life affirming.

True, this is a radically different vision from the orgiastic, Dionysian vision of liberation proclaimed in the immediate aftermath of Stonewall. To those wedded to that idea, sexual ecology must indeed seem like a step backward. But for gay men, Dionysus is the god who failed. Any future with him will have to look much like the despairing present. Indeed, any future with him will probably grow more despairing, because while AIDS the accident was one thing, AIDS the deliberate and permanent lifestyle will be something entirely different.

The good news is that AIDS can be contained, and that if it is, the future for homosexual people is brighter than it has ever been. Never before in human history has there been such a growth in the understanding of human sexuality and its mysterious twin, gender, and of the fact that some people are impelled to love members of the same sex. Never before has there been such a detailed understanding of ecology, including sexual ecology. These two elements of progress have created the radical possibility that homosexuality may finally be accepted for what it is: a natural variation of the human experience; the left-handedness of love. As understanding deepens that an openly gay world can also be a healthy and affirming world, ancient taboos against homosexuality could erode, opening up a future in which gay people will be free to express themselves as full, equal, healthy members of the human race.

The dual vistas stretching before us offer a future of almost unimaginably stark contrasts. On the one side is a vista of pain, entangled with self-hatred, despair, endless infection, and death. On the other a vision in which homosexual people accept themselves and are accepted by others for who they are. With the continuation of epidemic AIDS, the worst predictions of gaydom's most implacable enemies may not only be fulfilled but exceeded. But with its containment, the fondest dreams of those who fought for gay liberation may be surpassed.

A sustainable gay culture will not be easy to attain. To achieve it will require a reversal, or at least a modification, of many of the core tenets of gay liberation as they were expressed in the years after Stonewall. People will have to accept the fact that the unlimited, unstructured pursuit of absolute sexual freedom, whether it was psychologically good, bad, or indifferent, was biologically disastrous for gay men. We will also have to accept that the idea that unlimited sexual freedom could continue with a simple technological fix was mistaken. The use of condoms and the use of newer, better drugs must be augmented with behavioral changes based in ecological self-knowledge. We need to accept that such changes do not happen through education alone, but can only come about when we construct a new gay social order that explicitly encourages these changes in the individual lives of gay men. To construct such a new social order will require discipline, faith, understanding, study. It will require a belief in our ability to change, and a desire to survive as a healthy and positive people. And that desire will ultimately stem from our belief in ourselves, and our rejection of the homophobic myth that we are by nature shameful, diseased, and doomed.

Whether this very tall order will be achieved is an open question. But we will never know until we try, and that attempt will begin with each of us, and proceed one person at a time.

Notes

Chapter 1: The Birth of AIDS

PAGE

21   For an interesting discussion of the concept of blame as applied to AIDS, Sabatier's book is excellent.

22   Cindy Patton, *Inventing AIDS* (Routledge, 1990), p. 83.
      Robert Gallo, "The AIDS Virus," *Scientific American*, 256(1), (1987), p. 56.
      For a thorough overview of the hypothesis that HIV recently arose from a pool of primate SIVs, see Gerald Myers, Kersti MacInnes, and Bette Korber, "The Emergence of Simian/Human Immunodeficiency Viruses," *AIDS Research and Human Retroviruses* 8(3)(1992), pp. 373–86. Another interesting overview of Myers's views on the subject is contained in his chapter "Phylogenic Moments in the AIDS Epidemic," in *Emerging Viruses*, S. S. Morse, ed. (Oxford University Press, 1993), pp. 120–37.

23   Personal communication.
      Randy Shilts, *And the Band Played On* (St. Martin's, 1987), p. 3.

24   For the most extensive discussion of the problems with the concept of HIV's recent emergence, see Mirko D. Grmek, *History of AIDS: Emergence and Origin of a Modern Pandemic*, translated by Russell C. Maulitz and Jacalyn Duffin (Princeton University Press, 1990).

26   Personal communication.
      Perhaps the high point of the non-HIV AIDS hype was the *Time* magazine cover story "Losing the Battle," August 3, 1992. Papers debunking non-HIV AIDS and showing the cases to be nonrelated began appearing the following winter. See Dick Sheridan, "Studies Crush Fears of New AIDS Virus," *Daily News*, Feb. 11, 1993.

27 Harold P. Katner and George A. Pankey, "Evidence for a Euro-American Origin of Human Immunodeficiency Virus," *Journal of the National Medical Association*, 79(10), (1987). Again, the best discussion of this issue is found in Grmek.

28 Laurie Garrett, "Killer Found: Herpes Type Causes 2 AIDS-Linked Cancers," *New York Newsday*, Thursday, May 4, 1995. The discovery was made by the husband-and-wife team Drs. Patrick Moore and Yuan Chang of Columbia University. They named the virus "Kaposi's sarcoma–associated herpevirus," or KSHV.

An even earlier case, that of David Carr, a twenty-five-year-old British sailor, is now suspected of being a fraud. See Lawrence Altman, "Earliest AIDS Case Is Called into Doubt," *New York Times*, Thursday, April 4, 1995, p. C1.

30 Grmek, p. 145.

Francine McCutchan et al., "HIV Genetic Diversity," International Conference on AIDS (abstract no. Mo.02.).

32 Patton, p. 27. Also see Patton's excellent *Sex and Germs*. Patton's use of the techniques of deconstruction to analyze the way society responds to AIDS is illuminating.

New diseases continue to be noticed almost monthly. For the best overview of the subject of emerging diseases, see Laurie Garrett, *The Coming Plague: Newly Emerging Diseases in a World Out of Balance* (Farrar, Straus and Giroux, 1994).

33 Personal communication.

36 National Research Council, *The Social Impact of AIDS in the United States* (National Academy Press, 1993), p. 272.

Chapter 2: Gay Sexual Ecology

40 George Chauncey, *Gay New York: Gender, Urban Culture, and the Making of the Gay Male World 1890–1940* (Basic Books, 1994), p. 13. Anyone interested in this subject is strongly urged to read the entire volume.
Chauncey, p. 16.

41 Chauncey, pp. 21–22.
Allan Bérubé, "The History of the Baths," in *Coming Up*, 6:3 (December 1984), p. 16.

43 Allan Bérubé, *Coming Out under Fire: The History of Gay Men and Women in World War Two* (Free Press, 1990), p. 153.

44 Jonathan M. Mann, ed., *AIDS in the World: A Global Report* (Harvard University Press, 1992), p. 177.

46 Ibid, p. 14.

47 For a succinct discussion of core groups, see *AIDS in the World*, Chapter 5. *AIDS in the World*, p. 176.

The concept of synergy was developed in R. Wallace, "A Synergism of Plagues: 'Planned Shrinkage,' Contagious Housing Destruction and AIDS in the Bronx," *Environmental Research* 47 (1988), pp. 1–33.

For an interesting discussion of the concept of herd immunity generally, see Peter Gould, *The Slow Plague: A Geography of the AIDS Pandemic* (Blackwell, 1993), pp. 190–200.

50   Chauncey, p. 86.

Ibid.

Seymour Kleinberg, *Alienated Affections: Being Gay in America* (Warner, 1980), p. 285.

One of the more interesting, if somewhat sensational, discussions of the discrepancies in rates of STDs before and after Stonewall, and between men and women, is found in Robert Root-Bernstein, *Rethinking AIDS: The Tragic Cost of Premature Consensus* (Free Press, 1993), Chapter 8. While Root-Bernstein's thesis questioning HIV's role in AIDS is dubious, his research is solid, and his book remains an excellent source.

51   Chauncey, p. 13.

Michel Foucault, *The History of Sexuality: Volume 1: An Introduction*, trans. Robert Hurley (Vintage, 1990), p. 43.

52   The now classic work on this development is Bérubé, *Coming Out Under Fire.*

Chauncey, pp. 21–22.

55   Perhaps the best anthology of these views is found in Karla Jay and Allen Young, eds., *Out of the Closets: Voices of Gay Liberation* (Douglas, 1972).

56   The paper was Canada's *The Body Politic*. It is cited by Ian Young in his book *The Stonewall Experiment: A Gay Psychohistory* (Cassell, 1995), p. 89. Young, p. 77.

58   Chauncey, 212.

"Gay baths were few in number and served a more limited—and generally more affluent—clientele than most of the other spaces gay men appropriated in the early twentieth century." Chauncey, p. 223.

59   Ibid.

Ibid.

60   Ibid. Also Shilts, p. 19.

61   John L. Martin, "The Impact of AIDS on Gay Male Sexual Behavior Patterns in New York City," *American Journal of Public Health* 77 (5), pp. 579–80.

62   Yony, "A Foolish Young Circuit Queen Finds Out What It Means to Be Wise," *PWA Coalition Newsline*, October 1987, pp. 29–30. Cited in Ian Young, *The Stonewall Experiment*, p. 114.

Michael, Gagnon, Laumann, and Kolata, *Sex in America: A Definitive Survey* (Little Brown, 1994), p. 209.

63   Garrett, *The Coming Plague*, p. 271.

Douglas Sadownick, *Sex Between Men* (Harper San Francisco, 1996, p. 120.

64   Young, p. 124. Citing John Preston.

Chapter 3: The Synergy of Plagues

67   H. Most. "Manhattan: A Tropic Isle?" *American Journal of Tropical Medical Hygiene* 17 (1968), pp. 333–45.

Randy Shilts, p. 39.

For the best discussion of the emergence of drug-resistant strains of gonhorrhea, see Laurie Garrett, *The Coming Plague*.

The best source of information on the spread of STDs remains the Centers for Disease Control and Prevention. These figures are from CDC "Summary of Notifiable Diseases, United States," for 1980, 1981, 1988, and 1989.

68   Dr. Nahmias's work is cited by Robert Root-Bernstein in *Rethinking AIDS*, p. 289.

69   Shilts, p. 39.

Garrett, p. 270.

Root-Bernstein, 285.

Michael Callen, *Surviving AIDS* (HarperCollins 1990), p. 12. The late Michael Callen is widely deemed a hero among many who consider themselves sex positive in the classic seventies sense. Yet Callen was among the most brutally honest when it came to discussing the reality of gay fast lane life in the seventies. "No one asked what the cumulative consequences might be of continually wallowing in what was, to put it bluntly, an increasingly polluted microbiological sewer," he wrote in a passage in *Surviving AIDS* that would probably have been blasted as sex negative if it had been written by almost anybody else. "Rumors that the Health Department had been able to culture cholera and other exotic microbes from the greasy stairs of the Mineshaft (a notorious Manhattan sex club) were dismissed as apocryphal."

70   Garrett, 273.

Root-Bernstein, 164.

The most comprehensive overview of this subject, including prevalence infection charts, is found in Root-Bernstein, pp. 163–70. Also Garrett.

71   Callen, *Surviving AIDS*, pp. 5–6.

72   Garrett, p. 263.

74   For data on San Francisco, see Nancy A. Hessol et al., "Prevalence, Incidence and Progression of Human Immunodeficiency Virus Infection in Homosexual and Bisexual Men in Hepatitis B Vaccine Trials, 1978–1988," *American Journal of Epidemiology* 130(6) (1989), pp. 1167–75. See also James W. Curran et al., "The Epidemiology of AIDS: Current Status and Future Prospects," *Science* 229 (1985), pp. 1352–57. Also Warren Winkelstein Jr. et al., "Sexual Practices and Risk of Infection by the Human Immunodeficiency Virus," *JAMA*, 257(3) (1987), pp. 321–25.

New York data is found in Cladd E. Stevens et al., "Human T-Cell Lymphotropic Virus Type III Infection in a Cohort of Homosexual Men in New York City," *JAMA* 255(16) (1986), pp. 2167–2172.

MMWR supplement, vol. 36, no. 5–6, Dec. 18, 1987, Table 1, pp. 22–23.

75   Michael Callen, "Dinosaur's Diary," *QW* magazine, July 26, 1991.

77   David F. Greenberg, *The Construction of Homosexuality* (The University of Chicago Press, 1988), p. 26.

Carl Wittman, "A Gay Manifesto," reprinted in *Out of the Closets: Voices of Gay Liberation* (Douglas, 1972), p. 337.

78   For a discussion of the effects of versatility, see D. Trichopoulos, L. Spiros, and E. Petridou, "Homosexual Role Separation and the Spread of AIDS," *Lancet 2* (1988), p. 966.

The most thorough discussion of the difference between serial and concurrent multiple partners is contained in an unpublished paper by Martina Morris, Columbia University.

80   One study by Dr. Ann C. Collier of the University of Washington in Seattle found HIV in the semen of 22 percent of HIV-infected subjects but could find no predictors of who would be shedding virus.

82   Esther Newton, *Cherry Grove, Fire Island: Sixty Years in America's First Gay and Lesbian Town* (Beacon Press, 1993), p. 78.

Duncan Osborne, *Outweek* magazine 77, p. 38.

83   Ann Guidici Fettner and William A. Check, *The Truth About AIDS* (Holt, Rinehart and Winston, 1984), p. 69.

Garrett, *The Coming Plague*, p. 653.

85   J. A. Sonnabend, "The Etiology of AIDS," *AIDS Research* 1:1 (1983), pp. 2–3.

86   J. R. Thompson, "AIDS: The Mismanagement of an Epidemic," *Computer Math Applications*, Vol. 18, No. 10/11 (1989), pp. 965–72. Thompson's quote is from *The Houston Chronicle*, July 14, 1987.

88   *AIDS in the World*, p. 185.

89   Berridge and Strong, eds., *AIDS and Contemporary History* (Cambridge University Press, 1993), p. 23.

Chapter 4: The Birth of the Condom Code

92   Cited in Fee and Fox, eds., *AIDS: The Burden of History* (University of California Press, 1988), p. 155.

Shilts, p. 67.

93   *New York Evening Post*, cited in *AIDS: The Burdens of History*, p. 43.

94   Ronald Bayer, *Private Acts, Social Consequences* (Rutgers University Press, 1989), p. 24.

Harold W. Jaffe et al., "National Case Control Study of Kaposi's Sarcoma and Pneumocystis Carinii Pneumonia in Homosexual Men: Part 1, Epidemiological Results," *Annals of Internal Medicine* 99 (1983), pp. 145–52.

Kaposi's Sarcoma in Gay Men (Bay Area Physicians for Human Rights, San Francisco, 1982). Also *Towards a Healthier Gay Lifestyle: Kaposi's Sarcoma, Opportunistic Infections and the Urban Gay Lifestyle, What You Need to Know Know to Ensure Your Good Health* (Citizens for Human Equality, Houston, 1982). Also Nathan Fain, "More on Safe Sex," *The Advocate*, April 17, 1984, pp. 20–21.

95   CDC, "Prevention of Acquired Immune Deficiency Syndrome (AIDS): Report of Inter-Agency Recommendation, *MMWR* 32(8) (1983), pp. 101–103.

Cited in Ralph Bolton, "AIDS and Promiscuity: Muddles in the Models of HIV Prevention," *Medical Anthropology* 14 (1992), p. 168.

Bolton, p. 176.

96   Victor de Gruttola et al., "AIDS: Has the Problem Been Adequately Assessed?" (editorial), *Review of Infectious Diseases* 8(2) (1986), pp. 295–305. Cited in King, p. 39.

97   Cited in Neil Miller, *Out of the Past: Gay and Lesbian History from 1869 to the Present* (Vintage, 1995), pp. 442–43.

Cited in Bayer, p. 25.

98   John L. Martin, "The Impact of AIDS on Gay Male Sexual Behavior Patterns in New York City," *American Journal of Public Health* 77(5) (1987), pp. 578–81.

100   Richard Berkowitz and Michael Callen, *How to Have Sex in an Epidemic: One Approach* (New York: News from the Front Publications, 1983).

David L. Chambers, "Gay Men, AIDS, and the Code of the Condom," *Harvard Civil Rights Civil Liberties Law Review* 29:2 (Summer 1994).

101   Cited by King, p. 46. "The Netherlands provides a case-study of a country in which gay men were actively discouraged from using condoms for anal sex, in favor of giving up fucking altogether. . . . It seems clear that in Holland, use of condoms played at most a small role in stopping the spread of HIV among gay men."

Joseph Sonnabend, "Looking at AIDS in Totality: A Conversation," *New York Native*, October 7, 1985.

Michael Callen, "In Defense of Anal Sex," *PWA Coalition Newsline* 41 (1989), pp. 37–43.

102   Chambers, 360.

103   John L. P. Thompson, "Estimated Condom Failure and Frequency of Condom Use Among Gay Men," *American Journal of Public Health* 83:10 (October 1993), p. 1409.

MMWR 43:30 (August 6, 1993).

Jeffrey Perlman et al., "HIV Risk Difference Between Condom Users and

Nonusers Among U.S. Heterosexual Women," *Journal of AIDS* 3 (1990), pp. 155–65.

King, p. 93.

107   Chambers, p. 366.

Ibid.

Cited by Chambers, p. 366.

109   King, p. 86.

110   Risa Denenberg, *Applying Harm Reduction to Sexual and Reproductive Counseling: A Health Provider's Guide to Supporting the Goals of People with HIV/AIDS*, SIECUS Report, Oct./Nov. 1993.

111   Frank Browning, *The Culture of Desire: Paradox and Perversity in Gay Lives Today* (Crown Publishers, 1993), pp. 119–20.

112   Bayer, p. 26.

Maria L. Ekstrand et al., "Maintenance of Safer Sexual Behaviors and Predictors of Risky Sex: The San Francisco Men's Health Study," *American Journal of Public Health* 80(9) (1990), pp. 973–77.

Warren Winkelstein, Jr., et al., "The San Francisco Men's Health Study: Continued Declines in HIV Seroconversion Rates among Homosexual/Bisexual Men," *American Journal of Public Health* 78(11) (1988), pp. 1472–74.

113   John L. Martin et al., "The Impact of AIDS on a Gay Community: Changes in Sexual Behavior, Substance Use, and Mental Health," *American Journal of Community Psychology* 17(3) (1989), pp. 269–93.

The best discussion of degaying is found in Edward King, who devotes an entire chapter to the subject, and another to the subject of "regaying" AIDS.

114   Cited in *AIDS: The Burden of History* (1988), p. 205.

115   Cited in Fumento, p. 188.

Cited by Elizabeth Fee in her essay "Sin Versus Science: Venereal Disease in Twentieth-Century Baltimore," in *AIDS: The Burden of History*, p. 140.

Fumento, p. 211.

117   Cindy Patton, *Inventing AIDS*, p. 46.

Douglas Crimp, "How to Have Promiscuity in an Epidemic," in *AIDS: Cultural Analysis, Cultural Activism*, October, 43. p. 253. "Gay male promiscuity should be seen instead as a positive model of how sexual pleasures might be pursued by and granted to everyone if those pleasures were not confined within the narrow limits of institutionalized sexuality," wrote Crimp. "Indeed, it is the lack of promiscuity and its lessons that suggests that many straight people will have a much harder time learning 'how to have sex in an epidemic' than we did."

Chapter 5: The "Second Wave"

119   H. H. Handsfield et al., "Trends in Gonorrhea in Homosexually Active Men— King County, Washington, 1989," *MMWR* 38(44) (1989), pp. 762–64.

John B. F. deWit et al., "Safe Sexual Practices Not Reliably Maintained by Homosexual Men," (letter), *American Journal of Public Health* 82(4) (1992), pp. 615–16; V. C. Riley, "Resurgent Gonorrhea in Homosexual Men," (letter), *The Lancet* 337 (1991), p. 375; J. A. R. van den Hoek et al., "Increase in Unsafe Homosexual Behaviour," (letter), *The Lancet* 336 (1990), pp. 179–80.

Ron Stall et al., "Relapse from Safer Sex: the Next Challenge for AIDS Prevention Efforts," *Journal of AIDS* 3 (1990), pp. 1181–87.

120   S. Maurice Adib et al., "Relapse in Sexual Behavior among Homosexual Men: A 2-Year Follow-Up from the Chicago MAC/CCS," *AIDS* 5 (1991), pp. 757–60.

Project SIGMA, Update, London, March 1992. Cited in King, pp. 140–41.

Jeffrey A. Kelly, et al., "Acquired Immunodeficiency Syndrome/HIV Risk Behavior Among Gay Men in Small Cities," *Archives of Internal Medicine* 152 (Nov. 1992), pp. 2293–97.

NIAID AIDS Agenda, "Young Gay Men Not Heeding AIDS Messages, Rates of Infection Remain High," Summer, 1993, p. 5. (Cited in AAPHR Summit report.)

121   Ibid.

Donald R. Hoover et al., "Estimating the 1978–1990 and Future Spread of Human Immunodeficiency Virus Type 1 in Subgroups of Homosexual Men," *American Journal of Epidemiology* 134(10) (1991), pp. 1190–1205.

122   Graham Hart et al, " 'Relapse' to Unsafe Sexual Behaviour," *Sociology of Health and Illness* 14:2 (1992), p. 225.

King, p. 144.

123   Marshall H. Becker et al., "AIDS and Behavioral Change to Reduce Risk: A Revivew," *American Journal of Public Health* 78, pp. 394–410. Also, Ron Stall, et al., "Behavioral Risk Reduction for HIV Infection Among Gay and Bisexual Men: A Review of Results from the United States," *American Psychologist* 43 (1988), pp. 878–85.

125   M. Morris and L. Dean, "Effect of Sexual Behavior Change on Long-Term Human Immunodeficiency Virus Prevalence among Homosexual Men," *American Journal of Epidemiology* 140(3) (1994), pp. 217–32.

127   Most of this information is from unpublished data emanating from vaccine preparedness studies, which researchers say consistently show higher levels of unsafe sex as the nineties continue. Unfortunately, there are few ongoing studies the follow gay male behavior and infection rates.

128   A discussion of Farr's Law and other related theoretical ways of predicting the crest of the AIDS epidemic, including the theories of Alexander Langmuir, is found in Fumento, p. 312. Langmuir's predictions have proven remarkably accurate.

129   Nancy A. Hessol et al., "Prevalence, Incidence and Progression of Human Immunodeficiency Virus Infection in Homosexual and Bisexual Men in

Hepatitis B Vaccine Trials, 1978–1988," *American Journal of Epidemiology* 130(6) (1989), pp. 1167–75.

130 Alan P. Bell and Martin S. Weinberg, *Homosexualities: A Study of Diversity Among Men and Women* (Simon and Schuster, 1978).

131 Bolton, p. 30.

132 For an excellent discussion of the geography of HIV epidemiology, see Peter Gould, *The Slow Plague: A Geography of the AIDS Pandemic*, 1993.

Chapter 6: Surfing the Second Wave

136 For good summaries of the reported reasons why gay men often do not use condoms, see NIAID AIDS Agenda, "Young Gay Men Not Heeding AIDS Message, Rates of Infection Remain High," Summer 1993, p. 5. See also Robert A. Jones, "Dangerous Liaisons: Young Gay Men Know All About AIDS and HIV, Yet They Persist in Having Unprotected Sex," *Los Angeles Times Magazine*, July 25, 1993. The story of prevention subjects giving tips to prevention workers was presented off the record at the Dallas Prevention Summit.

The self-disclosure trend began with speeches at the Dallas Prevention Summit. It continued in the national press, both gay and mainstream. See Michelangelo Signorile, "Unsafe Like Me," *Out* magazine, Oct. 1994, and Michael Warner, "Why Gay Men Are Having Risky Sex," *The Village Voice*, Jan. 13, 1995.

137 New York's GMHC largely discontinued its condom distribution in NYC gay bars in 1995, to virtually no public protest.

138 R. B. Hays, S. Kegeles, T. Coates. "Understanding the High Rates of HIV Risk-Taking among Young Gay and Bisexual Men: The Young Men's Survey," CAPA, International Conference on AIDS, June 16–21, 1991 (abstract no. m.c. 101) 7(1), p. 48.

J. Stokes, R. Burzette, D. McKirnan, "Bisexual Men: Social Characteristics and Predictors of AIDS-Risk Behavior," International Conference on AIDS, 1991 (abstract no. M.D. 4048); J. S. Saint Lawrence, T. L. Brasfield "Factors Which Predict Relapse to Unsafe Sex by Gay Men," International Conference on AIDS, 1990 (abstract no. F.C. 725); J. A. Kelly, J. S. Saint Lawrence, T. L. Brasfield, "Predictors of Vulnerability to AIDS Risk Behavior Relapse," *Journal of Consulting Clinical Psychology* 59(1) (Feb., 1991), pp. 163–66.

139 Doug Sadownick, *Sex Between Men*, p. 230.

"Crystal Meth and You," *Out* magazine, Dec./Jan. 1996.

An overview of the debate between substance abuse as a causal marker or the cause of unsafe behavior is found in Ron Stall, "Intertwining Epidemic? A Short History of Research on the Relationship between Substance Use and the AIDS Epidemic Among Gay Men," presented at the Dallas AIDS

Prevention Summit. See also R. Bolten et. al., "Alcohol and Risky Sex: In Search of an Elusive Connection," *Medical Anthropology* 14(2–4) (1992), pp. 323–63; J. McKusker et al., "Use of Drugs and Alcohol by Homosexually Active Men in Relation to Sexual Practices," *Journal of AIDS* 3 (1990), pp. 729–36; M. J. Perry et al., "High-Risk Sexual Behavior and Alcohol Consumption among Bar-Going Gay Men," *AIDS* 8(9) (Sept. 1994), pp. 1321–24.

141   Walt Odets, "AIDS Education and Harm Reduction for Gay Men: Psychological Approaches for the 21st Century," *AIDS and Public Policy Journal* 9(1) (Spring 1994), pp. 1–15. Walt Odets, "Psychosocial and Educational Challenges for the Gay and Bisexual Male Communities," abstract presented at the Dallas AIDS Prevention Summit, 1994.

Walt Odets, *In the Shadow of the Epidemic: Being HIV-Negative in the Age of AIDS* (Duke University Press, 1995), p. 123.

Odets, *In the Shadow of the Epidemic*, p. 196.

Walt Odets, "AIDS Education and Harm Reduction for Gay Men: Psychological Approaches for the 21st Century," *AIDS and Public Policy Journal* 9(1), p. 3.

Odets, *In the Shadow of the Epidemic*, pp. 102–103.

143   Martin P. Levine and Karolynn Siegel, "Unprotected Sex: Understanding Gay Men's Participation," in *The Social Context of AIDS,* Joan Huber and Beth E. Schneider, eds. (Sage, 1992), pp. 47–71.

144   *The Social Context of AIDS*, p. 52.

146   "Infected Couples Still Spurn Condoms," *New York Times*, Aug. 10, 1995. The study, conducted by Dr. Isabelle de Vincenzi and published in the *New England Journal of Medicine*, tracked the cases of 256 men and women whose partners were infected and found that only 48 percent used condoms consistently. Of the 121 who did not, 12 became infected, leading to a projected infection rate of 5 percent a year.

148   Cited in Thomas J. Coates and Jeff Stryker, "HIV Prevention, Looking Back, Looking Ahead," *CAPA* (1994), p. 5.

150   Gil Gerald & Associates et al., "The Silent Crisis: Ongoing HIV Infections Among Gay Men, Bisexuals and Lesbians at Risk." Report of the GLMA/AAPHR Summit on HIV Prevention for Gay Men, Bisexuals, and Lesbians at Risk, July 15–17, 1994, Dallas, Texas (1995).

154   Ronald Bayer, "Sounding Board: AIDS Prevention—Sexual Ethics and Responsibility," the *New England Journal of Medicine* 354(23) (June 6, 1996), pp. 1540–42.

155   Walt Odets, "Psychosocial and Educational Challenges for the Gay and Bisexual Male Communities," abstract presented at the Dallas AIDS Prevention Summit, 1994, p. 6.

156   Eric Rofes, Address to the Dallas AIDS Prevention Summit, 1994.

157   Both the studies by Koopman and Samuels came to this conclusion, even

though they used different methods and studied different populations of gay men.

158   *The Social Context of AIDS*, p. 49.

160   Lawrence K. Altman, "Monkey Study Accents Risks of Oral Sex," *New York Times*, June 7, 1996, p. A18.

161   Walt Odets, "AIDS Education and Harm Reduction for Gay Men: Psychological Approaches for the 21st Century," *AIDS and Public Policy Journal* 9(1), p. 15.
      Odets, *In the Shadow of the Epidemic*, p. 253.

162   Walt Odets, "AIDS Education and Harm Reduction for Gay Men: Psychological Approaches for the 21st Century," *AIDS and Public Policy Journal* 9(1), p. 9.
      Walt Odets, "AIDS Education and Harm Reduction for Gay Men: Psychological Approaches for the 21st Century," *AIDS and Public Policy Journal* 9(1), p. 8.
      Odets, *In the Shadow of the Epidemic*, pp. 262–63.

Chapter 7: The Ecology of "Heterosexual AIDS"

163   Elizabeth Mehren and Victor Zonona, "Krim's Crusade: In the Fight Against AIDS, She Is a Scientist, a Socialite, a Strategist, a Spokeswoman and Sometimes a Cheerleader in Sensible Shoes," *Los Angeles Times*, Nov. 27, 1988.

164   *Life* magazine, July 8, 1985.
      "Women Living with AIDS," transcript of Feb. 18, 1987, *Oprah Winfrey Show*. Cited in Michael Fumento, *The Myth of Heterosexual AIDS: How a Tragedy Has Been Distorted by the Media and Partisan Politics* (Regnery Gateway, 1990), p. 3.
      Department of Health and Human Services, *AIDS Prevention Guide*.
      Testimony of Dr. John Seale to the California Senate Health and Human Services Committee, Sept. 29, 1986. Cited in Fumento, p. 181.

165   William H. Masters, Virginia E. Johnson, and Robert C. Kolodny, *Crisis: Heterosexual Behavior in the Age of AIDS* (Grove, 1988), p. 62.
      Cited in Fumento, p. 253.

166   Fumento, p. 178.
      Edward King, *Safety in Numbers*, p. 241.
      King, p. 239.

167   National Research Council, *The Social Impact of AIDS in the United States* (National Academy Press, 1993), p. 9.

170   Relative risks of infection are from World Health Organization, *AIDS Analysis in Africa* 5(6) (April/May, 1995). Further information is contained in Scott D. Holmberg et al., "Biologic Factors in the Sexual Transmission of Human Immunodeficiency Virus," *Journal of Infectious Diseases* 160(1)

(July 1989), pp. 116–25. Also N. S. Padian et al., "The Effect of Number of Exposures on the Risk of Heterosexual HIV Transmission," *Journal of Infectious Diseases* 161 (May 1990), pp. 883–87.

171   Michael, Gagnon, Laumann, and Kolata, *Sex in America; A Definitive Survey* (Little Brown, 1994) and Samuel S. Janus, Cynthia L. Janus, *The Janus Report on Sexual Behavior* (John Wiley & Sons, 1993).

Turner, Miller, and Moses, *AIDS, Sexual Behavior and Intravenous Drug Use* (National Academy Press, 1989), p. 1120.

172   Alan P. Bell and Martin S. Weinberg, *Homosexualities: A Study of Diversity among Men & Women* (Simon and Schuster, 1978).

Michael Callen, "Come One, Come All!" *QW* magazine, May 10, 1992.

175   The data on oral sex and crack is found in Joyce I. Wallace et al., "Sexual and Drug Practices and HIV Infection Among Streetwalking Prostitutes in New York City" (Foundation of Research on Sexually Transmitted Diseases, 1995). Among its conclusions: "The most surprising finding in our study is the apparent relationship between non-injecting prostitutes who perform mainly fellatio and an increased risk of HIV infection."

Data on midwestern crack users is from R. G. Carlson and H. A. Siegel, "The Crack Life: An Ethnographic Overview of Crack Use and Sexual Behavior among African-Americans in a Midwest Metropolitan City," *Journal of Psychoactive Drugs* 23, pp. 11–20.

177   "Growing Fast As a Factor in AIDS: Drugs," *New York Times*, May 16, 1996.
AIDS in the World, p. 29. See also pp. 97–98 for data on when HIV first entered Northeast Asia. Quote is from p. 37.

178   *The Slow Plague*, pp. 88–92.

179   *The Slow Plague*, p. 106.
James C. McKinley Jr., "A Ray of Light in Africa's Struggle with AIDS," *New York Times*, April 7, 1996.

180   *AIDS in the World*, p. 63.

181   The best overview of the emergence of new subtype E virus in Thailand is Jon Cohen, "A Shot in the Dark," *Discover* magazine, June 1996, pp. 66–73.

Chapter 8: Holisitic Prevention

186   The ecological association between technological fixes and air pollution was discussed by Bill McKibben in "Not So Fast," *New York Times Magazine*, July 23, 1995, pp. 24–25.

187   A full exploration of the statistical effect of technology on sexual mores is found in Laurie Garrett, *The Coming Plague*, particularly chapters 10 and 11.

188   For sources on deep ecology, see Arne Naess, *Ecology, Community and Lifestyle*, translated and edited by David Rothenberg (1989). Also Bill Devall and George Sessions, *Deep Ecology: Living as if Nature Mattered* (1985).

190   Ford Hickson et al., "Perceptions of Own and Partner's HIV Status and
       Unprotected Anal Intercourse Among Gay Men," paper presented at AIDS
       Impact: Second Conference of Biopsychosocial Aspects of HIV/AIDS,
       Brighton, 1994. "Most men who know they are positive who fuck without
       condoms do so with other men they know or believe to be positive."

       See also Mark Schoofs, "Can You Trust Your Lover? Gay Couples Weigh
       the Risk of Unprotected Sex," *The Village Voice,* Jan. 31, 1995. "Studies show
       that men in relationships where both partners have the same serostatus are
       much more likely to have unprotected anal sex than men in sero-discordant
       couples or men who don't know whether their partner is infected."

       However, not every study has verified this claim. See, for example,
       Samuel Perry et al., "Voluntarily Informing Others of Positive HIV Test
       Results: Patterns of Notification by Infected Gay Men," *Hospital and Com-
       munity Psychiatry* 41(5) (May 1990). "Sixty-six percent of subjects [who
       had just tested positive] notified every current sexual partner, although
       notification was not associated with a greater likelihood of safer sex prac-
       tices." Not all of these partners, of course, were long-term lovers.

198   Garrett Hardin, *Living Within Limits: Ecology, Economics and Population
       Taboos* (Oxford University Press, 1993), p. 202.

199   Gay Men's Health Crisis, "Policy Statement on Commercial Sex Establish-
       ments," adopted April 24, 1995.

200   Warren Winkelstein Jr. et al., "Selected Sexual Practices of San Francisco
       Heterosexual Men and Risk of Infection by the Human Immunodefi-
       ciency Virus," (letter), *JAMA* 257(11) (1987), pp. 1470–71. Winkelstein's
       report was based on data collected from the San Francisco Men's Health
       Study.

201   Laura Dean, "Sex in Public Places, HIV and New York's Gay Community,"
       presented at the Columbia University Workshop on Sex in Bathhouses,
       Dec. 11, 1995.

203   Ian Young, *The Stonewall Experiment*, pp. 138–39.

204   Michael Bronski, "Sex in the '90s: The Problems of Pleasure," *Steam* 2(2)
       (Summer 1994), pp. 132–34.

Chapter 9: Imagining a Sustainable Culture

217   Estimates are by the U.S. Public Health Service. An account of the furor
       over New York City's reestimate of AIDS cases by Joseph himself is found in
       Stephen C. Joseph, *Dragon within the Gates: The Once and Future AIDS
       Epidemic* (Carroll & Graf 1992), p. 169.

219   Ms. Haynes-Sanstad's comparison was contained in the Center for AIDS
       Prevention's peer-review of the manuscript of this book.

221   For the best examination of these arguments, see Robert Wright, *The Moral*

Animal: Why We Are the Way We Are, The New Science of Evolutionary Psychology (Vintage, 1994).

224 David Greenberg, *The Construction of Homosexuality* (University of Chicago Press, 1988), p. 151.

Michael Foucault, *The Use of Pleasure: The History of Sexuality Volume 2* (Vintage, 1990), pp. 49–50.

David Halperin, *One Hundred Years of Homosexuality* (Routledge, 1990), p. 69.

225 Foucault, p. 81.

The Pseudo-Lucian quote is from John Boswell, *Christianity, Social Tolerance and Homosexuality* (University of Chicago Press, 1980), p. 153.

The samurai quote is from Greenberg, p. 260.

Chapter 10: Building Incentives into Gay Culture

234 Garrett Hardin, *Living Within Limits: Ecology, Economics and Population Taboos* (Oxford University Press, 1993), p. 198.

235 Garrett Hardin, "The Tragedy of the Commons," *Science* 162 (1968), pp. 1243–48.

237 Paul Ehrlich and Anne Ehrlich, *The Population Explosion.* They point out five requisites to reduce fertility: (1) nutrition; (2) sanitation; (3) basic health care; (4) education of women; (5) women's rights. Women in traditional societies apply education to the home, which brings about improvements in sanitation and food, which reduce child mortality, making women receptive to smaller families. In addition, when women have rights they have access to sources of status other than large families, again making them receptive to smaller families.

239 Hardin, *Living Within Limits*, p. 218.

Chapter 11: The Stakes

264 Data about the effects of antibiotics on syphilis and gonorrhea are found in Laurie Garrett, *The Coming Plague*, chapters 10 and 11.

272 Eric Rofes, *Reviving the Tribe: Regenerating Gay Men's Sexuality and Culture in the Ongoing Epidemic* (Harrington Park, 1995), pp. 184–87.

286 *Harvard Gay and Lesbian Review*, Fall 1995, vol. ii, no. 4, p. 7.

287 Appuzzo, summit speech.

Selected Bibliography

Ackerman, Diane. *A Natural History of Love.* Random House, 1994.

Adam, Barry D. *The Rise of a Gay and Lesbian Movement.* Twayne, 1987.

Altman, Dennis. *Power and Community: Organizational and Cultural Responses to AIDS.* Taylor and Francis, 1994.

———. *AIDS and the New Puritanism.* Pluto, 1986.

———. *Homosexual Oppression and Liberation.* Avon, 1971.

Auerbach, Judith D., Christina Wypijewska, and H. Keith Brodie, eds. *AIDS and Behavior: An Integrated Approach.* National Academy Press, 1994.

Bateson, Mary Catherine, and Richard Goldsby. *Thinking AIDS: Social Responses to the Biological Threat.* Addison-Wesley, 1988.

Bayer, Ronald. *Private Acts, Social Consequences: AIDS and the Politics of Public Health.* Rutgers University Press, 1991.

Bell, Alan P., and Martin S. Weinberg. *Homosexualities: A Study of Diversity Among Men and Women.* Simon and Schuster, 1978.

Bell, Alan P., and Martin S. Weinberg and Sue Kiefer Hammersmith. *Sexual Preference: Its Development in Men and Women.* Indiana University Press, 1981.

Bernarde, Melvin A. *Our Precarious Habitat: An Integrated Approach to Understanding Man's Effect on His Environment.* Norton, 1970.

Berridge, Virginia, and Philip Strong, eds. *AIDS and Contemporary History.* Cambridge University Press, 1993.

Bérubé, Allan. *Coming Out Under Fire: The History of Gay Men and Women in World War Two.* Free Press, 1990.

Boswell, John. *Christianity, Social Tolerance and Homosexuality.* University of Chicago Press, 1980.

———. *Same-Sex Unions in Premodern Europe.* Villard, 1994.

Brandt, Allan. *No Magic Bullet: A Social History of Venereal Disease in the United States Since 1880.* Oxford University Press, 1985.

Browning, Frank. *The Culture of Desire: Paradox and Perversity in Gay Lives Today.* Crown, 1993.

Bullough, Vern L. *Science in the Bedroom: A History of Sex Research.* Basic Books, 1994.

Burkett, Elinor. *The Gravest Show on Earth: America in the Age of AIDS.* Houghton Mifflin, 1995.

Campbell, Bernard. *Human Ecology.* Aldine de Gruyter, 1983.

Callen, Michael. *Surviving AIDS.* HarperCollins, 1990.

Chambers, David L. "Gay Men, AIDS, and the Code of the Condom." *Harvard Civil Rights, Civil Liberties Law Review,* Vol. 29, No. 2, Summer, 1994.

Chauncey, George. *Gay New York: Gender, Urban Culture, and the Making of the Gay Male World 1890–1940.* Basic Books, 1994.

Crimp, Douglas, ed. "AIDS: Cultural Analysis Cultural Activism," in *October* 43 (Winter 1987).

Davies, P. M., and F. C. I. Hickson, P. Weatherburn, and A. J. Hunt, eds. *Sex, Gay Men and AIDS.* Falmer, 1993.

Eblen, Ruth A., and William R. Eblen, eds. *The Encyclopedia of the Environment.* Houghton Mifflin, 1994.

d'Arcangelo, Angelo. *The Homosexual Handbook.* 1968.

D'Emillio, John. *Sexual Politics, Sexual Communities: The Making of a Sexual Minority in the United States, 1940–1970.* University of Chicago Press, 1983.

Ewald, Paul W. *The Evolution of Infectious Diseases.* Oxford University Press, 1994.

Fee, Elizabeth, and Daniel Fox, eds. *AIDS: The Burden of History.* University of California Press, 1988.

———. *AIDS: The Making of a Chronic Disease.* University of California Press, 1992.

Fettner, Ann Giudici, and William A. Check. *The Truth About AIDS: The Evolution of an Epidemic.* Holt, Rinehart and Winston, 1984.

Fisher, Jeffrey A. *The Plague Makers.* Simon and Schuster, 1994.

Fisher, Helen. *Anatomy of Love: The Mysteries of Mating, Marriage, and Why We Stray.* Fawcett Columbine, 1992.

Foucault, Michel. *The History of Sexuality: An Introduction: Volume 1.* Trans. Robert Hurley. Vintage, 1990.

——. *The Use of Pleasure: The History of Sexuality, Volume 2.* Trans. Robert Hurley. Vintage 1990.

——. *The Care of the Self: The History of Sexuality, Volume 3.* Trans. Robert Hurley. Vintage, 1988.

Fumento, Michael. *The Myth of Heterosexual AIDS.* Regnery Gateway, 1990.

Gallo, Robert, M.D. *Virus Hunting—AIDS, Cancer, and the Human Retrovirus: A Story of Scientific Discovery.* Basic Books, 1991.

Garrett, Laurie. *The Coming Plague: Newly Emerging Diseases in a World Out of Balance.* Farrar, Straus and Giroux, 1994.

Gould, Peter. *The Slow Plague: A Geography of the AIDS Pandemic.* Blackwell, 1993.

Greenberg, David F. *The Construction of Homosexuality.* University of Chicago Press, 1988.

Grmek, Mirko D. *History of AIDS: Emergence and Origin of a Modern Pandemic.* Trans. Russell C. Maulitz and Jacalyn Duffin. Princeton University Press, 1990.

Halperin, David M. *One Hundred Years of Homosexuality.* Routledge, 1990.

Hardin, Garrett. *Living Within Limits: Ecology, Economics, and Population Taboos.* Oxford University Press, 1993.

Huber, Joan, and Beth E. Schneider, eds. *The Social Context of AIDS.* Sage, 1992.

Janus, Samuel S., and Cynthia L. Janus. *The Janus Report on Sexual Behavior.* John Wiley & Sons, 1993.

Jay, Karla, and Allen Young. *Out of the Closets: Voices of Gay Liberation.* Douglas, 1972.

Johnston, William I., *HIV-Negative: How the Uninfected Are Affected by AIDS.* Insight Books, 1995.

Joseph, Stephen C. *Dragon Within the Gates: The Once and Future AIDS Epidemic.* Carroll & Graf, 1992.

King, Edward. *Safety in Numbers: Safer Sex and Gay Men.* Routledge, 1993.

Kinsella, James. *Covering the Plague: AIDS and the American Media.* Rutgers University Press, 1989.

Kramer, Larry. *Reports from the Holocaust: The Story of an AIDS Activist.* St. Martin's, 1994.

————. *Faggots.* Warner, 1978.

Kleinberg, Seymour. *Alienated Affections: Being Gay in America.* Warner, 1980.

Mann, Jonathan, et al., eds. *AIDS in the World.* Harvard University Press, 1992.

Masters, William H., Virginia E. Johnson, and Robert C. Kolodny. *Heterosexuality.* HarperCollins, 1994.

————. *Crisis: Heterosexual Behavior in the Age of AIDS.* HarperCollins, 1988.

McElroy, Ann, and Patricia K. Townsend. *Medical Anthropology in Ecological Perspective.* Westview, 1989.

Michael, Robert T. et al. *Sex in America: A Definitive Survey.* Little Brown, 1994.

National Research Council. *The Social Impact of AIDS in the United States.* Albert R. Johnsen and Jeff Stryker, eds. National Academy Press, 1993.

Newton, Esther. *Cherry Grove, Fire Island: Sixty Years in America's First Gay and Lesbian Town.* Beacon, 1993.

Odets, Walt. *In the Shadow of the Epidemic: Being HIV-Negative in the Age of AIDS.* Duke University Press, 1995.

Patton, Cindy. *Inventing AIDS.* Routledge, 1990.

Perrow, Charles, and Mauro F. Guillen. *The AIDS Disaster: The Failure of Organizations in New York and the Nation.* Yale University Press, 1990.

Philipson, Thomas J., and Richard A. Posner. *Private Choices and Public Health: The AIDS Epidemic in an Economic Perspective.* Harvard University Press, 1993.

Radetsky, Peter. *The Invisible Invaders: The Story of the Emerging Age of Viruses.* Little Brown, 1991.

Reamer, Frederic G. *AIDS & Ethics.* Columbia University Press, 1991.

Rechy, John. *The Sexual Outlaw: A Documentary.* Dell, 1977.

Root-Bernstein, Robert S. *Rethinking AIDS: The Tragic Cost of Premature Consensus.* Free Press, 1993.

Sabatier, Renee. *Blaming Others; Prejudice, Race and Worldwide AIDS.* Panos, 1988.

Sadownick, Douglas. *Sex Between Men.* HarperSanFrancisco, 1996.

Shilts, Randy. *And the Band Played On: Politics, People and the AIDS Epidemic.* St. Martin's Press, 1987.

Sontag, Susan. *Illness as Metaphor and AIDS and Its Metaphors.* Anchor, 1989.

Walker, Robert Searles. *AIDS Today and Tomorrow: An Introduction to the HIV Epidemic in America*, second ed. Humanities Press, 1991.

Weinberg, Martin S., and Colin J. Williams. *Male Homosexuals: Their Problems and Adaptations.* Penguin, 1975.

Wright, Robert. *The Moral Animal: Evolutionary Psychology and Everyday Life.* Vintage, 1994.

Young, Ian. *The Stonewall Experiment: A Gay Psychohistory.* Cassell, 1995.

Index

activists, 3, 5, 25, 99, 104, 157, 230, 278–79, 282
  degaying promoted by, 114–15, 116
  epidemiological controversies and, 217
  lesbian, 287–88
  new prevention strategies promoted by,
    140–42, 146
  "relapse" and, 122
  sexual libertarianism and, 151–52
  unsafe behavior in, 136
ACT UP, 25, 152, 159, 279
adaptation, in natural selection, 11–12
addiction, rewards vs. consequences in, 233
Addison, Dick, 40–41
Advocate, 94
Africa, 21–24, 25, 27, 33–34, 114, 165, 177,
    179, 181, 182
  social changes in, 33
age:
  intergenerational interaction and, 247–48
  valuing of, 248–49
AIDS:
  awareness of, 136–37, 277, 279–80
  conferences on, 26, 30, 34, 111, 122, 181,
    262, 273, 274
  degaying of, 113–17, 165–66, 177, 181,
    278; *see also* heterosexual AIDS
  destigmatization of, 160
  discovery of, 31–32, 92–93
  drug therapies for, *see* drug therapies
  ecology of, 1–2, 4, 17–18, 175, 183; *see
    also* gay sexual ecology
  epidemiology of, 4–5, 6, 8
  fear of, *see* fear of AIDS
  gay men blamed for, 5, 25, 32, 48, 91–92,
    115, 217

  in heterosexuals, *see* heterosexual AIDS
  initial denial of, 93
  as manageable syndrome, 240–41, 267, 268
  myths about, 8–10
  non-HIV, 26
  origin of, 19–37
  predicted future course of, 121–22, 125
  pre-epidemic, retrospective diagnosis of,
    25–28
  prevention of, *see* prevention
  as restraining moral factor, 115, 165–66,
    176
  role of gay sexual behavior in, *see* gay
    sexual ecology
  Second Wave of, *see* Second Wave
  suspended extinction and, 208–9
  see also HIV
AIDS Action Committee, 160
AIDS and Contemporary History (Weeks),
    89
AIDS Cover-up, The (Antonio), 164–65
alcohol use, 41, 53, 61, 82–83, 137–40, 144,
    246, 247
Alexander the Great, 223
Alienated Affections (Kleinberg), 43, 69
American Association of Physicians for
    Human Rights, *see* Gay and Lesbian
    Medical Association
American Journal of Public Health, 103
*American Journal of Tropical Medical
    Hygiene*, 66
amplification, 32
analingus (rimming; oral-anal sex), 58,
    68–69, 89, 104, 105, 166
anal sex, 34, 92, 101, 129–30, 145, 168

anal sex *(cont.)*
  avoidance of, 97, 98, 101, 102, 190
  and avoidance of transformative change,
    109–10
  in bathhouses and sex clubs, 195–96
  as central to gay life, 76, 101, 188–89
  condom code and, 104–5, 188–89; *see
    also* condoms, condom code
  in earlier decades, 42, 43, 49
  multipartner, 9, 42, 57–58, 66–73, 75–76,
    89; *see also* core groups, gay; promis-
    cuity, gay male
  oral sex as substitute for, 155–60, 270–75
  oral sex risk masked by, 106
  parasites and, 68, 105
  poppers and, 83
  unsafe, *see* unsafe sex
  versatile, 57–58, 76–78, 89
And the Band Played On (Shilts), 6, 23, 84,
  278
antibiotic-resistant STDs, 187, 267
  gonorrhea, 7, 67, 105, 264, 272, 273
antibiotics, 58, 82, 89, 93, 186–87, 188,
  263–64, 266, 267
Antonio, Gene, 164–65
Appuzzo, Virginia, 287–88
Aristotle, 224
Aswan High Dam, 14
AZT, 165

bars and discos, 53, 55, 56, 60–62, 82, 152,
  159
  alternatives to, 246–47
  concurrent multipartnerism in, 79–80
  condoms in, 137
  gay opposition to regulation of, 196–202
bathhouses and sex clubs, 49, 53, 55, 56,
  58–62, 71, 76, 89, 268, 269
  anal sex in, 195–96; *see also* anal sex
  camaraderie of, 201
  closures of, 98, 199–202, 278
  concurrent multipartnerism in, 79–80, 89
  door-removal proposal for, 282–83
  gay opposition to regulation of, 196–202,
    282–83
  mixing of core group and rest of popula-
    tion in, 87–88
  oral sex in, 159, 195–96; *see also* oral sex
  prevention directed at, 195–96
  see also core groups, gay
Bayer, Ronald, 154
Beachy, Stephen, 280
Bell, Alan P., 171
Berkowitz, Richard, 100
Bérubé, Allan, 41, 43, 59, 65
birth control, 187, 188, 263
  condoms used for, 146–47
  population control and, 213, 233, 234,
    237, 238
Black Party, 63–64
blame, 230

directed at gay men, 5, 25, 32, 48, 91–92,
  115, 217, 276–79
  epidemiology and, 217
  within gay community, 48–49, 205, 287
Blaming Others (Sabatier), 21
blood transfusions and blood products, 20,
  34–35, 114, 168, 273
Blow Buddies, 271–72, 274
body image, 248, 253–54, 268
Body Politic, 111–12
Bolton, Ralph, 95
Borrowed Time (Monette), 226
Bronski, Michael, 203–4
Browning, Frank, 111
Buchanan, Patrick, 92

Callen, Michael, 69, 71, 75, 85, 100, 101–2,
  172, 204, 223
cancer, 15
Centers for Disease Control (CDC), 26, 72,
  176, 177
  *Morbidity and Mortality Weekly Report
    of*, 92, 103, 119
Chambers, David L., 100–101, 102, 106, 107
Chauncey, George, 40, 41, 49, 50, 51, 52
Cherry Grove (Newton), 53, 82
Chesley, Robert, 97
children:
  interaction with, 247–48
  raising of, 255–57
China, population growth in, 237–38
cigarette smoking, 209–10
closet, 285
  ecology of, 39–43
  HIV-negativity and, 242
  safe sex and, 137–38
CMV (cytomegalovirus), 70, 85, 100, 104, 105
Coates, Thomas, 112
cocaine, crack, 9, 47, 48, 173–75, 209
Coming Out Under Fire (Bérubé), 43
Coming Plague, The (Garrett), 26, 32, 71–72
Commentary, 284
Communication Technologies study, 158
community centers, 247
concurrency, 78–80, 85, 89
  in heterosexuals, 171
  viral load and, 80–81
  see also promiscuity
condoms, condom code, 9–10, 44, 45, 75, 94,
  97, 98, 99, 100–113, 116, 148, 149–51,
  163, 190, 206, 207, 209, 227, 245
  anal sex encouraged by, 188–89
  availability of, 102, 137, 192, 278
  and avoidance of transformative change,
    109–12, 134, 135, 148–49, 156, 185, 207
  consequences of, 106–8
  ecology ignored by, 104–5, 109, 123, 156,
    184–85, 188, 207
  education about, 136–37
  efficacy of, 102–4
  as harm reduction, 110–11

heterosexual use of, 146–47
HIV-positive status and, 107–8, 241–42
HIV transmission promoted by, 188–89
moralism and, 259
multipartnerism validated by, 111–12,
135, 148–49, 156, 194, 204
and new prevention approaches, 140–42,
146
non-use of, 118, 119, 120, 122–23,
126–27, 130, 134, 135–49, 151, 189–90;
see also unsafe sex
oral sex and, 105–6
rise of, 100–102
self-defense and, 108–9
as sole prevention method, 102, 106, 123
success or failure of, 112–13, 123, 124–27,
130, 132, 134
as technological fix, 188–89
see also safer sex
conscious evolution, 209, 211, 231
Construction of Homosexuality, The
(Greenberg), 76–77, 224
contact rate, 45–46, 189, 194, 207, 276
bathhouse closures and, 200–202
core groups, 46–50, 173, 195
bridging between rest of population and,
48, 86
of drug users, 35–36, 48, 168, 173–74,
175; *see also* injection drug users
dynamics of, 47–49
heterosexual, 172–73
marginalization of, 86
in Thailand, 178
core groups, gay, 9, 47, 48–49, 50, 57–58,
61, 62–63, 85–89, 175, 206, 245
anal sex in, 9, 42, 57–58; *see also* anal sex
bridging between rest of gay population
and, 9, 58, 86–88
escalation of sexual activities in, 63–64,
195–96
gay identity and, 202–5
group immunity in, 58
multipartner anal sex in, 75–76; *see also*
anal sex; promiscuity, gay male
multiple reinfection in, 71
and opposition to regulation of sex establishments, 196–202
oral sex in, 104–5; *see also* oral sex
partner reduction strategy and, 95
pre-Stonewall culture and, 49, 50
prevention programs targeted to, 88–89,
195–202; *see also* prevention
STDs in, 66–73
Thompson's models of, 86
see also bathhouses and sex clubs;
promiscuity, gay male
crack cocaine users, 9, 47, 48, 173–75, 209
Crimp, Douglas, 117
*Crisis: Heterosexual Behavior in the Age of
AIDS* (Masters, Johnson, and Kolodny),
165

crossover theory, 8, 21–24
cultural adaptation, 11–12
cultural incentives and rewards, 233–36
connection between behavior and reward
in, 253
in gay culture, 244–57
population control and, 237–39
safe sex and, 239–44
sexual restraint and, 222–23, 250–53,
254–57, 287
culture(s):
gay, *see* gay culture, sustainable; gay
sexual ecology
sexual behaviors shaped by, 38
sexual ecosystems in, 45–46
Culture of Desire, The (Browning), 111
cytomegalovirus (CMV), 70, 85, 100, 104,
105

Dallas, summit in, 149–51, 153, 160
Darwin, Charles, 11
Dean, Laura, 125–27, 201, 235
deep ecology, 187–88, 190
de Gruttola, Victor, 96
discos, *see* bars and discos
diseases, 8
drug-resistant, *see* drug-resistant diseases
medical ecology and, 12–15
microbes in, 13, 15
sexually transmitted, *see* sexually transmitted diseases
unnoticed, 32
drug-resistant diseases, 7, 8, 187, 267
gonorrhea, 7, 67, 105, 264, 272, 273
HIV, 7
drug therapies, 6, 7, 99, 107, 204–5, 240–41,
262–63, 264, 265–67, 268, 269, 275
increase in unsafe sex tied to, 268–69, 276
as prevention, 275–76
drug use:
crack cocaine, 9, 47, 48, 173–75, 209
among gays, 53, 58, 82–83, 89, 137–40,
144, 197, 246, 247, 268
public attitude toward, 282
see also injection drug users
Duberman, Martin, 65
Dubos, René, 4, 258

ecocide, 12
ecology, 4, 11–12
deep, 187–88, 190
defined, 11
of HIV, 1–2, 4, 17–18, 175, 183; *see also*
gay sexual ecology; HIV
of homosexuality, *see* gay sexual ecology
medical, 12–15; *see also* epidemiology
minimum change principle and, 185
morality and, 57, 260
origin of word, 4
and proof of cause and effect, 198–99
restoration, 206–8

ecology *(cont.)*
　scale and, 57, 58, 260
　of sexuality, *see* sexual ecology
　shallow, 187, 188
　technological fixes and, 185–87, 211, 267
　"think globally, act locally" precept in, 4,
　　258
ecosystems, 11
　sexual, 45–46
education, 214–18
　about condoms, 136–37
　self-, 215–18
"Effect of Sexual Behavior Change on Long-
　Term HIV Prevalence among Homo-
　sexual Men" (Morris and Dean),
　125–27, 201, 235
Egypt, schistosomiasis in, 13–14
Ehrlich, Paul, 211
Elkstrand, Maria, 112
environmentalism, 187
　AIDS prevention and, 211–15
　conscious evolution and, 211
　minimum change principle and, 185
　and proof of cause and effect, 198–99
　self-education in, 215, 216
　technological fixes and, 185–87, 211
　"think globally, act locally" precept in, 4,
　　258
　see also ecology
epidemics, 6, 32–33
　contact rate in, *see* contact rate
　core groups in, *see* core groups
　defined, 43
　development of, 127–28, 129
　infectivity and, 44, 189
　initial denial of, 93
　prevalence in, 44–45, 189, 207
　reproductive rate of, 43–44
　saturation point of, 128–29
　spread of, 43–46
　tipping point and, 44
epidemiology, 13–14, 215
　controversy and, 216–18
　ignorance of, 4–5, 6, 8, 215
　see also sexual ecology
Epstein-Barr virus, 70, 104, 105
Essex, Max, 181
evolution, 11, 209
　conscious, 209, 211, 231
　of HIV, 84–85, 180–82
　suspended extinction and, 208–9
Evolution of Infectious Diseases, The
　(Ewald), 84
Ewald, Paul, 84
"Exit the Rubberman" (O'Hara), 242
extinction, suspended, 208–9

"fairies," 40–41, 51, 52, 77, 226
Farr's Law, 128–29
fear of AIDS, 119–20, 122–23, 125, 134, 158,
　208, 245, 269

　abatement of, 268–70
　in prevention strategies, 160–61
　fidelity, honoring of, 245–46
Foucault, Michael, 51, 224
Friedman-Kien, Alvin, 97
Fumento, Michael, 115, 116, 165–67

Gallo, Robert, 22, 24
Gardner, Murray, 22
Garrett, Laurie, 26, 32, 62, 71–72
Garry, Robert, 28
Gay and Lesbian Medical Association
　(American Association of Physicians for
　Human Rights), 160, 270, 273–74
　Dallas summit of, 149–51, 153, 160
gay culture, sustainable, 10, 17, 18, 189, 209,
　211–32, 233–61, 289–91
　and ability to change, 218, 220–27
　age valued in, 248–49
　alternative meeting spaces in, 246–47
　avoidance of, 109–12
　education and, 214–18
　environmentalism and, 211–15
　historical record and, 223–27, 231–32
　intergenerational interaction in, 247–48
　and logic of unsafe sex, 239–44
　marriage and childrearing in, 255–57
　relationships and fidelity in, 245–46
　self-invention and, 249
　social incentives in, 244–49, 253–54
　social rewards in, 249–57
　spirituality in, 247
　"think publicly, act personally" precept in,
　　257–58
　tragedy of the commons and, 234–36, 276
　victimization and, 229–31
　and will to change, 218–20
　youth in, 227–29, 248–49
gay liberation, 10, 17, 18, 20–21, 51–55, 65,
　226–27, 276, 288–89
　AIDS prevention and, 89–90, 91–92, 93–94,
　　97, 99, 101, 102, 103–4, 107–8, 110–12,
　　148, 150, 153, 183, 196–205, 207–8
　bathhouses and, 59, 196, 201
　behavior changes and, 57–58
　continued HIV transmission and, 283–86
　contradictions in, 55–56
　HIV-positives and, 242–43
　and homosexuality as deviance, 51
　morality and, 259–60
　promiscuity and, 56, 59–63, 92, 219
　role-playing rejected in, 77
　STDs and, 72–73
　Stonewall and, 54–55, 204
　see also homophobia
"Gay Manifesto, A" (Wittman), 77
gay men:
　backlash against, 281–82, 286–88
　blamed for AIDS, 5, 25, 32, 48, 91–92, 115
　closet and, *see* closet
　erosion of political arguments of, 279–83

heterosexual AIDS and, 182–83
political defenses of, 276–83
prejudice against, 52–53, 278; *see also*
 homophobia
promiscuity in, *see* promiscuity, gay male
self-identity of, 5, 39–41, 50–51, 123,
 202–5, 249
sexual culture of, *see* gay culture, sustainable; gay sexual ecology
social acceptance of, 283–86
straight-identified sexual partners of,
 40–41, 42, 49–50, 52, 58, 59, 77
Gay Men's Health Crisis (GMHC), 94, 97,
 156, 199, 200, 274
door-removal proposal and, 282–83
"Safe Sex for HIV Positives" pamphlet of,
 107
Substance Use Counseling & Education
 program of, 139
Gay New York (Chauncey), 40, 41, 49, 50,
 51, 52
gay sexual ecology, 1–2, 3, 6, 7, 8, 9, 17–18,
 38–64, 66–85, 89, 93, 123, 183, 189,
 210, 232
anal sex in, *see* anal sex
and avoidance of transformative change,
 109–12, 134, 135, 148–49, 156, 185,
 207, 239
bathhouses in, *see* bathhouses and sex clubs
changes in, pre-epidemic, 9, 38, 39, 57–58
of the closet, 39–43
concurrency in, 78–80, 85, 89; *see also*
 promiscuity, gay male
condom code's ignoring of, 104–5, 109,
 123, 156
core groups in, *see* core groups, gay
and degaying of AIDS, 116
in earlier decades, 39–43, 49–50
factors that influenced HIV transmission,
 74–85
geography and, 132
ignorance and avoidance of, 6–7, 99–100,
 104–5, 109, 184–85, 188, 231, 269–75
importance of, 6–7
insertive/receptive versatility in, 76–78, 89
mid-century shift in, 50–55
morality and, *see* morality
multipartner anal sex in, 75–76; *see also*
 anal sex; promiscuity, gay male
opposition to change in, 218–20
oral sex in, *see* oral sex
outlaw aspect of, 53, 218
as preventative tool, 116–17
prevention summit's ignoring of, 150
promiscuity in, *see* promiscuity, gay male
self-education about, 215–18
sex clubs and, *see* bathhouses and sex
 clubs
in small cities, towns, and rural areas,
 130–32
STDs and, 66–73

sustainable, *see* gay culture, sustainable
"think publicly, act personally" precept
 and, 257–58
tragedy of the commons and, 236, 276
transformation of, *see* gay culture,
 sustainable
as unchangeable, 218, 220–27
viral load and, 80–81
see also prevention
geography, in sexual ecology, 132
Global AIDS Policy Coalition, 46, 178
GMHC, *see* Gay Men's Health Crisis
gonorrhea, 44–45, 46, 47, 67, 88, 104, 105,
 119, 186, 263, 264
antibiotic-resistant, 7, 67, 105, 264, 272, 273
rectal, HIV transmission compared with,
 133–34, 135
Gould, Peter, 179
government, 1, 2, 5, 6, 98, 99, 115, 136,
 277–78, 280–81
and degaying of AIDS, 116
partner reduction recommended by,
 94–95
Greece, ancient, 223–25, 226
Greenberg, David, 76–77, 223–24, 225
Grmek, Mirko, 23–24, 25–26, 27, 34
Gross, Jane, 118–19
gun ownership, 200
gym culture, 248, 253–54, 268

Haiti, 83, 114, 181
Halperin, David M., 224
Hardin, Garrett, 57, 198, 234–35, 239
harm reduction strategy, 110–11, 184–85,
 192, 202, 239
Hart, Graham, 122
*Harvard Civil Rights Civil Liberties Law
 Review*, 100
Harvard Gay and Lesbian Review, 286
Hay, Harry, 218
Haynes-Sanstad, Katherine, 219
health and research establishments, 2, 5, 6,
 99
heart disease, 14–15
hemophiliacs, 9, 35, 83
hepatitis, 69, 70, 104, 105
 B, 70, 72, 73–74, 93
 C, 7
heroin, 35, 178
see also injection drug users
herpes, 7, 16, 68, 74, 104, 105, 187, 272
Kaposi's sarcoma and, 27
heterosexual AIDS, 9, 114, 116–17, 163–83,
 278, 281
absence of epidemic of, 3–4, 9, 209
in drug users, *see* crack cocaine users;
 injection drug users
and evolution of HIV, 180–82
exaggerated risk of, 176–77
factors affecting transmission of, 169–72,
 180

heterosexual AIDS *(cont.)*
  gay men and, 182–83
  increased rates of, 175–76
  man-to-woman vs. woman-to-man trans-
    mission and, 169–70
  mid-eighties panic about, 164–65
  partner change and, 170–72
  possibility of future epidemic of, 180–82
  risk groups in, 172–73
  secondary transmission of, 168, 173
  tertiary transmission of, 168, 172–73
  in Third World, *see* Third World
  transmission of, 167–68, 169–73
  unsafe sex and, 146, 148
heterosexuals:
  condom use in, 146–47
  improper sexual behaviors in, 145–47, 148
  sexual ecology of, 4, 163–64, 169, 171,
    180, 181, 182, 209
Hethcote, Herbert, 47
History of AIDS (Grmek), 25
HIV:
  AIDS without, 26
  anal sex and, *see* anal sex
  behavior shifts and, 34–36
  concurrency and, 78–80, 85, 89; *see also*
    promiscuity, gay male
  crossover theory and, 8, 21–24
  decline in transmission of, 127–29, 130,
    132, 134
  drug-resistant strains of, 7
  in drug users, *see* injection drug users
  ecology of, 1–2, 4, 17–18, 175, 183; *see*
    also gay sexual ecology
  estimate of New Yorkers infected with, 217
  evolution of, 84–85, 180–82
  gay rights and, 283–86
  genetic sequencing of, 25, 29–31
  gonorrhea transmission compared with,
    133–34, 135
  hepatitis B vaccine trials and, 73–74
  in heterosexuals, *see* heterosexual AIDS
  highly-infectious period of, 87, 96
  historical existence in humans, 8, 20,
    25–32
  incubation period of, 240–41
  insertive/receptive versatility and,
    76–78, 89
  Kaposi's sarcoma and, 27–28
  as manageable syndrome, 240–41, 267,
    268
  mid-eighties drop in new infections,
    9–10
  multipartner anal sex and, 75–76; *see also*
    anal sex; promiscuity, gay male
  mutations and differing strains of, 7,
    84–85, 108, 180–82, 241–42, 262, 264,
    265–67, 273, 274
  myths about, 8–10
  oral sex and, *see* oral sex
  poppers and, 83, 93
  prevention of, *see* prevention
  recombinant, 30–31
  saturation point of, 128–30, 132, 134, 173,
    175
  in small cities, towns, and rural areas,
    130–32
  spread of, 72, 73–74, 97–98, 99
  STDs and, 33–34, 81–82
  tests for, 106–7, 108, 164, 269, 273
  tests for, on stored tissue samples, 25,
    28–29
  tragedy of the commons and, 57, 235–36,
    276
  transmission of, 4, 8, 20, 73–85, 168; *see*
    also gay sexual ecology
  transmission rates of, 10, 112–13, 124,
    127–29, 130, 132, 134, 275–76
  travel and, 83–84, 89
  type E, 180–81, 182, 265, 273, 274
  type O, 273
  viral load and, 80–81
  see also AIDS
HIV-2, 22, 23–24
HIV-positives, 49, 154–55, 241–42
  backlash against, 282
  moral obligations of, 107–9, 154–55
  prejudice against, 160, 193
  self-defense and, 108, 155, 193–94,
    241–42
  societal attitudes toward, 242–43
Holland, 101
Holleran, Andrew, 119
homophobia, 183, 203, 229–30, 284
  AIDS epidemic as result of, 1, 2, 230,
    277–78
  AIDS prevention and, 92, 93–94, 97, 102,
    103–4, 107–8, 110–12, 122, 140,
    141–42, 146, 148, 150, 160, 167, 203,
    204, 230–31, 253, 277, 283, 286
  HIV-positives and, 242–43
  political defenses against, 276–79
  shame fostered by, 205, 228, 259
  STDs and, 72–73
  victimization and, 229–31
  youth and, 228–29
  see also gay liberation
Homosexualities (Bell and Weinberg),
  171–72
homosexuality, *see* gay men; lesbians
Hoover, Donald R., 121–22, 125
Hudson, Rock, 113–14, 164

ICL (idiopathic CD4 T-lymphocytopenia), 26
IDUs, *see* injection drug users
immune system, 93, 105
  crack cocaine and, 174
  poppers and, 83, 93
immunization programs, 20, 22, 33
incentives, *see* cultural incentives and
  rewards
"In Defense of Anal Sex" (Callen), 101–2

India:
    AIDS in, 177, 179, 182
    population growth in, 237, 238–39
infectivity, 44, 189
injection drug users (IDUs), 3, 4, 9, 20–21,
    34, 35–36, 114, 116, 163, 168
    core groups of, 35–36, 48, 173–74
    gay male, 83
    harm-reduction rehabilitation and, 110, 184
    needle sharing by, 35, 36, 168, 173, 178,
        192
    in Thailand, 178
insertive/receptive versatility, 57–58, 76–78,
    89
intestinal parasites, 67, 68–69, 70, 104, 105
In the Shadow of the Epidemic (Odets), 162
intravenous drug users, *see* injection drug
    users
Inventing AIDS (Patton), 21–22, 31–32, 117
Italy, population control in, 237, 238
IV drug users, *see* injection drug users

Janus Report, 170–71
Japan, feudal, 225, 226
Johnson, Virginia, 165
Joseph, Stephen, 217
Journal of AIDS, 103, 119
Journal of the American Medical Association, 28
Journal of the National Medical Association, 27

Kaposi, Moritz, 27
Kaposi' sarcoma (KS), 7, 16, 27–28, 70
    herpes and, 27
Katner, Harold P., 27
King, Edward, 109–10, 122, 166
Kinsey Report, 171
Kleinberg, Seymour, 43, 50, 69
Kolodny, Robert, 165
Kramer, Larry, 97, 117
Krim, Mathilde, 163

Laga, Marie, 34
law enforcement, 200, 202
lesbians, 284–85, 287–88
    fidelity honored by, 245–46
    gay liberation and, 51–53
Levine, Martin P., 142–46, 148, 268
lifestyle, gay, *see* gay culture, sustainable;
    gay sexual ecology
Living Within Limits (Hardin), 198
Lynch, Michael, 111–12

MACS (Multicenter AIDS Cohort Study),
    103, 120
Malthus, Thomas, 212
marriage, 250–53, 255
    same-sex, 255–57
Mass, Lawrence D., 92–93, 94
Masses, Edmund, 115

Masters, William, 165
masturbation, 41, 42, 101
media, 2, 5, 6, 92–93, 98, 99, 115, 230, 278,
    280
medical and scientific establishments, 2, 5,
    6, 99
medical ecology, 12–15
    see also sexual ecology
microbes, 13, 15, 23, 32
    amplification of, 32
    see also epidemics
military, 43, 51, 252, 256
Mineshaft, Black Party at, 63–64
*MMWR (Morbidity and Mortality Weekly
    Report)*, 92, 103, 119
Monette, Paul, 226
monkeys, SIV in, 8, 21–24, 160
monogamy, 84, 96, 98, 102, 172, 207,
    250–52, 256
    alternative to, 246
    in heterosexuals, 170–72
    marriage, 250–53, 255–57
    serial, 78, 81, 246
Montagnier, Luc, 22
morality, 115, 166, 176, 259–61
    ecological scale and, 57, 260
    gay liberation and, 259–60
    HIV-positive status and, 107–9, 154–55,
        259
*Morbidity and Mortality Weekly Report
    (MMWR)*, 92, 103, 119
Morris, Martina, 125–27, 201, 235
Morse, Stephen, 23, 29, 32
Multicenter AIDS Cohort Study (MACS),
    103, 120
multipartnerism, *see* core groups, gay;
    promiscuity, gay male
Myers, Gerald, 22–23
Myth of Heterosexual AIDS, The (Fumento),
    116, 165–67

Naess, Arne, 187, 188
Nahmias, Andre, 68
National Academy of Sciences, 167
National Environmental Policy Act, 199
National Research Council, 36, 167
natural selection, 11, 12
    HIV and, 84–85
negotiated safety, 190–92, 206
New England Journal of Medicine, 154
Newport scandal, 43, 49
Newton, Esther, 53, 65, 82
New York Native, 92–93, 94, 97, 101
New York Newsday, 167
New York Times, 118–19
New York Times Magazine, 280
NIH, 62, 72
nitrate inhalants (poppers), 83, 93

Odets, Walt, 140–42, 155, 161–62
O'Hara, Scott, 242

oral-anal sex, *see* analingus
oral sex, 101
  in bathhouses and sex clubs, 195–96
  crack cocaine and, 174–75
  discrediting of PWAs infected through,
    157–58
  in earlier decades, 41, 42–43, 49, 50, 77
  riskiness of, 49, 50, 104–5, 105–6, 145,
    155–60, 270–75
Osborn, June, 62–63, 72
Osborne, Torie, 288
Out, 157, 274
OutWeek, 167
ozone layer, 198

Pankey, George A., 27
parasites, intestinal, 67, 68–69, 70, 104, 105
partner reduction, 94–96, 97, 98, 99, 100,
  101, 102, 111–12
party circuit, 82, 83–84, 197
Patton, Cindy, 21–22, 31–32, 65, 117
Pattullo, E. L., 284–85
penicillin, 67, 263, 264, 266, 267, 269, 276
People with AIDS Newsline, 62
P-FLAG, 229, 231
Plato, 224, 225
poppers (nitrate inhalants), 83, 93
population control, 212–14, 233, 234
  cultural rewards for, 237–39
  education and, 214–15
pornography, 55, 76
Preston, John, 63–64
prevalence, 44–45, 189, 207, 275
prevention, 91–117, 135–62, 269–70
  abstinence, 97, 98, 101, 102, 104, 190
  activists and, *see* activists
  in casual or anonymous sex, 190, 192–94,
    206
  condom code as entire message of, 102,
    106, 123; *see also* condoms, condom
    code
  core groups as target of, 88–89, 195–205;
    see also core groups, gay male
  Dallas summit on, 149–51, 153, 160
  and defining survival, 161–62
  and differing models of risk behaviors,
    145
  dissidents and, 97
  education in, 136–37, 214–18
  environmentalism and, 211–15
  fear as counterproductive to, 160–61
  gay culture as positive factor in, 116–17
  gay liberation, homophobia and, 89–90,
    91–92, 93–94, 97, 99, 101, 102, 103–4,
    107–8, 110–12, 122, 140, 141–42, 146,
    148, 150, 153, 160, 167, 183, 196–205,
    207–8, 230–31, 253, 277, 283, 286
  harm reduction philosophy of, 110–11,
    184–85, 192, 202, 239
  holistic, 10, 184–210, 218; *see also* gay
    culture, sustainable

  long-term, 206–9
  lost window of opportunity in, 97–100
  marriage and, 256
  monogamy and, *see* monogamy
  morality and, 107–9, 154–55, 259
  negotiated safety strategy in, 190–2, 206
  new approaches to, 140–42, 146, 152–62,
    259
  openness about unsafe sex in, 152–54
  oral sex and, 105–6, 155–60, 270–75
  partner reduction, 94–96, 97, 98, 99, 100,
    101, 102, 111–12
  permanent, 206; *see also* gay culture,
    sustainable
  population control compared with,
    213–15, 233, 234
  and projection of future AIDS trends,
    121–22, 125
  proof of sexual transmission and, 98,
    197–99, 274
  relapse and, *see* unsafe sex
  in relationships, 190–92, 206
  restoration ecology in, 206–8
  self-defense in, 108–9, 155, 193–94
  self-education in, 215–18
  separate campaigns for HIV-negatives and
    positives in, 154–55
  sexual libertarianism vs., 151–52, 202, 219
  success and failure of, 112–13, 123,
    124–27, 130, 132, 134
  "think publicly, act personally" precept in,
    257–58
  transformative change avoided in,
    109–12, 134, 135, 148–49, 156, 185,
    207, 239
  treatment as, 275–76
  see also gay sexual ecology; safer sex;
    unsafe sex
primary transmission, 168
Project SIGMA, 120
promiscuity, 9
  concurrency and, 78, 85
  contact rate and, *see* contact rate
  in heterosexuals, 170–72
promiscuity, gay male (multipartnerism), 1,
  49, 92, 93, 94, 171–72, 194, 207
  alternative to, 246
  anal sex and, 9, 42, 57–58, 66–73, 75–76,
    89; *see also* anal sex
  bathhouse closures and, 199–202
  bathhouse society and, 201
  concurrent, 78–80, 85, 89
  condom code and justification of, 111–12,
    135, 148–49, 156, 194, 204
  contact rate and, 45–46, 189, 194,
    200–202, 207, 276
  gay liberation and, 56, 59–63, 92, 219
  as inherent trait, 220–27
  oral substitution strategy and, 156
  partner reduction and, 94–96, 97, 98, 99,
    100, 101, 102, 111–12

as positive factor in prevention, 116–17
serial, 78, 81
in small cities and towns, 131–32
see also core groups, gay
prostitutes, 33, 46, 47, 49–50, 67, 68, 129,
171, 179
crack cocaine used by, 174
in Thailand, 178
Pseudo-Lucian, 225
PWA Coalition Newsline, 101

"queers," 40–41, 51, 52, 77, 226

Rechy, John, 203
Redfield, Robert, 165
relationships, honoring of, 245–46
religious organizations, gay, 247
research and health establishments, 2, 5,
6, 99
restoration ecology, 206–8
Reviving the Tribe (Rofes), 271–72
rewards, *see* cultural incentives and rewards
rimming, *see* analingus
risk groups, *see* core groups
Rofes, Eric, 155–56, 271–72
rural areas, small cities, and towns, 130–32

Sabatier, Renee, 21
Sadownick, Doug, 63, 139
safer sex, 5–6, 44, 86, 91, 92, 183
closet and, 137–38
condom code as sole strategy in, 102,
106, 123; *see also* condoms, condom
code
cultural incentives for, 239–44
education about, 136–37
"know one's partner" strategy in, 94, 96
and new prevention approaches, 140–42,
146
oral sex as, 105–6, 155–60, 270–75
partner reduction in, 94–96, 97, 98, 99,
100, 101, 102, 111–12
relapse in, 118–23, 126–27; *see also*
unsafe sex
in small cities, towns, and rural areas,
130–32
success and failure of, 112–13, 123,
124–27, 130, 132, 134
see also prevention; unsafe sex
saturation point, 128–29
of HIV, 128–30, 132, 134, 173, 175
schistosomiasis, 13–14
Science, 160, 234
Scientific American, 22
scientific and medical establishments, 2, 5,
6, 99
Seal, John, 164
secondary transmission, 168, 173
Second Wave, 6, 118–19, 129, 135, 147, 148,
183, 202, 204, 268, 270, 280, 282
AIDS awareness and, 136

denial of, 133, 134, 135
selection principle, 233
self-education, 215–18
serial monogamy, 78, 81, 246
Sex Between Men (Sadownick), 63
sex clubs, *see* bathhouses and sex clubs
Sex in America survey, 170
sexual ecology, 163–64, 169, 178
core groups in, *see* core groups
of crack cocaine users, 9, 174–75
defined, 16–17
ecosystems in, 45–46
of gay males, *see* gay sexual ecology
of heterosexuals, 4, 163–64, 169, 171, 180,
181, 182, 209; *see also* heterosexual
AIDS
ignorance about, 6–7
of Thailand, 178–79
sexuality:
culture and, 38
voluntary control of, 222–23, 250–53,
254–57, 287
sexually transmitted diseases (STDs), 15–17,
89, 93, 104–5, 133, 160, 172, 241
antibiotics and, 58, 82, 89, 93, 186–87,
188, 263–64, 266, 267
and changes in gay behavior, 39, 58
condom code and, 104–5
contact rate of, 45–46, 189, 194
core groups and, *see* core groups
crack cocaine and, 174
in gay core groups, 66–73
gonorrhea, *see* gonorrhea
hepatitis, *see* hepatitis
herpes, *see* herpes
HIV, *see* HIV
HIV transmission and, 33–34, 81–82
infectivity and, 44, 189
intestinal parasites, 67, 68–69, 70, 104,
105
male vs. female rates of, 50, 68
oral sex and, 49, 50, 104–5
prevalence of, 44–45, 189
prostitutes and, 46, 47, 49–50, 67, 68
as restraining moral factor, 115
spread of, 43–46
syphilis, *see* syphilis
in Third World, 33–34
transmission differences in, 44, 169
travel and, 71–72, 89
see also sexual ecology
sexual orientation, concept of, 39–40,
50–51, 52
sexual revolution, 20–21, 54, 187, 263–64
see also gay liberation
shallow ecology, 187, 188
shame, 205, 228, 259, 288–89
Shilts, Randy, 6, 23, 69, 84, 111, 117
Siegel, Karolynn, 142–46, 148, 268
SIV (simian immunodeficiency virus), 8,
21–24, 160

small cities, towns, and rural areas, 130–32
snails, schistosomiasis and, 13–14
*Social Impact of AIDS in the United States,
    The*, 35–36, 167
social incentives and rewards, *see* cultural
    incentives and rewards
Sonnabend, Joseph, 85, 97, 100, 101
special K, 139, 197
spirituality, 247
Stall, Ron, 119
state vs. trait, 220
STDs, *see* sexually transmitted diseases
Steam, 242
Stonewall Experiment, The (Young), 56
Stonewall Riots, 54–55, 204
Stop AIDS Project, 113
substance abuse, *see* alcohol use; drug use
Surviving AIDS (Callen), 71
suspended extinction, 208–9
synergism of plagues, 47
syphilis, 16, 33, 45, 46, 67, 104, 186, 263,
    264, 267, 276

TB (tuberculosis), 27, 36
technological fixes, 185–87, 211, 267
    condoms as, 188–89
tertiary transmission, 168, 172–73
Thailand, 83, 165, 177, 178–79
    HIV mutation in, 180–81, 182, 265, 273,
        274
Third World, 33–34, 114, 163, 168, 177–82
    blood products from, 34
    population growth in, 237
    see also Africa; Thailand
Thompson, James, 85–86
towns, small cities, and rural areas, 130–32
"Tragedy of the Commons, The" (Hardin),
    57, 234–36, 276
travel, 71–72, 83–84, 89
treatment, AIDS, *see* drug therapies
tuberculosis (TB), 27, 36
Turner, Thomas B., 115

Uganda, 177, 179
"Unprotected Sex: Understanding Gay
    Men's Participation" (Levine and
    Siegel), 142–46, 148, 268
unsafe sex, 118–23, 126–27, 135–49, 150–51,
    205, 206, 253

activists' confessions of, 136
AIDS treatments tied to increases in,
    268–69, 276
crack cocaine and, 174
dispersal theory of, 199–202
heterosexual conduct compared with,
    145–47, 148
human condition and, 147–49
justifications and excuses for, 143–45,
    268–69
Levine and Siegel's study of, 142–46, 148,
    268
logic of, 239–44
openness about, 152–54
oral substitution strategy and, 159
and regulation of commercial sex estab-
    lishments, 196–202, 282–83
rewards for, 243–44
set point of, 194, 207
in sex clubs, 195–96
substance abuse related to, 137–40, 144
weak negative consequences of, 240–43
    see also prevention; safer sex
USA Today, 114

vaccination programs, 20, 22, 33
Vaid, Urvashi, 286
venereal diseases, *see* sexually transmitted
    diseases
versatility, insertive/receptive, 57–58,
    76–78, 89
Victoria AIDS Council/Gay Men's Health
    Centre, 190–91
viral load (viremia), 80–81

Wall Street Journal, 176, 177
Weeks, Jeffrey, 89
Weinberg, Martin S., 171
Winfrey, Oprah, 164
Winkelstein, Warren, 112
Wittman, Carl, 77
World Health Organization, 169, 177

Yokoyama, S., 30
Yorke, James, 47
Young, Ian, 56, 203
Young Men's Study, 138
youth, gay and lesbian, 227–29, 248–49,
    284–85